T0323631

Advance praise for *Adolescent Co-Occurring Substance Use and Mental Health Disorders*

"Winters and Ingwalson write with passion, compassion, and authority in this incisive and eminently practical textbook. Adolescence substance abuse is an enormous problem in its own right, and sadly and all-too-commonly, the beginning of a pattern continuing into adult life. As these expert authors make clear throughout, the adolescent development of substance abuse can only truly be understood and managed in the context of underlying, comorbid psychological disorders. I highly recommend this book to anyone wanting to better understand substance abuse, especially students."—**Robert E. Emery**, PhD, Professor of Psychology, Director of the Center for Children, Families, and the Law, Department of Psychology, University of Virginia, co-author of *Abnormal Psychology* now in its 9th edition

"This comprehensive textbook provides an excellent overview of co-occurring substance use and mental health in youth. Engaging case vignettes and informative side bars highlight a chapter's key points. This reader-friendly textbook is the ideal teaching tool for students seeking a degree or certificate as an addiction counselor."—**Tammy Chung**, PhD, Professor of Psychiatry, Rutgers, The State University of New Jersey

"*Adolescent Co-Occurring Substance Use and Mental Health Disorders* is a clearly written textbook appropriate for trainees and treatment providers learning about the specific needs of youth with dual diagnoses. It provides a straight forward, research-based account of adolescent development, psychopathology, and developmentally appropriate assessment and treatment modalities. As an educator, I appreciate the inclusion of case vignettes, discussion questions, and additional resources to use in fostering student discussion and engagement with the material. All around a comprehensive introduction to the field."—**Kristen G. Anderson**, PhD, Professor of Psychology, Adolescent Health Research Program (Principal Investigator), Reed College

"Drs. Ken C. Winters and Ann Ingwalson's new textbook, *Adolescent Co-Occurring Substance Use and Mental Health Disorders*, is comprehensive and compelling in content, yet concise and accessible in style. The book's 13 chapters are well sequenced, and iteratively increase readers' knowledge about co-occurring substance use and mental health problems among teenagers. Each chapter concludes with helpful mini-review bullet lists, discussion points, and suggestions for seeking more information. The authors do a particularly job summarizing current knowledge regarding cannabis use and mental health and are to be commended for their excellent coverage of process addictions and recovery programs. The book includes informative illustrations, figures, and photos, thoughtfully selected sidebar highlights, and a highly usable Learner's Test Question Bank. Winters and Ingwalson's *Adolescent Co-Occurring Substance Use and Mental Health Disorders* is an excellent choice for coursework in programs training professional addiction counselors."—**Eric F. Wagner**, PhD, Director, Community-Based Research Institute, Professor, Florida International University, Licensed Psychologist, State of Florida

"The intersection of psychiatric disorders and substance use disorder is arguably the most foundational area in the prevention and treatment of addictions. Winters and Ingwalson provide essential coverage of core etiological factors predicting substance use disorders and process addictions. Throughout, there are explanations of the roles of psychiatric disorders, developmental trends, and brain development in the etiology of substance use disorders and process addictions. Current evidence-based treatment and prevention models for substance use disorders are explored in depth to provide the reader with information on important trends in the intervention and prevention field in addiction. Using foundational coverage of best clinical practices in treatment and delivery of care, this text fills an essential need in training the next generation of mental health and addiction professionals."—**Serena M. King**, PhD, Professor and Chair, Department of Psychology, Hamline University

Adolescent Co-Occurring Substance Use and Mental Health Disorders

KEN C. WINTERS

AND

ANN INGWALSON

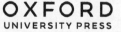

OXFORD
UNIVERSITY PRESS

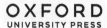

Oxford University Press is a department of the University of Oxford. It furthers
the University's objective of excellence in research, scholarship, and education
by publishing worldwide. Oxford is a registered trade mark of Oxford University
Press in the UK and certain other countries.

Published in the United States of America by Oxford University Press
198 Madison Avenue, New York, NY 10016, United States of America.

Library of Congress Cataloging-in-Publication Data
Names: Winters, Ken C., editor. | Ingwalson, Ann, editor.
Title: Adolescent co-occurring substance use and mental health disorders /
Ken C. Winters and Ann Ingwalson.
Description: New York, NY : Oxford University Press, [2023] |
Includes bibliographical references and index.
Identifiers: LCCN 2022010873 (print) | LCCN 2022010874 (ebook) |
ISBN 9780190678487 (hardback) | ISBN 9780190678500 (epub) | ISBN 9780190678517
Subjects: LCSH: Teenagers—Substance use. | Substance abuse—Treatment. |
Teenagers—Mental health. | Teenagers—Mental health services. | Comorbidity.
Classification: LCC RJ506.D78 A358 2023 (print) | LCC RJ506.D78 (ebook) |
DDC 616.8600835—dc23/eng/20220602
LC record available at https://lccn.loc.gov/2022010873
LC ebook record available at https://lccn.loc.gov/2022010874

DOI: 10.1093/med-psych/9780190678487.001.0001

9 8 7 6 5 4 3 2 1

Printed by Integrated Books International, United States of America

CONTENTS

Ken C. Winters, PhD, is a Senior Scientist at the Oregon Research Institute (MN location) and a Research Associate Professor, Office of Research and Economic Development, Florida International University. Dr. Winters retired in 2016 as a Full Professor in the Department of Psychiatry at the University of Minnesota, where he founded and directed the Center for Adolescent Substance Abuse Research for 25 years. Dr. Winters received his BA from the University of Minnesota and a PhD in Psychology (Clinical) from the State University of New York at Stony Brook. His primary research interests are the assessment and treatment of addictions, including adolescent drug abuse. He is on the editorial boards of the *Journal of Substance Abuse Treatment*, *Journal of Child and Adolescent Substance Abuse*, and the *Psychology of Addictive Behaviors*. Dr. Winters has received numerous research grants from the National Institutes of Health and various foundations, and has published over 155 peer-reviewed articles and over 50 book chapters.

Ann Ingwalson, PsyD, LADC, LPCC, DBTC, is a long-standing faculty member and instructor in the Master of Professional Studies in Integrated Behavioral Health and Addiction Studies programs at the University of Minnesota. She received her PsyD from Capella University. She has worked with youth and families in a variety of clinical settings for over 25 years. Her clinical emphasis for the last 15 years has been specifically working with youth who have mental health and substance use co-occurring disorders. Ann serves as the Assistant Training Coordinator for the Doctoral Internship Program at the Natalis Counseling & Psychology Solutions in St. Paul, MN. She is a member of the Minnesota Psychological Association, American Psychological Association, Minnesota Association of Resources for Recovery and Chemical Health, and the Minnesota Association for Children's Mental Health.

Both authors express gratitude to our editors at Oxford University Press, Sarah Harrington and Hayley Singer, for their support and guidance with the preparation of this book. Appreciation also to Mary K. Winters for researching topics.

Introduction

CHAPTER OUTLINE

INTRODUCTION

Welcome to the first edition of *Adolescent Co-Occurring Substance Use and Mental Health Disorders*. The writing of this book is based on the both the absence of a textbook on adolescent substance abuse and coexisting disorders that is aimed at students seeking a degree or certificate as an addiction counselor and acknowledgment that, despite improvements in prevention and treatment services, adolescent substance abuse and co-existing disorders continue to be a major public health problem. The national 2017 survey conducted in the United States indicated that 4.0% of adolescents ages 12–17 years (~990,000 adolescents) met diagnostic criteria for at least one current (within the past year) substance use disorder (Substance Abuse and Mental Health Services Administration, 2018). It is estimated that between 60 and 90% of adolescents with a substance use disorder also suffer from a coexisting mental or behavioral disorder (Armstrong & Costello, 2002; Chan et al., 2008). The negative impact of the lockdown resulting from the COVID-19 pandemic has strained the mental health of adolescents, and future studies are likely to indicate elevated rates of mental disorders attributed to the "COVID effect" (Panchal et al., 2021).

Mental illnesses are on the rise

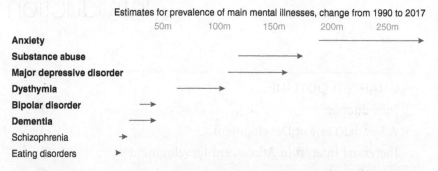

Estimates for prevalence of main mental illnesses, change from 1990 to 2017

Guardian Graphic | Source: Institute for Health Metrics Evaluation, Global Burden of Disease 2017

Are mental illnesses on the rise? This chart would seem to indicate the answer is yes. But the increases are only slightly higher than the rise in global population since 1990. According to Harvey Whiteford, Professor of Population Mental Health at the University of Queensland (Australia), there have been two big changes in the past 20 years. The first is that recognition and destigmatization have resulted in a huge surge of people seeking help. The second is that surveys repeatedly show that more young people are reporting mental distress. The latter point may be due to the greater ease in talking about mental health issues among young people.
Copyright Guardian News & Media Ltd 2020

The fact that, in the United States, substance use is typically initiated during adolescence further highlights the importance of this textbook. Moreover, those who suffer from a substance use disorder early in life are four to five times more likely to have a shorter life span than the general public, and life expectancy is even shorter if the person has a coexisting behavioral or mental disorder (Fridell et al., 2019). Therefore, it is vital that service providers in the addiction treatment field who wish to work with adolescents be familiar with the developmental issues and current trends in adolescent substance use and mental health disorders. In this light, the scope of this textbook is to provide service providers with an updated, comprehensive, and clinically oriented resource.

A SPECIAL TIME OF DEVELOPMENT

A core emphasis of the textbook is that adolescence is a unique developmental period. It is a time of dramatic change in the life of every person, in every corner of the world. The relatively uniform growth of childhood is suddenly shifted to an increase in the speed of growth and is characterized by rapid changes in terms of hormones, physical characteristics, cognition, and emotional behavior, and for some, gender identity issues. In this context, a young person is influenced by many external factors, including parents, peers, school, culture, and the media. There are a number of different ways of looking at adolescent development, including how to define when adolescence begins (which we discuss below) and how different theories provide a basis for understanding its characteristics. Whereas no two teenagers negotiate the adolescent years identically, just about every adolescent faces numerous developmental challenges during these years (Steinberg & Morris, 2001).

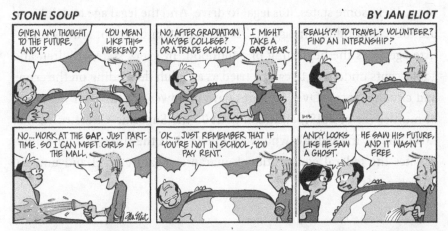

STONE SOUP   **BY JAN ELIOT**

Yet, when does adolescence begin and end? As summarized by Casey (2019), the answer to this depends on what point of view is advanced.

A *developmental perspective* indicates that the child is learning skills to be relatively independent from one's parents or caregivers and in preparation for functioning in the future as a productive adult. These new skills include meeting demands, often without the help of an adult, on an intellectual, emotional, social, physical, and sexual level.

From a *societal perspective*, adolescence involves financial dependence on parents and the continuation of formal academic or vocational training. When financial independence and completion of education are achieved and the person starts their own family, most cultures regard this as the start of adulthood. One sign that the period of adolescence is being extended is that in the United States, the median age of marriage in the 1950s was 22 years, whereas in 2019 it is 28 years (Statista Research Department, 2022).

Legally what constitutes adolescence is complicated. In the United States, the legal age of majority (adulthood) varies considerably depending on the privilege or right under consideration. At age 18, an individual can vote, serve in the military, get married, gamble (with some limitations), and sign legal documents without parental permission or consent. Prior to age 18, in some states, it is legal to drive. And the legal age to drink and use tobacco products in age 21. The legal system does not always recognize age 18 as the beginning of adulthood. In every state, children and adolescents under age 18 can be tried as an adult depending on the crime and circumstances. Over 20 states have no lower age limit for the crime of murder (as of 2018), although in 2005 the Supreme Court ruled that execution of individuals who were under 18 at the time of their crimes violates the federal constitutional guarantee against cruel and unusual punishments.

Under the Supreme Court's ruling, minors can still get life without parole sentences—just not automatically after a conviction; instead, a judge will need to decide, taking into account the minor's youth.

Why is a young person considered an adult in most of the world at age 18? There was no science to set this as the key age. Historians note that society long viewed this age when most humans reached a level of maturity and base knowledge to be responsible for themselves and their own actions. It was legally and social inconvenient to not have a baseline age, so age 18 was picked, even if it is not ideal in all cases and contexts.

A final perspective is the *brain maturation* point of view. As we discuss in detail in Chapter 3, neuroscientists have intensively studied the maturation process of a young person's brain. The authors (we) are struck by how common age 25 is cited in research and pop culture publications as the "maturation point." Pinpointing when the brain reaches maturity is problematic; the brain is a dynamic organ that changes and adapts on the basis of new information and experiences throughout the life span. But there are important and unique brain changes during the teenage years, and these developmental processes have implications for how adolescence is viewed.

These different developmental perspectives regarding the transition from adolescence to adulthood raise many important clinical questions, which we will discuss throughout this book. Suffice it to say that when providing services to adolescents, it will be important to consider your client's maturity based on developmental, societal, legal, and brain maturation perspectives.

INCREASED INTEREST IN ADOLESCENT DEVELOPMENT

This textbook is capitalizing on the expansion of research about and clinical implications of adolescent development. Numerous journals are devoted to this age group (e.g., *Journal of Adolescence, Journal of Child and Adolescent Substance Abuse, Developmental Psychology*) and a substantial number of pages are devoted to adolescence in long-standing health-related research journals (e.g., *Abnormal Psychology, American Journal of Public Health*). The

Society for Research on Adolescence, the major professional association for researchers on adolescent development, had their inaugural meeting in 1986 and now has over 1,000 members. The current diagnostic manual for behavioral and mental disorders published by the American Psychiatric Press, the *Diagnostic and Statistical Manual of Mental Disorders, Fifth Edition (DSM-5),* provides detailed descriptions of the numerous mental disorders that adolescents suffer from. (A revised edition, the *Diagnostic and Statistical Manual of Mental Disorders, Fifth Edition, Text Revision (DSM-5-TR),* will be published sometime in 2022). Of note, on a scholarly level is the recent report by a committee convened by the National Academies of Sciences, Engineering and Medicine (NASEM), *The Promise of Adolescence: Realizing Opportunity for All Youth* (National Academies of Sciences, Engineering, and Medicine, 2019). This publication synthesizes the latest research on the science of adolescent development, with a focus on the neurobiological and sociobehavioral processes that characterize maturation during the adolescent years. The clinical implications of the committee's findings are included throughout this book.

BOOK STRUCTURE

Adolescent Co-Occurring Substance Use and Mental Health Disorders consists of three overarching sections, comprising the book's next 12 chapters. Each chapter includes core content, sidebar points of interest, summary highlights, discussion questions, and test questions. Several chapters include case vignettes. The textbook's sections and chapters are listed below.

    Section 1: Adolescent Development
        Physical and Psychosocial Development (Ch. 2)
        Adolescent Brain Development (Ch. 3)
    Section 2: Co-Occurring Disorders
        Overview of Psychoactive Substances (Ch. 4)
        Substance Use Disorders (Ch. 5)

REFERENCES

Armstrong, T. D., & Costello, E. J. (2002). Community studies on adolescent substance use, abuse, or dependence and psychiatric comorbidity. *Journal of Consulting and Clinical Psychology, 70,* 1224–1239.

Casey, B. J. (2019). Healthy development as a human right: Lessons from developmental science. *Neuron, 102,* 724–727.

Chan, Y. F., Dennis, M. L., & Funk, R. R. (2008). Prevalence and comorbidity of major internalizing and externalizing problems among adolescents and adults presenting to substance abuse treatment. *Journal of Substance Abuse Treatment, 34,* 14–24.

Fridell, M., Bäckström, M., Hesse, M., Krantz, P., Perrin, S., & Nyhlén, A. (2019). Prediction of psychiatric comorbidity on premature death in a cohort of patients with substance use disorders: A 42-year follow-up. *BMC Psychiatry, 19,* 1–13.

National Academies of Sciences, Engineering, and Medicine. (2019). *The promise of adolescence: Realizing opportunity for all youth.* The National Academies Press.

Panchal, U., Salazar de Pablo, G., Franco, M., Moreno, C., Parellada, M., Arango, C., & Fusar-Poli, P. (August 18, 2021). The impact of COVID-19 lockdown on child and adolescent mental health: Systematic review. *European Child & Adolescent Psychiatry,* 1–27. doi:https://doi.org/10.1007/s00787-021-01856-w

Steinberg, L., & Morris, A. S. (2001). Adolescent development. *Annual Review of Psychology, 52,* 83–110.

Statista Research Department. (January, 2022). Median age of U.S. Americans at their first wedding, by sex 1998–2019. https://www.statista.com/statistics/371933/med ian-age-of-us-americans-at-their-first-wedding/#:~:text=This%20statistic%20conta ins%20data%20on%20the%20estimated%20median,United%20States%20from%201 998%20to%202019%2C%20by%20sex

Substance Abuse and Mental Health Services Administration. (2018). *Key substance use and mental health indicators in the United States: Results from the 2017 National Survey on Drug Use and Health.* NSDUH Series H-53, HHS Publication No. (SMA) 18-5068. Rockville, MD, Center for Behavioral Health Statistics and Quality. https://store.samhsa.gov/sites/default/files/d7/priv/sma18-5068.pdf

ADOLESCENT DEVELOPMENT

Physical and Psychosocial Development

CHAPTER OUTLINE

INTRODUCTION

This chapter focuses on the physical and psychosocial developmental features that are hallmarks of adolescence. In a subsequent chapter (Chapter 3) we will focus on the emerging science of brain maturation during adolescence, a topic that deserves its own chapter.

Adolescence is a time when physical and psychosocial changes are happening at an accelerated rate. The adolescent will experience the onset of puberty and negotiate the completion of physical growth, including the development of their sexually dimorphic body shape. These physical changes influence the youth's development of a sense of personal and sexual identity, how one thinks, and how one relates to outside factors such as parents, peers, and the community close at home and the larger one of school and society at large. And there is tentative evidence that pubertal hormones might influence the structure and function of the developing human brain (Spear, 2000). In terms of psychological development, general theories have been advanced since the beginning of the 1900s. As we summarize in Box 2.1, each of these theorists focus on specific aspects of human development (e.g., cognitive development, moral development, and identity development). Whereas each theory has a unique focus, they all share the theme that each adolescent is an individual with a unique personality and interests, but with numerous developmental issues that just about every teenager faces during the adolescent years.

Below we first address the issue of the relative influences of genetics and environment on development. We then delve into the specifics of physical and psychological development during adolescence, followed by related topics of how development can be affected by physical activity, sleep, and the digital age (social messaging and smartphones).

RELATIVE INFLUENCE OF GENETICS AND ENVIRONMENT ON DEVELOPMENT

There is growing interest in understanding the joint influence of biology and environment on physical and psychological development. The branch of research known as behavioral genetics research provides some insights into the relative influence of these three sources of influences on adolescent development: genetic (or biological), shared environment, and nonshared environmental. Some interesting trends have emerged from this body of work. Briefly, there is a wealth of data suggesting that genetic factors strongly influence several personality traits, such as aggression, antisocial behavior, and delinquency, as well as internalizing problems in

BOX 2.1

Four Prominent Developmental Theories of Adolescence

The beginning of modern theories on adolescent development is traced to Jean Piaget's theory during the 1920s of children's *cognitive development* and a related theory of children's moral development. Piaget contended that children's cognitive abilities developed in a sequential, step-wise fashion and their cognitive development subsequently influenced their social awareness and moral maturity.

In the late 1950s, Lawrence Kohlberg extended Piaget's *moral development theory*. Unlike Piaget, who under-emphasized the influence of social environment, Kohlberg believed that social relationships and culture were central to understanding children's cognitive and moral development.

A *psychosocial theory of human development* was advanced by a contemporary of Kohlberg, Erik Erikson. Erikson's theory posited that individuals must pass through sequential developmental stages, or "crises," during which they either develop the necessary skills to become successful, happy members of society or they fail to successfully navigate the crisis and remain "stuck" at that developmental stage.

The *identity status theory* was theorized in the mid-1960s by James Marcia. Marcia focused on the way adolescents develop their own individual identity within the framework of their *families and larger culture*.

adolescence, such as risk for suicide and depressed mood (Blumenthal & Kupfer, 1988; Jacobson & Rowe, 1999). Interestingly, female adolescents may be more influenced by genetic factors than male adolescents with respect to both internalizing and externalizing problems. When the relative influences of shared and nonshared environmental factors are examined, the following general trends have been observed: nonshared factors, such as parental differential treatment, peer relations (a topic we address later in this chapter), and school experiences, are particularly strong in adolescence, whereas shared environmental factors, such as socioeconomic status, neighborhood quality, and parental psychopathology, appear to be less influential (e.g., McGue et al., 1996).

STAGES OF PHYSICAL DEVELOPMENTAL

Puberty Onset

Before puberty, children grow approximately 2 to 3 inches a year and gain around 5 pounds a year. But during adolescence, which traditionally begins at about age 12, the velocity of growth significantly increases for the only time in life. This rapid growth spurt, known as *puberty*, represents a period of profound transition in terms of drives, emotions, motivations, social life, and physical changes.

These physical changes are triggered by an increase in estrogen and testosterone hormonal activity and most obviously contribute to the maturation of the sex organs. However, these maturational changes occur with great variability among youths, and thus adolescents of a given chronological age may vary widely in physical development (Tanner, 1981). Several factors can influence either early or delayed puberty. Factors that contribute to early puberty are genetics, obesity (girls), and abnormalities in the central nervous system that disrupt hormonal activity. Delayed puberty can be caused by poor nutrition, chronic illness, eating disorder, exposure to trauma, and disruption in hormonal activity.

Nutrition is particularly important during adolescence (Spear, 2002b). The dramatic increase in physical growth and development during adolescence creates a great demand for nutrients. To complicate matters, changes in lifestyle and food habits may create health issues.

Because of the wide variability in growth rates, physical activity, and metabolic rate, estimates of specific nutrient requirements for adolescents is problematic. Yet, there is solid research on the relationship between growth and energy intake (Berkey et al., 2000). On average, boys tend to increase their energy intake steadily to approximately 3,470 food calories (kcal) per day at 16 years of age. From 16 to 19 years of age, the intake decreases to approximately 2,900 kcal per day. In girls, the rise in energy intake increases at age 12 with a peak level of 2,550 kcal per day, followed by a decline in energy intake through to 18 years of age, with intakes averaging 2,200 kcal per day (Spear, 2002b).

The issue of adolescent nutrition includes the need for minerals and vitamins. Sufficient vitamins can be provided by a well-chosen diet without necessitating the use of vitamin supplements. Overreliance on "convenience" snacks and foods will result in low intake of minerals and vitamins.

Development During Puberty

Both boys and girls pass through identifiable stages of development of sex characteristics. The change from prepuberty to full reproductive capacity may take as little as 18 months or as long as 5 years. But there are significant sex differences. Girls seem to enter puberty long before boys. Their first sign of puberty—development of breast buds—tends to occur about 6 months prior to the earliest sign for boys—increasing testicular volume. On average, these first signs occur at 11.5 years of age for girls and at 12 years of age for boys.

Because the growth spurt is also more rapid in girls, girls seem considerably more developed in the early teenage years compared to boys. For girls, the defining event of puberty is menarche. The mean age at menarche has shown substantial decline in most developed countries through the first half of the 20th century, stabilizing in the 1960s in most countries at around 13 years for white girls and 12.5 years for African American girls.

Table 2.1 Summary of Tanner Stages of Adolescent Development

Boys	Girls
Stage 1: no maturation of genitalia	*Stage 1:* no maturation of genitalia
Stage 2: small amount of pubic hair; increased activity of sweat glands	*Stage 2:* small amount of pubic hair; increased activity of sweat glands; growth spurt
Stage 3: voice begins to change; facial hair begins; growth spurt	*Stage 3:* end of growth spurt; beginning of acne
Stage 4: voice deepens; end of growth spurt; acne may be severe	*Stage 4:* acne may be severe; menarche begins
Stage 5: adult-type genitalia; muscle mass increases significantly	*Stage 5:* adult-type genitalia and breasts; increase in fat and muscle mass

The stages of sexual maturation in adolescents, known as the *Tanner stages*, were first described by James Tanner, a British pediatrician, based on his research in the mid-1900s. An accompanying Tanner Scale was developed by him (Tanner, 1981); this measurement system defines sexual maturation in adolescents based on external primary and secondary sex characteristics (size of the breasts, genitals, testicular volume, and development of pubic hair). Rating assignments for each characteristic range from 1 (prepubertal) to 5 (adult); Table 2.1 provides a summary of these Tanner stages of adolescent physical growth for girls and boys.

Impact of Puberty on Brain Development

Recent preliminary evidence from developmental brain imaging studies has suggested that puberty hormones (most notably testosterone and estrogen) might significantly influence the structure and function of the developing human brain. Some experts think hormones' influences may be stronger than chronological age. Whereas this emerging science is relatively new, a wealth of evidence from nonhuman animal studies supports this view. Studies indicate that the hormonal events of puberty exert significant effects on brain maturation and a range of behaviors associated with reproductive activity and behavior related to seeking independence from parents (Sisk & Foster, 2004). Future research on this topic will benefit from combining behavioral, hormonal, and neuroimaging measures in order to clarify how puberty hormones influence the development of brain structure and function, which in turn affects adolescent behaviors.

Can Connection with the Family Affect Puberty?

An interesting issue among developmental psychologists is the possible causal link between pubertal development and family climate (Steinberg & Morris, 2001). The general finding of several studies is that that reproductive development in adolescence can be influenced by the extent and nature of the teenager's relationship with parents. For example, earlier and faster maturation has been observed among adolescents raised in homes characterized by less closeness and more conflict (Kim & Smith, 1998). Among girls from homes in which their biological father is not present, earlier maturation is more likely (Surbey, 1990).

Puberty's Impact on Psychological Health

The timing of puberty has been shown to be linked to a teenager's well-being. Late-maturing boys have relatively lower self-esteem and stronger feelings of inadequacy, whereas early-maturing boys are more popular and have a more positive self-image (Petersen, 1988). At the same time, however, early-maturing boys are more likely than their late-maturing peers to engage in delinquency, including drug use, truancy, and precocious sexual activity (e.g., Williams & Dunlop, 1999). Like boys, early-maturing girls are more popular and more likely to become involved in delinquent activities, use substances, have problems in school, and engage in early sexual activity (e.g., Flannery et al., 1993; Ge et al., 1996). These patterns may be due to the tendency for early maturers to affiliate with older peers

(Silbereisen et al., 1989), including that early-maturing females spend more time with older boys. Also, early-maturing girls have a tendency to have more emotional problems, a lower self-image, and higher rates of depression, anxiety, and disordered eating than their late-maturing peers (e.g., Ge et al., 1996). These effects among girls seem to be particularly pronounced in Westernized countries where cultural beliefs about attractiveness emphasize thinness.

In many ways, body dissatisfaction has emerged as a core aspect of young women's physical and mental health. Nearly half of American girls and young women report being dissatisfied with their bodies (Grabe et al., 2008), and these perceptions often begin to emerge during childhood. These feelings are not inconsequential; they have been linked to critical physical and mental health problems, including being a risk factor for eating disorders (Neumark-Sztainer et al., 2006).

Experts say that a major source of body-image dissatisfaction is that thin-bodied females are over-represented in print, film, and electronic-based media, and even thinner sometimes than the criteria for anorexia (Greenberg & Worrell, 2005). The media's consistent depiction of a thin ideal may lead girls to see this ideal as normative and central to attractiveness.

Sexual Activity and Adolescence

Most adolescents initiate sexual activity during high school, and this early initiation is associated with a host of risk factors, including not using condoms, teen pregnancy, and sexually transmitted infection (STI; Ethier et al., 2018). Yet these health risks seem to be taken more seriously by adolescents of late. There has been in recent years an overall decrease in the prevalence of ever having sexual intercourse. During the 2005–2015 period, the decrease among all students in grades 9–12 was 46.8% to 41.2%. This pattern was observed for both males and females and for most ethnic groups. Of note is the large decrease among ninth graders (34.3% to 24.1%, respectively). These trend data are a positive change in the level of sexual risk among adolescents in the United States (Ethier et al., 2018).

PSYCHOSOCIAL DEVELOPMENT

Introduction

The physical changes that signal the start of adolescence occur alongside psychological and social changes that mark this period as a critical stage in becoming an adult. These *psychosocial changes or challenges* involve developing new cognitive skills, a clearer sense of personal and sexual and gender identity, and a desire for independence from parents on an emotional, personal, and financial level. Also, an important hallmark of changes during adolescence is the maturation of the teen's *abstract thinking capacities*. Abstract thinking is the ability to use internal symbols or images to represent reality. In contrast to concrete thinking, which is common during pre-adolescence, where objects have to represent "things" or "ideas" for solving problems, abstract thinking enables a person to think hypothetically about the future, to assess many possible outcomes, and to choose a verbal or behavioral response to a situation by considering multiple options. But the development of abstract thinking runs into an opposing force during youth—the pervasive belief in personal invulnerability. This mindset of being "bullet-proof" can lead an adolescent to take major risks in terms of health, including substance abuse (Christie & Viner, 2005).

The joys and challenges of puberty have not gone unnoticed by Hollywood. "Coming-of-age" movies include *Y Tu Mama Tambien, Eighth Grade, Lucas, Saint Ralph,* and *Puberty Blues.* Can you identify TV or streaming shows that focus on adolescence?

Another major hallmark of adolescence pertains to the social tasks associated with resetting the *balance between independence and dependence* with respect to the self and the teenager's spheres of influence (parents, peers, and the community) (Christie & Viner, 2005). Striving for independence is an essential developmental task of adolescence. It involves learning to take responsibility, choosing to make decisions that reflect independence, and forming values that the teenager is comfortable with. Signs of independence can take many forms—choice of music and fashion; what hobbies to spend time with; the friends with which one affiliates.

Social and cultural factors will influence the timing and nature of this process of "balancing" one's development of a self-identity with one's relationships with the environment. The dominant motivation to shape self-identity tends to create the tendency for the teenager to view others only through their self-lens. This self-absorption, at the expense of empathy, can translate to much frustration for parents and other adults because it looks like the teenager does not understand the impact of behavior on others. Too often, common sense and general knowledge are given only minimal value and even ignored, leading to "What were they thinking?" from puzzled adults. For adolescents, a common reaction is "You do not understand me!"

Our guiding model to understand these challenges of adolescence is the *biopsychosocial model*. This approach acknowledges the role of biology for pubertal changes but emphasizes that adolescence and its challenges have a wide range of psychological and social elements; it assumes that the greater part of psychological and social development will depend on environmental and sociocultural influences. Below we review the five major psychosocial developmental challenges of adolescence: developing personal identity (including gender), developing intimate sexual relationships with an appropriate peer, establishing independence and autonomy, taking risks, and dealing with change.

These challenges interact with physical changes and the social environment and create great variability among teenagers of the same age. There are infinite ways that these types of interactions contribute to such differences. Here is a simple example: Two unrelated 14-year-old teenagers, Tom and Frank, are the same age by a month, each has lived on the same block and gone to the same school for their whole life. Tom is raised in a multi-sibling home with two parents. Tom is surrounded by a very active social life consistent with a large family. Tom is physically precocious; he is significantly ahead of his peers in physical signs of adolescent development. This includes facial hair growth and the presence of a deep voice. His parents are very involved in Tom's life, as they are with all of their children. Family conversations about life's lessons are common. Tom's social acumen and physical traits contribute to him being very popular among students in his school. He is enjoying adolescence and not finding its challenges daunting. Frank is an only child and being raised by a single parent. His mother struggles to spend a lot of quality time with Frank; their conversations are cordial but typically do not delve deeply into topics about life. Frank's physical development is behind that of his peers and his social skills are weak. Frank struggles with many of the challenges of adolescence. He does not make friends easily, has trouble connecting to any extracurricular school activities, and feels intimated by opportunities to take on new interests. Adolescence looks quite different for Tom and Frank. An argument can be made that some of these differences may be biological in nature, but the contrasting environments in which each were raised likely plays a significant role as well. Imagine if we consider a teenager raised in a non-Westernized culture; the differences between a teenager from an underdeveloped country and a typical American are likely be even more extreme than the differences between Tom and Frank.

Developing a Personal Identity

A central focus during adolescence is on identity formation. From early to late adolescence, the young person reveals many behavioral and attitudinal changes that involve the process of figuring out who you are. Box 2.2 summarizes these changes throughout stages as the young person ages through adolescence.

During early and middle adolescence, the young person has not yet fully realized their social identity (e.g., What type of peers do I want to affiliate with? How do I want to spend my free time socially?) and not defined the personality traits that characterize one's attitudes, values, and behaviors (e.g., Am I a follower or a leader? How assertive am I comfortable being? How spiritual am I? What are my political beliefs?).

Identity foreclosure. Some teenagers actively seek to define their identity, a process called *identity foreclosure.* Described by the famous developmental psychologist Eric Erickson (1963), this psychological term describes the stage when a teenager is exploring options about self-identity. The "finding a sense of self" stage may involve the adolescent adopting different traits and qualities from friends and relatives. This can include exploring their values, beliefs, career interests, sexual orientation, gender identity, political leanings, and more to reach an identity that feels comfortable and uniquely their own. In some cases, a teenager may have a comfortable sense of self but then later in adolescence encounter new peers or a new environment and decide to re-evaluate their beliefs. This can be expected to happen to a lot of young people when they leave home for college and are introduced to new perspectives on life that may be quite different from what they experienced earlier. Erickson called this an *identity crisis* and argued that it is a common occurrence among teenagers.

One of the authors saw this identity crisis occur with his brother. Never very religious or spiritual during his childhood or early adolescence, he rather suddenly connected with a social group in college that was very religious. Soon he embraced very strong religious beliefs, focused most of his social life around the church, and changed his professional goals to work for the church.

Support from parents is critical to healthy adolescent identity formation. Not only can they encourage their teenager to not be a carbon copy of their parents when it comes to values and beliefs, but they can provide guidance as the teenager takes on more responsibility for their behavior

BOX 2.2

Primary Psychosocial Developmental Changes During Stages of Adolescence

Early Adolescence (approximately 10–14 years of age)

Seeking Independence

A tendency to express feelings by actions rather than by words; great interest in and influence by close friends and start of strong peer identification; growing distance from parents that may include bouts of rudeness to them; often resort to childish behavior in the face of stress

Interests

Increasing career interests; greater exploration; greater ability to be a reliable worker

Cognitive Development

Focus on present and near-term future; concrete thinking is predominant, but there is a growing capacity for abstract thought and early moral concepts

Sexuality

Progression of sexual identity development (sexual orientation); for some, same-sex peer interest; girls physically mature faster than boys; experimentation with body (masturbation); concerns and repeated self-assessment of body image

Behavioral and Attitude Hallmarks

Rule and limit testing; occasional experimentation with substances

Middle Adolescence (approximately 15–16 years of age)

Seeking Independence

More self-indulgence, often characterized by swings of feelings of failure and unrealistically high expectations; more introspective; extreme concern with appearance and one's body image; growing angst about parents, dominant interest in new peers and lack of interest in family activities; interest in social media; periods of mood swings

Interests

More focus on intellectual pursuits and activities; greater attention to creative and career interests

Cognitive Development

Self-assess one's school and academic performance and one's social skills; greater verbal skills; still view self as "bullet-proof"

Sexuality

Concerns about sexual attractiveness; more clearly defined sexual orientation; for those not comfortable with their sexual orientation or gender identity, distress may be experienced; tendency to change relationships frequently; feelings of tenderness, affection, love, and passion

Behavioral and Attitude Hallmarks

More concrete goal setting, including longer-term goals; more adept at abstract thinking; greater interest in moral reasoning; evidence of behavior and attitudes reflecting one's ideals and value system; greater ability to feel empathy; strong peer identification; increased health risk (smoking, alcohol, etc.)

Late Adolescence (approximately 17–21 years of age)

Seeking Independence

Self-identity more crystallized; development of social autonomy; greater skill in delaying gratification and resisting impulses; more use of humor in social settings; hobbies and use of free time become more defined; less self-absorbed, including greater use of compromise and more concern for others

Interests

Higher level of concern for the future; more attention to one's role in life and career choice

Cognitive Development

Greater ability to think through complex ideas; enhanced verbal skills; work habits become more stable

Sexuality

Clear sexual identity; interest in and capacity for tenderness, passion, and sensual love; signs of the establishment of long-term romantic relationship

Behavioral and Attitude Hallmarks

Greater use of insight to guide decision making; ability to set and act on realistic goals; more self-regulation of emotions and increased impulse control; development of vocational interests and capability; endorsement of and immersion in social institutions and cultural traditions; greater appreciation of the difference between law and morality; further development or rejection of religious and political ideology

Adapted from Spano, S. (2004). *Stages of adolescent development.* https://www.actforyouth.net/resources/rf/rf_stages_0504.pdf.

BOX 2.3

THREE BASIC PARENTING PRINCIPLES TO MAXIMIZE THE HEALTH AND WELL-BEING OF AN ADOLESCENT

1. **Nurture a positive relationship with your teenager.** Strive to promote interactions with your adolescent that are characterized by respect, warmth, and kindness. Be a good listener.
2. **Use mistakes by your teenager as lessons learned.** Be willing to tolerate "oops mistakes" by your teenager and use such instances as lessons in good decision making.
3. **Have genuine interest in your adolescent's hobbies and activities.** Demonstrate true interest in and support for the proclivities that your teenager is showing. These include hobbies and how free time is spent.

Adapted from Spano, S. (2004). *Stages of adolescent development*. https://www.actforyouth.net/resources/rf/rf_stages_0504.pdf.

and decisions, including, for the first time, adult-like responsibilities, such as getting a job and learning to drive a car. More details of how parents can optimize the health and well-being of their teenager are provided in Box 2.3.

Cognitive development. During adolescence, a period of cognitive maturity occurs in which the individual demonstrates a higher level the thinking, characterized by the ability of hypothetical and deductive reasoning and to think more deeply about abstract concepts. Piaget (1960) refers to this as the *formal operational stage* of cognitive development. During this time, people develop the ability to think about abstract concepts. Piaget contends that during childhood mostly concrete or *inductive reasoning* is used, which involves drawing general conclusions from personal experiences and specific facts. But the adolescent becomes capable of *deductive reasoning*, in which the teenager draws specific conclusions from abstract concepts using logic and can think hypothetically. A common manifestation of deductive reasoning is the expression of "what-if" type statements. Formal operational thinking contributes to a more realistic ascertainment of possible outcomes and consequences of actions, enhanced ability to reflect on one's thinking processes (i.e., meta-cognition), and improved problem solving.

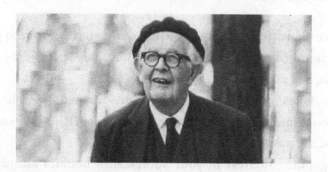

Jean Piaget, the famous theorist of cognitive development.

Establishing independence and autonomy in the context of one's social and cultural environment. A stage related to developing personal identity is expressing independence from one's surroundings. Behaviors and attitudes included in this stage are challenging authority, challenging the traditional moral and social structure of society, renegotiating rules at home and with adults, demanding opportunities for responsibilities and rights, and tendencies to venture away from the family and toward increasingly novel and adult-like activities.

Developmental psychologist Urie Bronfenbrenner emphasizes the importance of contextual influences from the environment, such as the family, peers, schools, and the media, on this stage (Bronfenbrenner, 1994). Bronfenbrenner believed that a child's development was affected by everything in their surrounding environment, which he divided into five different levels: the microsystem (e.g., the family, peers or caregivers), the mesosystem (e.g., the relationship between the child's peers and the family), the exosystem (e.g., the links between the child's microsystem and social settings in which the individual does not have an active role, such as the parent's experiences at work), the macrosystem (e.g., the culture in which the child lives), and the chronosystem (e.g., the patterning of environmental events and transitions over the life course, such as going to college).

Developing intimate sexual relationships with an appropriate peer. The important stage of sexuality during adolescence consists of developing relationships with a peer or peers with whom one feels an attraction, understanding one's sexuality, and engaging in sexual activity (Brown, 1999). The onset of puberty changes a focus on the need for friendship to a heightened interest in sexual expression. The extent to which a teenager is sexually attractive and accepted by opposite- or same-sex peers becomes a major source of one's self-worth. Over-attention to sexuality can distort this self-view, and often conflicts with parents arise as the teenager's expressions of sexuality are not met with parental approval. Nonetheless, truly intimate relationships emerge during this period, characterized by intimacy, openness, self-disclosure, and trust.

There have been changes in the median age at first marriage for both men and women in the United States. In 2018, the median age at first marriage was almost 30 for men and almost 28 for women. Historically, women married at an age that was about 3 years younger than men. But that gap has been slowly but steadily decreasing; now they are only separated on average by 2 years (Lake, 2022).

Teenagers often experience their first romantic experience in mixed-sex peer groups during late adolescence and young adulthood, an experience that addresses the dual need for friendship and sexual expression (Connolly & Goldberg, 1999; Carver et al., 2003). Romantic and sexual relationships develop into more serious and committed relationships, often leading to cohabitation, joint parenthood, and marriage (see Figure 2.1). Also, for some adolescents, their experience with sexual relationships involves identifying with a "desired" or "experienced gender" that is not the gender of the person assigned at birth.

Sex and intimacy. Sex often occurs as part of romantic experiences during adolescence; approximately 40% of all adolescents have intercourse before they graduate from high school (Ethier et al., 2018). Unintended teenage pregnancy and risk for HIV infections and other STIs

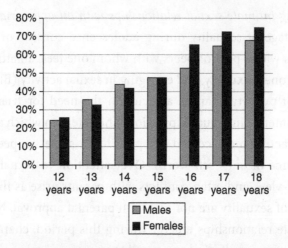

Figure 2.1 Percentage of adolescents reporting a romantic relationship within the past
18 months. Results from the National Longitudinal Study of Adolescent Health indicate that
it is relatively common for teenagers to have experienced a "special romantic relationship."
As the figure shows, that percentage increases to just under half of 15-year-olds, and then
leaps upward at age 16 to reach more than 70% by age 18 (Carver et al., 2003).
From Carver, K., Joyner, K., & Udry, J. R. (2003). National estimates of adolescent romantic
relationships. In P. Florsheim (Ed.), *Adolescent romantic relations and sexual behavior*
(pp. 37–70). Taylor Francis Group.

is a risk for teenagers who engage in sex. Youth (aged 13–24) accounted
for an estimated 22% of all new HIV diagnoses in the United States in
2015 (Centers for Disease Control and Prevention, 2016), and nearly half
of the nearly 20 million new STIs reported each year were among youth
in this age group (Centers for Disease Control and Prevention, 2016). As
adolescents extend their dating lives well into their 20s or forgo marriage
altogether, romantic relationships and sexual experience during the transition to adulthood have the potential to create a course of relationship
formation that may take on many different forms.

Cognitive changes during adolescence and intimacy. Cognitive changes
in adolescence are believed to have a significant impact on friendship
and intimacy. As we noted earlier in this chapter, the cognitive maturity during adolescence is characterized by a higher level of thinking
and a greater ability to think more profoundly about abstract concepts.
(*Abstract thinking* is the ability to use internal symbols or images to

represent reality. In contrast, *concrete thinking* involves objects to represent ideas.) Adolescence begins a period when the teenager better understands interpersonal relationships and communication, allowing them to have relationships with higher empathy, self-disclosure, and sensitivity. They are able to put themselves in "someone else's shoes," which is something that a child cannot do as well. Consider this contrast: to a child, friendship is more organized around activities and sharing play time; to an adolescent, relationships begin to build strong emotional bonds with another person. As the adolescent seeks and achieves more behavioral independence, they can be alone with friends and engage in intimate conversations. The structure of most high schools contributes to allowing teenagers to get closer to their peers, including coming in contact with older ones.

Taking risks. The teenage years mark a period when an individual is prone to take risks, as exemplified by drug use, unintentional injuries (especially car accidents), and unprotected sexual activity (Arnett, 1992). As discussed in Chapter 3, the remarkable findings from developmental neuroscience suggest that the way the brain matures during adolescence may contribute to this risk-taking proneness. Many researchers have argued that the basis for the link between neurobiology and risk behavior is the differential maturation rates of two brain development processes.

One process that emerges early in adolescence is the maturation of regions of the brain associated with emotion (amygdala) and motivation (nucleus accumbens) (Casey et al., 2008). These early-maturing "reward circuits" encourage the adolescent to venture away from the family and toward increasingly novel and sometimes risky activities (Spear, 2007). At the same time, researchers contend that the adolescent's prefrontal cortex (PFC), the "seat of sober second thought," has not yet matured to the point where risks can be adequately assessed and sufficient control can be exerted. Thus, this maturational gap in the development of the reward circuitry and the judgment region contributes to an inevitable period of risk for adolescents (Steinberg, 2008). In this light, adolescent risk-taking tendencies are more the result of normal development and the inevitable lack of experience associated with engaging in these novel behaviors. As we discuss in subsequent chapters, there is increasing interest among prevention and treatment programs to include content that aims to improve adolescent decision making when faced with temptations to engage in risky activities.

Risk-taking trends. Risk taking by teenagers can be moderated by the social and cultural environment, and trend data suggest some risk-taking behaviors are on the decline. One example is the decline of tobacco use by adolescents. Cigarette smoking rates among high school students have consistently dropped since the early 1990s. For example, the daily smoking rate among 12th graders in 1976 was 28.8% and in 2020 it was less than 2.0% (Meza et al., 2020). Experts point to several factors contributing to this decline: higher costs for tobacco products (for example, through increased taxes); prohibiting smoking in indoor areas, including public places and schools; mass media messages targeted toward youth to counter tobacco product advertisements; a focus of prevention programs in schools and communities that encourage tobacco-free environments and lifestyles; and in some regions, the raising of the minimum age of sale for tobacco products to 21 years.

The recent popularity of e-cigarettes and vaping is leading to an upward trend in use tobacco products. Now adolescents are more likely to use e-cigarettes than cigarettes. Based on the 2020 national Monitoring the Future survey data, 17 of 8th graders, 31% of 10th graders, and 35% of 12th graders reported vaping nicotine in the past year (National Institute of Drug Abuse, 2020).

Another example is the reported general decline in adolescent delinquency behaviors. Health data were analyzed from 12- to 17-year-old participants from the National Survey on Drug Use and Health, a representative survey of the household-dwelling population of the United States, across the 2003–2014 period (Grucza et al., 2018). Adolescent risk behaviors, including violence, crime, bullying and fighting, appear to have declined by as much as 34% during this period. The authors of the report further analyzed these data and concluded that these observed trends may be due to a corresponding downward trend in risk-taking tendencies and preferences. Yet the question remains as to why this decline in risk-taking has occurred. The authors note that given the relatively steep decline in the prevalence of these delinquency behaviors, the potential causes are likely to be environmental factors that have undergone relatively rapid changes in recent years. Possibilities include the expansion of school-based prevention programs that focus on bullying, the reductions in childhood lead exposure (Nevin, 2000), and the increased rates of use of medications for mental and behavioral conditions among pediatric populations (Finkelhor & Johnson, 2017).

The greater use of pharmacotherapy for adolescent behavioral and mental disorders includes medications for attention-deficit/hyperactivity disorder (ADHD) (e.g., Ritalin, Concerta, Stratera), depression and anxiety (e.g., Prozac, Lexapro, Zoloft), and early-onset psychosis (e.g., olanzapine, risperidone). However, there is considerable controversy that physicians are over-medicating adolescents. The authors want to emphasize a time-honored principle of adolescence: many of them will "mature out" of their teenage distress.

Influence of peers on psychosocial development. It has long been observed by developmental psychologists that peers have a wide-ranging influence during the teenage years. A famous book on the subject, *The Nurture Assumption*, first published by Judith Rich Harris (Harris, 2011), challenges the idea that the personality of adults is determined chiefly by the way they were raised by their parents. She reviewed a vast developmental psychology literature, and while acknowledging that parent genetic and socializing influences are significant, she points to the *peer group* as a major modifier of a child's behavior and attitudes. Her argument is that children and teenagers identify in important ways with their classmates and modify their behavior to fit with the peer group.

Neuroscientists also have weighed in on this issue of peer influences. Brain development that occurs during adolescence may contribute to tendencies to be influenced by same-aged peers. This topic is discussed below in detail in Chapter 3.

A common observation made by those studying the influence of peers is that adolescent risk behaviors often occur among peer groups and not as individual acts. But how might peers have a role in risk taking? Researchers are beginning to understand the causal role of peer influence. There are several explanations that fit a psychosocial-based perspective. A teenager affiliates with other risk-taking teenagers because the teen shares similar risk tendencies; group dynamics energize the peer members, contributing to "group think" and a pack mentality when seeking out and engaging in risk taking. Then there is the possibility that a non–risk taker affiliates with risk-taking peers and seeks social acceptance by engaging in risky behaviors that the non–risk taker would not normally do.

The influence of peers on *substance use* has received considerable attention in the research literature. Adolescents who report having substance-using friends and affiliating with peers who have attitudes that favor substance use indicate higher levels of substance use compared with those who deny having substance-using friends (Clark & Winters, 2002). The link between peer and personal substance use may be associated with underlying socialization and environmental influences, including the role of drug use in friendship selection (i.e., individuals already using drugs may tend to select friends with similar habits), certain members within the group modeling substance use (e.g., Dawes et al., 2000).

Biology and peer influences. There is also a biological explanation to consider when we examine peer influences. This position argues that the presence of peers may promote adolescent risk taking by sensitizing brain regions associated with the anticipation of potential rewards. One study supported this by examining brain activity in adolescents, young adults, and adults as they made decisions in a simulated driving task (Chein et al., 2011). Brain activity was measured using a type of brain imaging known as functional magnetic resonance imaging (fMRI). Participants completed one simulated driving task condition while alone, and one condition while their performance was observed by peers in an adjacent room. Risky types of driving behavior (e.g., risky driving decisions; simulated car crashes) measured during the *peer observation condition* indicated that adolescents revealed two patterns of brain activity that were not observed with the young adults and adults: greater brain activation in reward-related brain regions and less brain activation in brain regions related to cognitive control. These results suggest that the presence of peers increases adolescent risk taking by heightening sensitivity to the potential reward value of risky decisions.

Medical technology has advanced significantly with respect to imaging the brain, to better understand its structure and functions. One such technology is a functional magnetic resonance imaging (fMRI). This noninvasive test uses a strong magnetic field and radio waves to create detailed images of blood flow in the brain to detect areas of activity. These changes in blood flow, which are recorded on a computer, provide insights for scientists about how the brain works. Common uses of fMRI by neurologists and neuroscientists include detecting injured or diseased brain regions and brain mapping the brain's activity as the individual engages in a task (as was the case in the study by Chein et al., 2011).

Dealing with change. In addition to the major physical and psychological changes during adolescence, the teen years include various external or social changes. The major one that occurs for nearly all youths is changing schools and educational environment. Other youths may have to deal with moving to a new neighborhood or with family changes (e.g., new sibling; divorce by parents). These social challenges interact with psychological changes and may produce unique coping challenges.

Impact of use of drugs on psychosocial development. This important issue, which is discussed in more detail in Chapters 4 and 5, is typically viewed through the lens that adolescents' psychosocial development is arrested by use of drugs. Yet there is substantial evidence that deficits in psychosocial social functioning often precede and contribute to the development of a drug problem. Drug abuse may negatively impact several domains of youth functioning. For example, the following problems often follow after a teenager has been abusing drugs: lower academic success; lower vocational functioning; increased problems with family and other interpersonal relations; increased risk for trauma; elevated risk for sexual and blood-transmitted diseases (e.g., HIV, hepatitis B and C). And these problems can compound matters by interfering with social opportunities that would promote healthy development (e.g., engaging in prosocial behaviors, honing behavioral skills that will be useful in adulthood).

ADOLESCENCE AND PHYSICAL ACTIVITY

Adolescence is a period when habits associated with physical activity may be established, and these habits can affect future risk for cardiovascular disease. Cardiovascular risk factors of overweight, hypertension, increased blood lipids, and cholesterol levels are linked to physical inactivity (Heath et al., 1994). Whereas the early adolescent period often is often characterized by high physical activity, as adolescents move toward the end of the teenager years, there is a tendency toward a significant decline in participation in community and school-based recreation programs and overall vigorous activity (Spear, 2002a). Heath and colleagues (1994) showed that only 37% of students in grades 9 through 12 (approximate age range: 14 to 18 years) engaged in 20 minutes of vigorous physical activity three or more times per week. Although physical activity was higher among boys than girls, both had low participation levels. Even for the students who were enrolled in physical education classes, only 33% reported exercising 20 minutes or more in class three to five times per week. What are the specific cardiovascular health impacts of minimal physical activity? Sedentary adolescents have higher resting blood pressure and less favorable blood lipid profile, and, as expected, physically active adolescents have healthier blood pressure and lipid levels (Alpert & Wilmore, 1994).

What are optimal levels of activity? Experts do not agree on this issue, but a consensus panel from various countries developed these two guidelines for physical activity for adolescents: (1) be physically active every day as part of one's daily routine, and (2) engage in three or more sessions per week of activities that last 20 minutes or more at a time and that require moderate to vigorous levels of exertion (Sallis & Patrick, 1994).

SLEEP AND ADOLESCENCE

Sleep is vital to an individual's well-being. When sleep deprivation occurs, it can affect a person's mood, how well they do in school, and make them vulnerable to viruses (Short et al., 2011). Yet adequate and stable sleep can be a challenge during adolescence. Sleep pattern is generally stable during childhood (e.g., timing of sleep is relatively constant for all days in a week); this stability is marked by a stable circadian mechanism that helps a youngster to consistently wake up in the morning at the same time. However, the sleep patterns for adolescents are markedly different (Carskadon et al., 1998). It is common during adolescence to have different sleep patterns on weekdays from those on weekends. On weekends, the preference is to go to bed late and sleep; on weekdays, there is still the preference to stay up late but the requirement to wake up early often leads to feeling tired throughout the day. Experts say that teenagers need about 8 to 10 hours of sleep each night to function best. Yet most teens do not get this level of sleep, particularly during weekdays (it is natural for teenagers to not be able to fall asleep before 11:00 PM). One study found that only 15% reported sleeping 8 1/2 hours on school nights (Suni & Dimitriu, 2022).

Why the change in sleep pattern from childhood to adolescence? It is natural to point to psychosocial factors and demands that put a strain on getting enough sleep during the weekday: the teenager has greater academic demands; the school schedule does not accommodate good sleep; the teenager may have an evening job and increased involvement in social activities. But some researchers suggest that the onset of puberty unique to adolescence is a major contributing factor. How does puberty affect sleep? Experts believe that puberty causes a shift in the timing of circadian rhythms. A person's internal body clock controls the circadian rhythms in their body. *Circadian* means to occur within a daily period; a person's body clock makes them feel sleepy or alert at regular intervals within a 24-hour cycle. Everyone's body has this natural timing system. Prior to puberty, the body clock indicates it is time to sleep at typically around 8:00 or 9:00 PM. When puberty begins, this rhythm shifts a couple hours later; the teenage body clock kicks in with its "sleepy" feeling at around 10:00 or 11:00 PM.

This "sleep phase delay" means that the need for sleep during adolescence is delayed by roughly 2 hours. Yet an adolescent still needs a healthy amount of sleep, which is an average of 9 hours of sleep at night. Because most teens have to wake up early for school but cannot easily fall asleep early enough the previous night, many teenagers are sleep deprived during the weekdays. This situation causes them to fight a daily battle during school against sleepiness. A person is not at their best for thinking clearly and in control of one's emotions when tired. And a lack of sleep will also put them at greater risk of being in an accident in the car or on the job.

Exposure to any light—sunlight or artificial light—can dysregulate one's sleep. The hypothesized biological mechanism for this effect is that light suppresses a person's production of the hormone melatonin. Melatonin has a role in regulating body temperature, blood pressure, and glucose levels.

A solution to this problem is not easy. Some experts recommend that sleeping in much later on the weekend will help the teenager to catch up. But this response may further disrupt the body clock and make it even harder to get good sleep during the next school week.

Some school districts have moved the start of high school to later in the morning in an effort to address the problem of sleep deprivation in teenagers. The Minneapolis Public School District changed the starting times of seven high schools from 7:15 AM to 8:40 AM. A study by the University of Minnesota found that students benefited by obtaining 5 or more extra hours of sleep per week, improvement in attendance and enrollment rates, increased daytime alertness, and decreased student-reported depression.

Fortunately, many teenagers make changes and adjust to the new sleep schedule (e.g., avoid caffeine; take afternoon naps; begin to wind down and avoid high-level activity at 8 PM or so; avoid using a smartphone or laptop in the late evening because these machines' ultraviolet light can disrupt one's circadian rhythms). Also, parents can play a vital role in helping teens get the sleep they need by paying close attention to their adolescent's sleeping pattern and assisting with strategies cited above. For example, teenagers of parents who set and enforce bedtimes obtain more sleep and experience improved daytime wakefulness, less fatigue, and better emotional health (Palmer et al., 2018; Short et al., 2011).

PSYCHOLOGICAL HEALTH, SOCIAL MESSAGING, AND SCREEN TIME

Those individuals born in 1994 or later are known as the *i*Generation or Generation Z, and what distinguishes them is that they grew up with a smartphone and other electronic devices in hand. It is estimated that approximately 90% of teenagers in the United States have a smartphone or access to one in the home. As smartphones, laptops, and other electronic platforms become a staple of youth, there are many questions about their impact on the health of teenagers. A recent report by Statista indicates that these devices are contributing to provocatively high levels of social media usage by adolescents (see Figure 2.2).

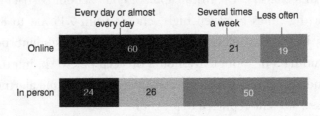

Six-in-ten teens spend time with their friends online on a daily or near-daily basis

% of U.S teens who say they get together with friends online or in person (outside of school or school-related activities)...

Note: Respondents who did not give an answer are not shown.
Source: Survey conducted March 7-April 10, 2018.
"Teens' Social Media Habits and Experiences"

PEW RESEARCH CENTER

Figure 2.2 Trends in Teenage Use of Social Media.
SOURCE: *"Teens' social media habits and experiences"* Pew Research Center, Washington, D.C. (NOVEMBER 28, 2018) https://www.pewresearch.org/internet/2018/11/28/teens-friendships-and-online-groups/

Jean Twenge's thoughtful book (Twenge, 2014) on the "Net Generation" makes the case that use of smartphones, and the habit of using them excessively on social media, exacerbates the common concern among teenagers about being left out. A she notes, when teenagers do congregate, they document their activity on Snapchat, Instagram, and Facebook. Those youths not invited become keenly—and perhaps painfully—aware of this and thus suffer more psychological distress. This trend has been especially steep among girls. Girls, who use social media more often than boys, are particularly prone to feeling excluded and lonely in the face of their classmates getting together without them (Twenge, 2014).

Another troubling trend is that more *overall screen time* is associated with greater distress. A U.S. survey of over 40,000 adolescents found that more than an average of 1 or more hours of screen time was associated with less psychological well-being, less self-control, and great difficulty making friends (Twenge & Campbell, 2018). For adolescents who report more than an average of 7 hours a day of screen time, they are twice as likely to have been diagnosed with a mental or behavioral disorder (Twenge & Campbell, 2018).

Other factors could be contributing to the association of screen time and psychological health. Kane and colleagues (2018) examined one likely confound—economic factors. They looked at several economic indicators (income equality, unemployment, median household income) and none of them correlated with changes in mood across the years 2007 to 2012.

Trend data point to similar findings. A recent study examined trend data on mood and media based on survey responses from roughly 1.1 million U.S. teenagers to examine trends in happiness and life satisfaction (Kane et al., 2018). Prior to 2012, adolescent ratings of mood were generally rising or at least stable, but that trend shifted in the downward direction in 2012. Perhaps this drop was associated with the sharp downturn in the economy around that time, or was there another contributing factor? A candidate suspect: the 2007 introduction of the smartphone. By 2012, approximately 37% of teens owned one, and this figure rose to at least 73% of teenagers by 2016. Also, when the researchers examined ratings of mood and self-reported time on their smartphone with all its online options, they found the same pattern as Twenge and Campbell (2018): adolescents' psychological well-being was lowest in years when, as a group, they spent more time with their smartphones and other electronic screens (on social media, texting, electronic games, the Internet) and when more of them owned smartphones. On the other hand, psychological well-being was highest in years when adolescents spent more time not online but with their friends in person, reading print media, and participating in exercise and sports (Kane et al., 2018; Schmuck, 2021).

Is there a sweet spot of screen time for psychological health? Experts do not agree on this question. For example, the American Academy of Pediatrics does not offer any specific recommendation for how much screen time is too much for a young person. A recent report from the

United Kingdom evaluated the link of health and amount of screen time among 120,000 teenagers (U.K. House of Commons Science and Technology Committee, 2019). Youth that used their smartphones no more than 2 hours a day or limited video games to no more than 6 hours a day reported slightly higher psychological health compared to those who used these screens less or not at all. Also, the high-end screen users reported slightly less well-being. Thus, perhaps moderation in screen time has benefits.

MINI-REVIEW

- Physical and psychosocial changes are happening at an accelerated rate during adolescence. Physical changes include the onset of puberty and the development of a sexually dimorphic body shape.
- The adolescent's view of their personal identity and how they relate to the outside world are greatly influenced by these physical changes.
- Genetic factors strongly influence several personality traits, including tendencies to engage in antisocial behavior and risk for depression. The influence of peers and parents will shape various features of a teenager's personality.
- The Tanner Scale provides a measurement system to define sexual maturation in adolescents.
- The critical psychosocial challenges of adolescence involve developing a clearer sense of personal and sexual identity and a desire for independence from one's parents.
- Other hallmarks of psychosocial development are involvement in romantic relations, risk-taking tendencies, changes in physical activity, and sleep deprivation.
- Psychological health can be adversely affected by indulgence in social messaging and too much screen time.

DISCUSSION POINTS

1. Research indicates that earlier and faster maturation has been observed among adolescents raised in homes with more discord and absence of a biological father. What might be the adaptive reasons for this?

2. Expressions of independence during adolescence can take many forms. What are some signs that you showed during your teenage years? Here are signs identified by experts:
   - Sudden change in peer groups
   - Isolating themselves from the family
   - No longer interested in hobbies and activities they once enjoyed
   - Distinct mood swings (more severe than moodiness)
   - Being unresponsive and/or defensive when confronted with parents' concerns and worries

3. Along with expressions of independence are tendencies to take unhealthy risks. What are some unhealthy risks that adolescents often take?

4. Developmental psychologists offer the view that the structure of high schools promotes connecting with peers and thus are favorable for a teenager's development. But what about the structure of high schools may also contribute to frustrations and emotional angst during the adolescent years?

5. Think back to your adolescence. Can you identify with the pattern during early adolescence of being very physically active but as you got into your later teen years your physical activity declined? What examples do you have?

6. Experts do not agree on whether or not it's best for a young person's health for them to use social media. What do you think about this? Could no use of social media lead to more distress? What about limiting social media use or strategies of media use?

7. The issue of gender identity is more front and center for teens than has been the case in years past. Why do think that is so? In what ways do current social factors contribute to a teen questioning one's gender identity?

Further Curiosity and Digging

Physical Development During Adolescence—Overview

McNeely, C., & Blanchard, J. (2009). *The teen years explained: A guide to healthy adolescent development.* Center for Adolescent Health at John Hopkins Bloomberg School of Public Health. https://www.jhsph.edu/research/centers-and-institutes/center-for-adolescent-health/_docs/TTYE-Guide.pdf

Puberty—Overview

MedicineNet. (n.d.). *Puberty.* https://www.medicinenet.com/puberty/article.htm

Puberty—How Do Hormones Work?

Bryce, M. (2018, June). *How do your hormones work?* [Video]. TED Conferences. https://www.ted.com/talks/emma_bryce_how_do_your_hormones_work?language=en

Importance of Sleep to Adolescents

Troxel, W. (2016, November). *Why school should start later for teens.* [Video]. TED Conferences. https://www.ted.com/talks/wendy_troxel_why_school_should_start_later_for_teens?language=en

References

Alpert, B. S., & Wilmore, J. H. (1994). Physical activity and blood pressure in adolescents. *Pediatric Exercise Science, 6,* 361–380.

Arnett, J. (1992). Socialization and adolescent reckless behavior: A reply to Jessor. *Developmental Review, 12,* 391–409.

Berkey, C. S., Rockett, H. R., Field, A. E., Gillman, M. W., Frazier, A. L., Camargo, C. A., & Colditz, G. A. (2000). Activity, dietary intake, and weight changes in a longitudinal study of preadolescent and adolescent boys and girls. *Pediatrics, 105,* e56–e56.

Blumenthal, S. J., & Kupfer, D. J. (1988). Overview of early detection and treatment strategies for suicidal behavior in young people. *Journal of Youth and Adolescence, 17,* 1–23.

Bronfenbrenner, U. (1994). Ecological models of human development. *Readings on the Development of Children, 2,* 37–43.

Brown, B. B. (1999). "You're going out with who?": Peer group influences on adolescent romantic relationships. In W. Furman, B. B. Brown, & C. Feiring (Eds.), *The development of romantic relationships in adolescence* (pp. 291–329). Cambridge University Press.

Carskadon, M. A., Wolfson, A. R., Acebo, C., Tzischinsky, O., & Seifer, R. (1998). Adolescent sleep patterns, circadian timing, and sleepiness at a transition to early school days. *Sleep, 21,* 871–881.

Carver, K., Joyner, K., & Udry, J. R. (2003). National estimates of adolescent romantic relationships. In P. Florsheim (Ed.), *Adolescent romantic relations and sexual behavior* (pp. 37–70). Psychology Press.

Casey, B. J., Getz, S., & Galvan, A. (2008). The adolescent brain. *Developmental Review, 28*, 62–77.

Centers for Disease Control and Prevention. (November, 2016). Diagnoses of HIV infection in the United States and dependent areas, 2015. *HIV Surveillance Report 2015,* vol. 27. https://www.cdc.gov/hiv/pdf/library/reports/surveillance/cdc-hiv-surveillance-report-2015-vol-27.pdf

Chein, J., Albert, D., O'Brien, L., Uckert, K., & Steinberg, L. (2011). Peers increase adolescent risk taking by enhancing activity in the brain's reward circuitry. *Developmental Science, 14*, F1–F10.

Christie, D., & Viner, R. (2005). Adolescent development. *British Medical Journal, 330*, 301–304.

Clark, D. B., & Winters, K. C. (2002). Measuring risks and outcomes in substance use disorders prevention research. *Journal of Consulting and Clinical Psychology, 70*, 1207–1223.

Connolly, J., & Goldberg, A. (1999). Romantic relationships in adolescence: The role of friends and peers in their emergence and development. In W. Furman, B. B. Brown, & C. Feiring (Eds.), *The development of romantic relationships in adolescence* (pp. 266–290). Cambridge University Press.

Dawes, M. A., Antelman, S. M., Vanyukov, M. M., Giancola, P., Tarter, R. E., Susman, E. J., Mezich, A., & Clark, D. B. (2000). Developmental sources of variation in liability to adolescent substance use disorders. *Drug and Alcohol Dependence, 61*, 3–14.

Erikson, E. H. (1963). *Childhood and society.* Norton.

Ethier, K. A., Kann, L., & McManus, T. (2018). Sexual intercourse among high school students—29 states and United States overall, 2005–2015. *MMWR. Morbidity and Mortality Weekly Report, 66*, 1393.

Finkelhor, D., & Johnson, M. (2017). Has psychiatric medication reduced crime and delinquency? *Trauma, Violence, & Abuse, 18*, 339–347.

Flannery, D. J., Rowe, D. C., & Gulley, B. L. (1993). Impact of pubertal status, timing, and age on adolescent sexual experience and delinquency. *Journal of Adolescent Research, 8*, 21–40.

Ge, X., Conger, R. D., & Elder Jr., G. H. (1996). Coming of age too early: Pubertal influences on girls' vulnerability to psychological distress. *Child Development, 67*, 3386–3400.

Grabe, S., Ward, L. M., & Hyde, J. S. (2008). The role of the media in body image concerns among women: A meta-analysis of experimental and correlational studies. *Psychological Bulletin, 134*, 460.

Greenberg, B. S., & Worrell, T. R. (2005). The portrayal of weight in the media and its social impact. In K. D. Brownell, R. M. Puhl, M. B. Schwartz, & L. Rudd (Eds.), *Weight bias: Nature, consequences, and remedies* (pp. 42–53). Guilford.

Grucza, R. A., Krueger, R. F., Agrawal, A., Plunk, A. D., Krauss, M. J., Bongu, J., Cavazos-Rehg, P. A., & Bierut, L. J. (2018). Declines in prevalence of adolescent substance use disorders and delinquent behaviors in the USA: A unitary trend?. *Psychological Medicine, 48*(9), 1494–1508.

Harris, J. R. (2011). *The nurture assumption: Why children turn out the way they do.* Simon and Schuster.

Heath, G. W., Pratt, M., Warren, C. W., & Kann, L. (1994). Physical activity patterns in American high school students: Results from the 1990 Youth Risk Behavior Survey. *Archives of Pediatrics & Adolescent Medicine, 148*, 1131–1136.

Jacobson, K. C., & Rowe, D. C. (1999). Genetic and environmental influences on the relationships between family connectedness, school connectedness, and adolescent depressed mood: Sex differences. *Developmental Psychology, 35*, 926.

Kane, H. S., Wiley, J. F., Dunkel Schetter, C., & Robles, T. F. (2018). The effects of interpersonal emotional expression, partner responsiveness, and emotional approach coping on stress responses. *Emotion, 19*, 1315–1328.

Kim, K., & Smith, P. K. (1998). Retrospective survey of parental marital relations and child reproductive development. *International Journal of Behavioral Development, 22*, 729–751.

Lake, R. (2022). What is the average age of marriage in the U.S.? *Brides*, February 25. https://www.thespruce.com/estimated-median-age-marriage-2303878

McGue, M., Sharma, A., & Benson, P. (1996). Parent and sibling influences on adolescent alcohol use and misuse: Evidence from a US adoption cohort. *Journal of Studies on Alcohol, 57*, 8–18.

Meza, R., Jimenez-Mendoza, H., & Levy, D. T. (2020). Trends in tobacco use among adolescents by grade, sex, and race, 1991–2019. *JAMA Network Open, 3*(12), e2027465. https://jamanetwork.com/journals/jamanetworkopen/fullarticle/2773464

National Institute of Drug Abuse (NIDA). (2020, December 15). *Study: Surge of teen vaping levels off, but remains high as of early 2020.* https://nida.nih.gov/news-events/news-releases/2020/12/study-surge-of-teen-vaping-levels-off-but-remains-high-as-of-early-2020

Neumark-Sztainer, D., Levine, M. P., Paxton, S. J., Smolak, L., Piran, N., & Wertheim, E. H. (2006). Prevention of body dissatisfaction and disordered eating: What next? *Eating Disorders, 14*, 265–285.

Nevin, R. (2000). How lead exposure relates to temporal changes in IQ, violent crime, and unwed pregnancy. *Environmental Research, 83*, 1–22.

Palmer, C. A., Oosterhoff, B., Bower, J. L., Kaplow, J. B., & Alfano, C. A. (2018). Associations among adolescent sleep problems, emotion regulation, and affective disorders: Findings from a nationally representative sample. *Journal of Psychiatric Research, 96*, 1–8.

Petersen, A. C. (1988). Adolescent development. *Annual Review of Psychology, 39*, 583–607.

Piaget, J. (1960). The general problems of the psychobiological development of the child. In J. M. Tanner & B. Inhelder (Eds.), *Discussions on child development* (vol. 4, pp. 3–27). Tavistock.

Sallis, J. F., & Patrick, K. (1994). Physical activity guidelines for adolescents: Consensus statement. *Pediatric Exercise Science, 6*, 302–314.

Schmuck, D. (2021). Following social media influencers in early adolescence: Fear of missing out, social well-being and supportive communication with parents. *Journal of Computer-Mediated Communication, 26*, 245–264.

Short, M. A., Gradisar, M., Wright, H., Lack, L. C., Dohnt, H., & Carskadon, M. A. (2011). Time for bed: Parent-set bedtimes associated with improved sleep and daytime functioning in adolescents. *Sleep, 34*, 797–800.

Silbereisen, R. K., Petersen, A. C., Albrecht, H. T., & Kracke, B. (1989). Maturational timing and the development of problem behavior: Longitudinal studies in adolescence. *Journal of Early Adolescence, 9*, 247–268.

Sisk, C. L., & Foster, D. L. (2004). The neural basis of puberty and adolescence. *Nature Neuroscience, 7*, 1040–1047.

Spear, B. A. (2002a). Adolescent growth and development. *Journal of the American Dietetic Association, 102*(Suppl), S23–S29.

Spear, B. A. (2002b). Nutrition in adolescence. In L. K. Mahan & S. Escott-Stump (Eds.), *Krause's food, nutrition, and diet therapy* (pp. 257–270). W.B. Saunders.

Spear, L. P. (2000). The adolescent brain and age-related behavioral manifestations. *Neuroscience & Biobehavioral Reviews, 24*, 417–63.

Spear, L. P. (2007). The developing brain and adolescent-typical behavior patterns: An evolutionary approach. In D. Romer, & E. F. Walker (Eds.), *Adolescent psychopathology and the developing brain: Integrating brain and prevention science* (pp. 9–30). Oxford University Press.

Steinberg, L. (2008). A social neuroscience perspective on adolescent risk-taking. *Developmental Review, 28*, 78–106.

Steinberg, L., & Morris, A. S. (2001). Adolescent development. *Annual Review of Psychology, 52*, 83–110.

Suni, E., & Dimitriu, A. (2022). *Teens and sleep.* Sleep Foundation. https://www.sleepfoundation.org/articles/teens-and-sleep

Surbey, M. K. (1990). Family composition, stress, and the timing of human menarche. In T. E. Ziegler & F. B. Bercovitch (Eds.), *Monographs in primatology, Vol. 13. Socioendocrinology of primate reproduction* (pp. 11–32). Wiley-Liss.

Tanner, J. M. (1981). Growth and maturation during adolescence. *Nutrition Reviews, 39*, 43–55.

Twenge, J. M. (2014). *Why today's young Americans are more confident, assertive, entitled—and more miserable than ever before.* Atria Paperback.

Twenge, J. M., & Campbell, W. K. (2018). Associations between screen time and lower psychological well-being among children and adolescents: Evidence from a population-based study. *Preventive Medicine Reports, 12*, 271–283.

U.K. House of Commons Science and Technology Committee. (2019). *Impact of social media and screen-use on young people's health.* https://publications.parliament.uk/pa/cm201719/cmselect/cmsctech/822/822.pdf

Williams, J. M., & Dunlop, L. C. (1999). Pubertal timing and self-reported delinquency among male adolescents. *Journal of Adolescence, 22*, 157–171.

Adolescent Brain Development

INTRODUCTION

New scientific discoveries based on neuroimaging data have refined our understanding of adolescent behavior. As we discussed in Chapter 2, adolescent development is characterized by major physical changes, and these changes influence behavioral tendencies during the teenage years. Research now suggests that the human brain is still maturing in significant ways during the adolescent years; it is the last major organ in the body to reach full maturity (Giedd, 2004). There have been exciting attempts to capitalize on brain imaging data in order to develop a human brain maturity index or growth curve, and experts believe this neurodevelopment may influence the way teenagers make decisions and have implications for health.

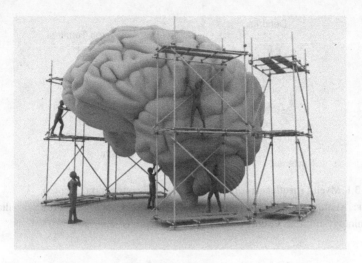

SOURCE: Science Photo Library/Alamy Stock Photo.

WORK IN PROGRESS

Advanced technologies in brain imaging now offer a unique opportunity to better understand the developing brain. This window into the teen brain has provided several insights. On a basic level, our brain develops by increasing the strength of neural connections that are intertwined throughout the brain. This is facilitated by the process of *myelination*, which is the wrapping of insulation—myelin sheath—around these neural connections (see Figure 3.1). This is like having rubber insulation around electrical wires. Myelination promotes fast neural connection.

But children and teenagers have more synapses than are necessary, creating a clutter of connections that impedes brain activity. Prior to adolescence, the brain's growth of connections between brain cells is robust. At about age 11 or 12 years, these connections begin to significantly disappear or "prune back." This reduction of connections is another important part of development by promoting myelination and the long-term health of the brain. Pruning clears out brain "wiring" that has not

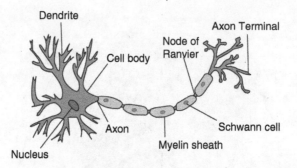

Figure 3.1 Myelin sheath surrounding the nerve cell connections (axons).
Source: "Anatomy and Physiology" by the US National Cancer Institute's Surveillance, Epidemiology and End Results (SEER) Program/Wikipedia.

yet been activated and provides room for the continuing strengthening of already functioning connections. This loss is healthy in the long run and is a vital part of growing up. The pruning process clears out unneeded wiring to make way for more efficient and faster information processing, and it promotes the building of the long chains of nerve cells that are required for the more demanding problem solving needed during adulthood (see Figure 3.2).

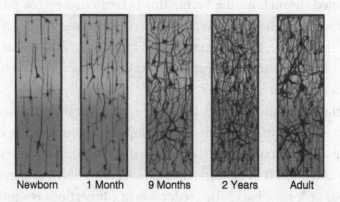

Figure 3.2 Synaptic density at five ages.
Adapted from Corel, J. L. The postnatal development of the human cerebral cortex. Cambridge, MA: Harvard University Press; 1975.

Brain Maturation Process

It is believed that the pruning process generally follows a "use-it-or-lose-it" principle. Neural connections that have already been activated are retained, while those connections that are not activated are pruned out. If you played soccer during your youth, it is likely that neural connections involved in foot and leg coordination are strengthened to a greater degree during pruning than in a teenager who played the piano as child, whose connections associated with finger coordination likely will have been more resistant to pruning. The eminent researcher Dr. Giedd describes this process accordingly: "Ineffective or weak connections are pruned in much the same way a gardener would prune a tree or bush, giving the plant the desired shape" (Giedd, 2004).

Another consideration of brain maturation is how different regions of the brain mature at different rates during adolescence. This discovery is important given regions of the brain are associated with different brain functions. The brain maturation process tends to occur in an uneven fashion—generally from the back of the brain to the front (see Figure 3.3).

Gray Matter Maturation

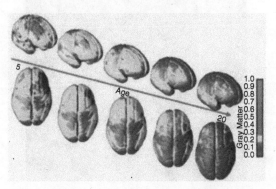

Figure 3.3 Maturation of the brain's gray matter from age 5 to 20 years.
From Gogtay, N., Giedd, J. N., Lusk, L., Hayashi, K. M., Greenstein, D., Vaituzis, A. C., . . .
Rapoport, J. L. (2004). Dynamic mapping of human cortical development during
childhood through early adulthood. *Proceedings of the National Academy of Sciences, USA,*
101(21), 8174–8179. Copyright (2004) National Academy of Sciences, U.S.A.

Located more to the back of the brain is the limbic system, or the "go for it" region. Brain structures here are associated with memory, motivation, and pleasure-based behaviors, such as the urge to eat when hungry and the desire to have sex. The frontal region of the brain, particularly the prefrontal cortex (PFC), is associated with regulating emotion, attention, and motivation and is believed to be the brain sector primarily responsible for suppressing risk taking, making decisions, and feeling empathy. The PFC is symbolically the "neurological brakes" for resisting impulses and delaying gratification, and it helps us to make good decisions. During the brain development of adolescence, it is believed that the limbic-related regions mature earlier than the frontal, PFC brain region (Giedd, 2004; Gogtay et al., 2004). As psychologist Laurence Steinberg sees it, a teenager's brain "has a well-developed accelerator but only a partly developed brake" (Steinberg, 2004).

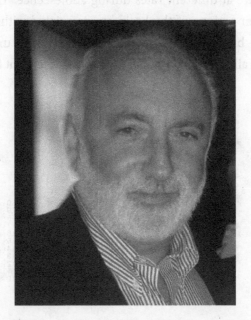

Laurence Steinberg, Ph.D. is one of world's leading experts on adolescent development. Photo courtesy of Laurence Steinberg.

Does brain maturation occur uniformly for all youth? Whereas it is accepted that the general pattern of prolonged development of prefrontal control circuitry and more rapid maturation of the limbic region is universal, evidence suggests neurodevelopmental variability is a function of sex (the brain maturation of girls tends to be ahead of that of boys) and environmental experiences (Kaufmann et al., 2017). For example, it appears that excessive exposure to emotionally arousing states or conditions will hamper brain maturation (Rudolph et al., 2017).

Plasticity principle. A key phenomenon that underlies brain development is plasticity. *Brain plasticity* describes the ability of the brain's structure and function to adapt in response to environmental demands, experiences, and physiological changes (Pascual-Leone et al., 2005). Whereas plasticity occurs throughout our lifetime—it's a key basis for learning throughout life—experts now believe that because adolescence is an active period of myelination and pruning, it's also a sensitive period of brain plasticity.

Research is accumulating that *early trauma* can alter brain development. One study is particularly noteworthy because of its strong research design. Lutz and colleagues (2017) compared postmortem brain tissue from 27 individuals who had suffered severe physical or sexual abuse before the age of 15 and had died by suicide. As controls, the team also examined postmortem data from 25 people who suffered from major depression and died by suicide but had no history of child abuse, as well as 26 psychiatrically healthy individuals with no history of child abuse. The investigators focused on the brain region involved in regulating mood and emotions. Their analysis determined that brain cells from people who had suffered abuse as children had less myelin sheath in this region; myelin sheath develops during childhood and is important for preserving electrical signals that must travel long distances across the brain. This structural difference could compromise a person's emotional regulation and their ability to handle stress.

Rate of development during adolescence. Brain changes in terms of structure and neurochemical functions are quite rapid during early to mid-adolescence. Yet the pace of neurodevelopment during late adolescence through the 20s is slower and more focused (Baker et al., 2015). These changes are concentrated on strengthening neural connections that support emotional regulation, problem solving, and future planning. Thus, neural connections between the emotional and thinking centers of the brain become stronger and provide greater capacity for planful thinking.

The Developing Brain and Its Possible Influence on Adolescent Behavior

Such heightened plasticity may result in not only increased opportunities for development but also increased vulnerabilities, and may influence numerous aspects of adolescent functioning. This complex issue has been the source of considerable discussion among experts. To what extent does brain development shape and alter adolescent behavior?

A long-standing test that presumably measures the ability to delay gratification is the so-called "marshmallow test." Pioneered in the 1960s by Stanford psychology professor, Walter Mischel, the marshmallow test involves leaving a child between the ages of 3 and 5 years alone in a room with two identical plates, each containing different quantities of a treat, such as a marshmallow. Before leaving the room "to do some work," the adult researcher instructs the child that they are free to eat the marshmallow at any time. But if the child waits for the adult to return before eating it, the child is told a second, bigger treat will be available. After the adult researcher leaves the room, the child's behavior is monitored on the other side of a two-way mirror to see how long they can hold out before licking or eating the treat.

Research over the years suggests that superior results on a delayed-gratification task during the toddler years is associated with better performance in school and in jobs, healthier relationships, and even fewer chronic diseases. A new study (Carlson et al., 2018) suggests that children are improving on this task compared to prior generations. Contemporary children, on average, are displaying more delay in gratification with the marshmallow test than children decades back. The authors reiterate the importance that delay of gratification is still a good bellwether of the self-regulation skills so important for achievement and success.

It is well established that when humans engage in thinking that is related to dealing with gratification or with impulses to act, the prefrontal region of the brain is called on. This region is primarily responsible for what your reactions will be when faced with highly emotional messages (such as, "This will be fun!") or when confronted by challenges from the environment to act quickly (such as, "Join us now!"). While scientists caution against definitive linkages between brain development and adolescent behavior, it believed that the relative imbalance between the slower-to-mature PFC (brake system) and the earlier developing limbic region (accelerator system) may significantly contribute to a developmentally normative increase in risk taking and novelty seeking by youth, particularly during the younger teenage years of 12 to 15.

Furthermore, certain conditions may be ripe for risk taking by teenagers. These include situations when the teenager is experiencing high emotion, is in the presence of intense peer pressure, or is faced with a perception that a positive or rewarding outcome will immediately be obtained. In this light, the still-maturing circuitry in the front part of the brain may be particularly overwhelmed in such situations and, thus, make it difficult for the teenager to engage in thoughtful decision making. Thus, given this neurological imbalance, adolescence may be a developmental period when controlling impulses is particularly difficult (Reyna & Farley, 2006). Experts say that even at ages 16 and 17, when compared to adults, adolescents on average are more inclined to be risk-takers, more aggressive, more emotionally volatile, and more vulnerable to peer influences (Dahl, 2004; Steinberg, 2004; Winters & Arria, 2011). We provide a list

---

BOX 3.1

BEHAVIORAL AND ATTITUDINAL TENDENCIES OF ADOLESCENCE THAT
MAY BE INFLUENCED BY BRAIN DEVELOPMENT

Particular interest in and preference for . . . .
. . . physical activity
. . . high excitement and rewarding activities
. . . social situations with peers
. . . novelty

Lapses in . . . .
. . . emotional control
. . . consideration of negative consequences

Tendencies to . . . .
. . . be attentive to social information
. . . take risks

---

in Box 3.1 of the prominent behaviors of adolescence that developmental
psychologists suggest have some link to brain development.

Risk taking. As we discussed in Chapter 2, adolescence is a developmental period that is marked by risk taking. It is tempting to view adolescent *brain development* in light of behaviors that teenagers are challenged
by, such as breaking rules, gaps in sound judgment, failure to experience
empathy, and high susceptibility to peer influences. These behaviors
can be the basis for a range of risk-taking behaviors. Studies show that
adolescents, compared to children and adults, react more strongly to
situations that offer reward and risk. When a teenager feels high emotion
or intense peer pressure, conditions are ripe for the still-maturing brain
to be overwhelmed, resulting in tendencies to be emotionally labile, make
poor judgments, and take risks (Dahl, 2004).

Also relevant is the role of peers on risk-taking behavior. Teenagers
are more susceptible to peer influences than other age groups. A study

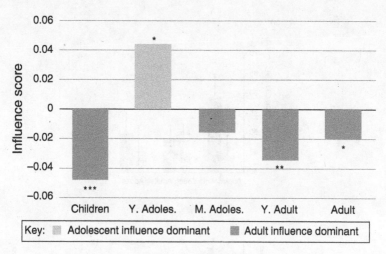

Figure 3.4 Effect of social influence on risk ratings (Knoll et al., 2015).
Source: Knoll, L. J., Magis-Weinberg, L., Speekenbrink, M., & Blakemore, S. J. (2015).
Social influence on risk perception during adolescence. *Psychological Science, 26*(5), 583–592. License: CC BY 4.0.

by Knoll and colleagues (Knoll et al., 2015) measured the extent of social influence on risk perception. Young adolescents were more influenced by the opinions of teenagers than by the opinions of adults, whereas all other age groups—including children, young adults, and adults—were more influenced by the adults' opinions about risk (see Figure 3.4).

A study was conducted in which the investigators had adolescents complete a simulated driving task under two conditions: one with an active adolescent "passenger" who had risk-taking tendencies and offered decision-making guidance during the driving task, and one with a passive adolescent (Centifanti et al., 2014). The risky driving decisions made by the adolescent driver during simulation were significantly greater in the presence of the active adolescent than with the passive one. A related study compared adolescents, young adults, and adults when playing a simulated driving task. All subjects played the game twice—once in an alone condition and once in a peer condition, in which participants were made aware that their performance was being observed on a monitor in a nearby room by two same-age, same-sex peers who had accompanied

(a)

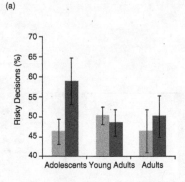

(b)

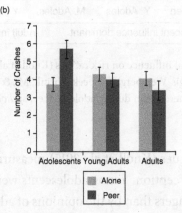

Figure 3.5 Susceptibility of adolescents, young adults and older adults to peer influences on performance in the Stoplight game (Chein et al., 2011). The graphs show (a) the mean percentage of risky decisions and (b) the number of crashes for participants playing the Stoplight game either alone or with a peer audience. Error bars indicate standard errors of the mean.
SOURCE: Peers increase adolescent risk taking by enhancing activity in the brain's reward circuitry, by Jason Chein, Dustin Albert, Lia O'Brien, Kaitlyn Uckert, Laurence Steinberg. *Developmental Science*, Volume 14, Issue 2, March 2011, Pages F1–F10.

them to the experiment. As predicted, adolescents, but not young adults and adults, took significantly more risks when they were being observed by peers than when they were alone (Chein et al., 2011) (see Figure 3.5). These studies are consistent with other research that has shown that adolescent risky behavior almost always occurs in the presence of familiar peers (Cohen & Prinstein, 2006; Crosnoe et al., 2004).

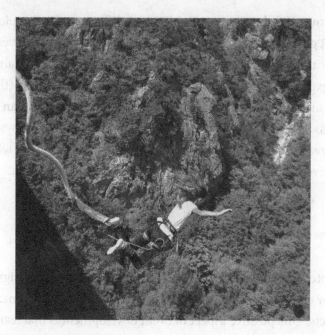

Of course, teenagers often make sound decisions; they are capable of self-control and frequently display good judgment. And some brain development is complete during the teen years; normal levels of language and spatial abilities are reached by adolescence and their capacity to learn is higher in adolescence than it is later in life. But some aspects of brain development likely contribute to risk-taking tendencies of youth. The part of the brain—the reward center—which is responsible for our response to reward and risk, is more active during adolescence, and the region of the brain that accounts for controlling impulses and thoughtful thinking—the PFC—is underdeveloped during the teen years. Thus, the teenager, with less-than-optimal impulse control mechanisms, may be prone to act impulsively and with gut instinct when confronted with high-emotion, peer-influenced situations, without fully appreciating the immediate consequences of their actions.

Gender differences. There are some differences in brain development between girls and boys. One big difference pertains to rate—on average, girls are approximately 2 years ahead of boys in the developmental trajectory.

Keeping in mind that there are individual differences, it is typical to ob-serve that girls during the early and mid-teen years are about 2 years ahead of boys with respect to emotional maturity and ability to plan ahead. This may be explained by the fact that, in general, the frontal lobe (the seat of decision making) of female brains reaches maturity sooner than the male brain. This brain maturation difference may also explain why boys typically display greater risk taking than girls; the basis of adolescent risk taking may be a relatively immature development of the frontal lobe region.

The Developing Brain and Life Experiences

As we noted above, the teenager's brain development can be significantly shaped by early experiences. This presents opportunities for amazing pos-itive effects. One positive aspect of brain development is that learning can be accelerated during this period, allowing a teenager to work on their strengths, try new things, and address weaknesses with great energy. But it also suggests that the teenage brain may be vulnerable to the effects of negative things, such as stress and the effects of drug use.

Brain Development and Learning

Adolescence is a sensitive period for memory. Studies suggest that our re-call of music, books, films, and public events from adolescence is superior to that for similar such stimuli experienced at other age periods (Rubin & Schulkind, 1997). Perhaps you have noticed this with your parents, who can show a remarkable ability to recall very specific autobiographical memories from their youth with more detail than of events that occurred during adulthood. Even mundane events that happened during youth in adolescence and early adulthood appear to be overrepresented in memory.

If memory is indeed to have a heightened impact during adolescence, then this is an opportunistic time for enhanced learning. Thus, the em-phasis on formal education during these years is critical to lifelong health and social development. Many regions of the world do not provide easy access to secondary school education; it is estimated that 40% of the world's teenagers do not have access to secondary school education (UNICEF, 2011). However, there are encouraging signs that his status quo is now changing (World Health Organization, 2014).

Brain Development and Mental Health

Based on a wealth of studies, experts now view most mental illnesses as a developmental disorder of the brain, and further point to the deleterious impact on early exposure of stress on brain maturation and risk for mental and behavioral disorders. One in four people at some point in their life span will experience at least one type of mental illness, and the majority of them have their onset during youth, including late childhood and the teenage years (Kessler et al., 2007). A longitudinal study showed that 74% of adults with a mental disorder received a diagnosis before 18 years of age and 50% before 15 years of age (Kim-Cohen et al., 2003). Alterations in neurodevelopment have been linked to several adolescent-onset mental and behavioral disorders, including attention-deficit/hyperactivity disorder, depression, anxiety disorders, autism, obsessive-compulsive disorder, and schizophrenia (Kaminer et al., 2019) (more on the onset of mental disorders in Chapters 6 and 7). These various neurodevelopmental disorders show similar features, including difficulties in sensor and motor systems, problems with speech and language, and impairments with learning and organizational skills (Martens & Van Loo, 2007). These facts place the adolescent years as a vulnerable time. By studying how the circuitry of the brain develops, and what factors may alter the circuitry, scientists hope to understand when and why brain development can result in mental illness.

Stress. One contributory factor regarding risk for future mental or behavioral problems being studied is stress. Teens' perception of stress and anxiety is actually amplified compared to that of adults, and social stress in particular is thought to have a disproportionate impact during adolescence (Andersen & Teicher, 2008). Understanding the changes taking place in the brain if the youth is repeatedly exposed to stress is an important area of research.

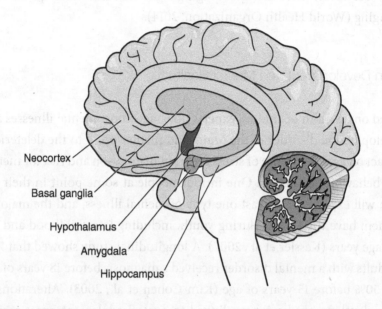

Neocortex

Basal ganglia

Hypothalamus

Amygdala

Hippocampus

Unfortunately, bullying is fairly common during adolescence. Experts estimate that about 25–50% of teenagers in the United States report have been a victim of bullying or have bullied others. Neuroscientists are learning that adolescents who bully other teens tend to display a different pattern of brain activity in response to certain facial expressions. Swartz and colleagues (Swartz et al., 2019) examined the brain activity among a group of adolescents in the brain region known as the amygdala, which plays a key role in emotional processing and responding to threats. The adolescents had their brain activity measured with functional magnetic resonance imaging technique while they completed an emotional face-matching task. The adolescents who reported engaging in more either physical bullying behavior or relational bullying (purposefully excluding a peer or spreading rumors) tended to display higher amygdala activity in response to angry faces and lower amygdala activity in response to fearful faces. The authors interpreted the finding as follows: higher amygdala activity to angry faces could suggest that these teens are more sensitive to signals of anger from other people (which may be a trigger to act as a bully), whereas lower amygdala activity to fearful faces could suggest that the brains of these teens are less responsive to signals of distress and thus are not sensitive to the concerns of the teen being victimized by the bullying.

SOURCE: Blamb/Shutterstock.

Many youth are exposed to traumatic experiences or to chronic stress (Russotti et al., 2021). This can include living in poverty; being victimized by physical, sexual, or emotional abuse; or living in a chaotic, threatening, or unpredictable environment. Mounting research from developmental psychologists tells us that severe and frequent stress alters brain maturation by overfocusing neurodevelopment on strengthening the ability to respond to threats at the expense of building capacity for emotional and cognitive self-control. Children who experience such adversity may be more challenged with respect to planning and managing impulse control as they grow older.

There is evidence that bullying in childhood has lasting negative effects into adulthood on physical and mental health (Takizawa et al., 2014). Exposure to physical or sexual abuse as a child is a known risk factor for adolescent drug abuse (Clark & Winters, 2002). One study showed that exposure to childhood neglect or physical abuse was associated with heavy episodic drinking from early adolescence into young adulthood, and that exposure to both was linked to a more severe trajectory than for those who experienced one of these sources of childhood maltreatment (Shin et al., 2013) (see Figure 3.6). Also, the experience of acculturation stress attributable to migration predicts longitudinally symptoms of depression and anxiety in adolescence (Sirin et al., 2013).

Stressful experiences early in life have been linked to how a teenager responds to stress later in life (Davidson & McEwen, 2012). For example, human studies suggest that early stressful experiences alter hormonal changes that later contribute to an imbalance in neural systems development: an increase in the growth of several sectors of the amygdala (which is involved in how we respond emotionally to stress) and a decrease in growth of both the hippocampus (memory center) and the PFC (judgment region). These downstream impacts on behavior are believed to be linked to low self-esteem, impulsiveness, poor executive function (decision-making skills), and aggression and anxiety (McEwen & Gianaros, 2011).

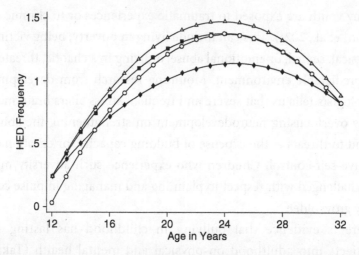

Figure 3.6 Projected pattern of heavy drinking as a function of type of childhood maltreatment.
SOURCE: Exposure to childhood neglect and physical abuse and developmental trajectories of heavy episodic drinking from early adolescence into young adulthood, by Sunny H. Shina, Daniel P. Miller, Martin H. Teicher, *Drug and Alcohol Dependence*, Volume 127, Issues 1–3, 1 January 2013, Pages 31–38.

How is an adolescent mouse defined? Adolescence in female mice lasts approximately from postnatal day (PND) 20 to 40, and in males, from PND 25 to 55 (Schneider, 2013).

Animal models. Studies using mice in the laboratory provide the opportunity to manipulate experimentally exposure to social stress and to potentially offer important insights about the harmful effects of stress during adolescence. A range of mice studies have shown that adolescent mice (1) subjected to repeated *stress*, as defined by being defeated repeatedly by a dominant individual, reveal more persistent avoidance behaviors than aggressive behaviors (Ver Hoeve et al., 2013); (2) faced with the absence of social stimulation, including social isolation, can show irreversible effects on some aspects of exploratory behavior (Einon, & Morgan, 1977); and (3) may not recovery well after a stress experience (Pattwell et al., 2012).

A significant takeaway from this body of work is that adolescence is a vulnerable age in the face of stress, including that it may be more difficult to recover from stress. But there are marked differences among youth in response to being exposed to the same stress event. Such variability implies that individual differences in genetic susceptibility might be a contributory factor. Thus, studies of how genes might interact with the environment have gained momentum. One prominent focus in this area is that variability in a gene that regulates a neurotransmitter believed to be important to how humans respond to the environment—serotonin—contributes to differences in sensitivity to stress (Caspi et al., 2003). Whereas exceptions exist, there are several studies supporting the view that individuals with an at-risk serotonin transporter genotype are at elevated risk to develop depression after life stress (Moffitt & Caspi, 2014).

Sleep. Another factor relevant here is the issue of sleep. Sufficient sleep is key to emotional health. Yet during teen brain development, the regulation of sleep is offset from normal cycles, and this contributes to the tendency to stay up late at night. Sleep deprivation can be a nagging source of fatigue and irritability; but at a more serious level, it also can contribute to depression and impulsive behaviors (Dahl & Lewin, 2002; Palmer et al., 2018).

Maternal support. The focus so far has been on how negative experiences can be harmful to brain development. But the environment can promote healthy brain development as well. The first formal discussion that environmental enrichment early in life results in enhanced brain development was provided by Hebb in the late 1940s, and this notion was empirically validated with animal models 20 years later (Greenough et al., 1987). Work in this area continues supporting the view that many early positive experiences and enrichments in the environment promote the healthy development of brain architecture and support the foundation for all future learning, behavior, and health.

Early maternal support is one such tangible environmental experience shown to support healthy structural brain development, and recent research in this area has honed in on the biological mechanisms that underlie the link between maternal support and brain development.

Maternal support provided early in life appears to promote the growth of neurons and adaptive stress responses. Also, much retrospective data suggest a link between early psychosocial factors, including maternal support, and hippocampal volumes in humans. To examine this notion with longitudinal data, Luby and colleagues investigated whether early maternal support predicted later hippocampal volumes (Luby et al., 2012). Maternal support observed in early childhood was strongly predictive of hippocampal volume measured at school age. As we noted above, healthy hippocampal volume is important for memory and learning, as well as the abilities to regulate emotions and deal with stress.

The Developing Brain and Drugs

Scientists are beginning to explore the issue of drug use and brain development. Adolescence is a time of heightened engagement in risky health behaviors, such as unsafe sexual behavior and dangerous driving, and it is also a period when teenagers are prone to experience with drugs and are sensitive to the effects of drugs (Steinberg, 2008). As we discussed above, peers can be influential during this period. Thus, the drug use tendency of youth may be partly influenced by the increase in time spent with friends rather than family and the accompanying propensity for adolescents to engage in risky behavior—including drug use—when with peers rather than when alone (Dishion & Tipsord, 2011; Simons-Morton et al., 2005). Adolescents whose friends regularly consume drugs are more likely to use them themselves (Clark & Winters, 2002).

As we discuss in more detail in Chapter 4, national surveys indicate that use of substances, particularly tobacco, alcohol, and cannabis, is relatively common during adolescence (e.g., Johnston et al., 2020). The majority of teenagers will try alcohol before the legal age of 21, and over half will try an illicit drug (usually cannabis) at least once during their teenage years. This early onset of drug use by many teenagers raises questions about the role of brain maturation in decisions to use and to what extent, if at all, drug use may *alter* brain development and impact its functioning. There are concerns that regular drug use can have widespread negative effects on brain development and stands to jeopardize a young person's chances of success in life.

Animal studies are limited in their application to the complex human brain, but such studies can more definitively assess the relationship between drug exposure and various outcomes. It would be unethical to give a drug to a child or teenager and measure its effects, and so animal models allow us to gain insights into the nature of drug use and addiction. Nonhuman primates, such as rats, mice, and monkeys, are valuable in behavioral studies and a wide range of biomedical research because of their many similarities to humans (Institute of Medicine, 1991). Animal experiments have produced valuable information on the acute and long-term effects of drug use, how drug abuse interacts with the environment, and the etiology and treatment of and recovery from addiction. We would know much less about numerous aspects of drug use without animal research. Continued animal research is essential if new ways are to be found to cope with addiction.

We will address this complex intersection of drug use and brain development by reviewing three lines research: (1) Does brain development contribute to drug-use seeking and using behavior? (2) Does brain development make the teenager more vulnerable to the risk for addiction compared to adults? (3) Does the developing brain suffer deleterious effects as a result of using alcohol or other drugs? The data pertaining to these questions come from both human and animal studies.

Does Brain Development Contribute to *Drug Involvement*?

On a general level, the way the teen brain develops may contribute to drug involvement and the effects that lead to addiction. Several scientific findings provide some clues to this question. As noted above, brain maturation during adolescence can give rise to taking risks and underappreciating negative consequences when risks are taken, to seeking novelty, and to being easily influenced by social pressures. In this light, adolescents will find drug use rather attractive. And we have already noted that because teenagers are particularly sensitive to peer influences, these can push a reluctant teenager to use drugs.

Brain development per se may also contribute to drug use. The teenage brain may be particularly sensitive to the effects of drugs on the brain. This position is linked to the now well-established principle that nearly all addictive drugs directly or indirectly target the brain's reward system by flooding the circuit with dopamine. Dopamine is a neurotransmitter present in regions of the brain that regulate movement, emotion, cognition, motivation, and feelings of pleasure. The overstimulation of this system, which rewards our natural behaviors, produces the euphoric effects sought by people who use drugs and teaches them to repeat the behavior. Experts contend that this acute surge in dopamine is more pronounced for a young, maturing brain than for an adult brain (Volkow et al., 2011). With this greater dopamine sensitivity to drugs, the drug experience is heighted and the risk to continue to use is elevated in adolescents compared to in adults (Nestler & Malenka, 2004). Moreover, continued and chronic drug use has the effect of *dampening* dopamine production in the brain, which may contribute to urges to use in between drug use experiences. Because the adolescent brain is thought to be particularly vulnerable to the dopamine dampening effect, teenagers who are using chronically may experience drug urges of greater intensity and length than an adult would (Fuhrmann et al., 2015) (more in Chapter 4 on the dopamine theory of drug addiction).

Research on brain development and alcohol adds further insight as to why alcohol might be particularly popular among adolescents. Studies using animal models suggest that an adolescent rat while intoxicated from alcohol will display more pronounced social behaviors compared to an adult rat that is similarly intoxicated (Spear, 2002). The generalization of this finding to humans is that alcohol may elicit a more pleasurable social experience for the adolescent (i.e., greater social disinhibition) than for adults. Also, adolescent rats are observed to be less sensitive to the acute (immediate) effects of alcohol intoxication (e.g., drowsiness; poor motor coordination) than adult rats. Adolescent rats can typically consume two to three times as much alcohol for their body weight as that consumed by adult rats (Spear, 2002). Adolescent humans also show this diminished sensitivity to intoxication; their higher metabolic rates allow them to consume greater amounts of alcohol (Spear, 2002). A lower sensitivity to alcohol's effects would be consistent with the observation that young people are capable of drinking large amounts of alcohol in the absence of these acute intoxication effects.

Another consideration is that brain development mediates the hormone surge during adolescence. Hormones encourage novelty seeking and promote social competitiveness. The revved-up hormonal production during adolescence may promote drug use of any kind, attributable to the intent to seek novel experiences and rewarded by the social approval from peers during the experience.

Does Brain Development Contribute to an Elevated Risk for a Substance Use Disorder?

Several cross-sectional and longitudinal studies have highlighted the reliable association between youth and risk for developing a drug use problem (Grant et al., 2004; Winters & Lee, 2008). Let's examine alcohol in more detail. National data from 2001–2002 indicate that among youth aged 15 20 years old, 12.2% met an official definition (American Psychiatric Association, 1994) of an alcohol abuse or dependence disorder within the past 12 months (National Epidemiological Survey of Alcohol and Related Conditions (https://catalog.data.gov/dataset/national-epidemiologic-sur vey-on-alcohol-and-related-conditions-nesarcwave-1-20012002-and). This rate was much higher than for the other age groups; for example, the rate of alcohol abuse/dependence was 4.1% for individuals in the 30 to 34 age group) (see Figure 3.7).

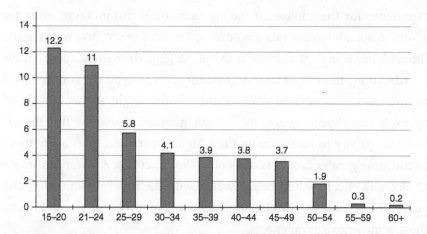

Figure 3.7 Prevalence of past-year DSM-IV alcohol d Use Disorder for age groups: United States, 2001–2002 (National Epidemiological Survey on Alcohol and Related Conditions; https://catalog.data.gov/dataset/national-epidemiologic-survey-on-alcohol-and-related-conditions-nesarcwave-1-20012002-and-).

This association is also apparent when we consider age of onset of use. There is a reliable association between early-onset drug use and elevated risk for future drug-related problems (Kessler et al., 2007; Winters & Lee, 2008). The finding has held up for over three decades of research and across diverse demographic groups and it applies to several drugs (see Figure 3.8). The earlier that use begins during adolescence, the greater the risk of developing a substance use disorder in one's lifetime (including during adolescence).

The association between early-onset use and elevated risk for drug addiction is most certainly influenced by the accumulating effect of extended exposure to drugs on a person's social and personal life; a drug habit can affect multiple spheres of a person. Then there is the issue that because adolescents can learn faster and build stronger connections and by nature are risk-takers, the way the brain develops is believed to further contribute to getting addicted faster. Finally, biological mechanisms also may play a role by virtue of brain changes associated with repeated drug use. As noted above, the teenager's dopamine system may create a two-fold vulnerability by elevating the acute rewarding effects of drugs and, if chronic use occurs, reducing dopamine level more intensely and heightening urges.

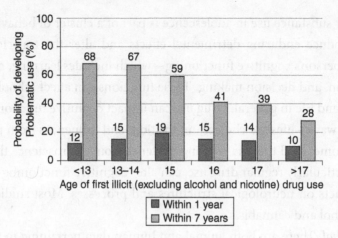

Figure 3.8 Earlier onset of illicit drug use is associated with a greater likelihood of future problematic use.

Does the Developing Brain Suffer *Deleterious Effects* as a Result of Using Alcohol or Other Drugs?

The bulk of the studies that examine links between drug use and health outcomes are based on cross-sectional studies. Interpreting results from such studies needs to proceed cautiously. In cases where drug use is reported to be associated with a negative health outcome, four possible scenarios are plausible:

1. The drug use directly causes the outcome.
2. The presence of a pre-existing risk factor or condition increased the likelihood of drug use.
3. Another variable that is not systematically accounted for in the study is responsible for the outcome.
4. Some combination of the aforementioned scenarios is responsible for the findings.

These caveats remind us of the importance of not overinterpreting the findings from one study, and the value of examining multiple studies with converging methodologies and of prospective large samples involving adolescent to adulthood subjects.

Regular substance use in adolescence is part of a cluster of behaviors that can produce enduring detrimental effects and alter the trajectory of a young person's cognitive functioning—which includes learning, memory, attention, and decision making. These functions can affect school performance and life in general. Drug use can impact cognitive functioning in a host of ways—lifestyle choices, motivation, and influences from peers, to name some. And there is growing evidence from neuroscience that drug use, particularly regular drug use, can alter cognitive functioning because of impacts on neurological structures and processes. Most studies focus on alcohol and cannabis.

Alcohol. There are both animal and human data pertaining to the possible impact of alcohol use during adolescence on memory and learning. Adolescent rats exposed to various amounts of alcohol have significantly more brain damage in their frontal cortex (important for decision making) and show greater damage to their working memory than their adult counterparts (Spear, 2002). With long-term use, adolescent rats have shown massive neuronal loss in other key parts of the brain, including the cerebellum (sensory perception and motor coordination), basal forebrain (learning), and neocortex (language) (Spear, 2002). In human studies, adolescents with an alcohol dependence disorder showed greater memory retrieval deficits compared to a nondependent control group (Brown et al., 2000) and were found to have reduced volume in the hippocampus, the memory region of the brain (Tapert & Schweinsburg, 2005). Because these studies were cross-sectional and did not have memory performance or hippocampus data on the participants prior to alcohol use, the link between heavy alcohol use and memory deficit is only suggestive. However, evidence from a longitudinal study also supports the association between adolescent drinking and memory impairment. A general population of adolescents who were *frequent binge drinkers* by the age of 15 were found to reveal moderately impaired working memory 3 years later (age 18), whereas non-drinking youth did not (working memory involves remembering very recent events and information just learned) (Mahedy et al., 2018).

Cannabis. The possible negative effects of cannabis use on adolescent cognitive functioning have received a great deal of attention of late. An important background issue is the role of the endocannabinoid system in humans. This system consists of brain receptors that bind to the active ingredients in cannabis—known as *cannabinoids*—and they encompass several regions of the brain important for neurodevelopmental processes related to cognition, as well as appetite, stress response, and emotional control (see Figure 3.9). A normal development of the endocannabinoid system is vital for healthy cognitive development (Lisdahl & Price, 2012). But this developing system is vulnerable to the effects of cannabis. The concern is that use of cannabis may deleteriously alter its growth and lead to cognitive impairments (Lisdahl & Price, 2012). Such interference might be a bigger problem for developing brains.

What do the data indicate? Converging evidence from animal and human studies supports the view that cannabis affects multiple cognitive systems in the developing brain, including attentional processing, several aspects of memory, and higher-order executive functioning (decision making) (Bara et al., 2021). *Animal studies* show that exposure to

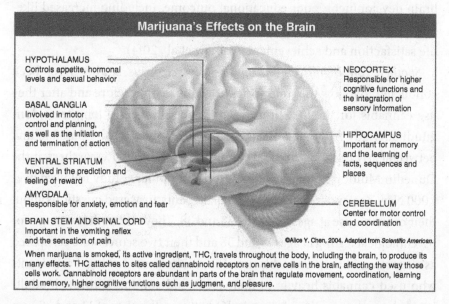

Figure 3.9 Cannabis binds to cannabinoid receptors located throughout the brain.
SOURCE: National Institute on Drug Abuse. https://www.drugabuse.gov/publications/research-reports/marijuana/how-does-marijuana-produce-its-effects.

the active ingredient in cannabis (THC) during adolescent development can cause long-lasting changes in the brain's hippocampus, a brain area critical for learning and memory (Schuster et al., 2018). A number of *human studies* have found evidence of brain changes in teens and young adults who smoke cannabis; these findings include both structural brain abnormalities and altered neural activity in cannabis users (Albaugh et al., 2021; Batalla et al., 2013). Of course, individual differences occur, but these negative effects can persist after recent use and the impact is more pronounced among heavy and chronic users. And the earlier the age of onset of regular cannabis use, the worse the negative neurocognitive outcomes (Schuster et al., 2018).

This issue of early onset of use was highlighted in a recent review of the literature by the Director of the National Institute on Drug Abuse, Dr. Nora Volkow, and colleagues (Volkow et al., 2014). That report identified seven adverse effects of "long-term or chronic" cannabis use, and the following five were further flagged as effects being strongly associated with adolescent-onset of cannabis use: risk for addiction; altered brain development; poor educational outcome, including increased likelihood of dropping out of school; cognitive impairment; and diminished life satisfaction and achievement (Volkow et al., 2014).

Spotlight on cognitive functioning. Few rigorous studies have been conducted to follow the trajectories of young people before and after they use cannabis for the first time. There is one impressive long-term, longitudinal study from New Zealand that sheds light on the possible link between early cannabis use and cognitive functioning. Researchers at the Dunedin Multidisciplinary Health and Development Study followed over 1,000 New Zealanders born in 1972. Participants answered questions about their cannabis use at ages 18, 21, 26, 32 and 38. They also underwent neuropsychological testing at ages 13 and 38 and their two scores were compared as a function of their cannabis use. The results were striking: Participants who used cannabis heavily in their teens and continued through adulthood showed a significant drop in IQ between the ages of 13 and 38—an average of eight points for those who met criteria for cannabis dependence (Meier et al., 2012). For context, eight IQ points is approximately a

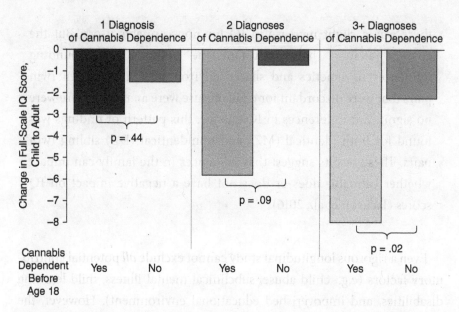

Figure 3.10 Changes in IQ score as a function of cannabis use (early or later onset of use; chronicity of use) (Meier et al., 2012).

Meier, M. H., Caspi, A., Ambler, A., Harrington, H., Houts, R., Keefe, R. S. E., ... Moffitt, T. E. (2012). Persistent cannabis users show neuropsychological decline from childhood to midlife. *Proceedings of the National Academy of Sciences, USA, 109*, E2657–E2664.

one-half standard deviation of IQ points; a loss of eight IQ points could drop a person of average intelligence into the lowest third of the intelligence range. By comparison, those who started using cannabis regularly or heavily after age 18 showed minor, nonsignificant declines, and those who *never used* cannabis showed no declines in IQ. Also, and strikingly, those who used cannabis heavily before age 18 showed mental decline even after they quit taking the drug (see Figure 3.10).

Another longitudinal look at cannabis and IQ was reported by Jackson and colleagues (2016). Because these investigators used a twin sample, they were able to compare co-twins who were discrepant on cannabis use (i.e., one twin uses and one twin does not). The overall finding was a decline in IQ scores from time 1 (late childhood) to time 2 (mid- to late-adolescence) for those who used cannabis, whereas there was a slight increase in IQ for non-cannabis users. But the co-twin analysis holds constant the potentially confounding influences of genetics and shared environment. Thus, when twin pairs that were discordant for cannabis use were analyzed, there were no significant differences in IQ change; this pattern of findings was found for both identical (MZ) and nonidentical (DZ) sibling twin pairs. These results suggest that influences in the family can impact whether cannabis does or does not have a negative impact on IQ scores (Jackson et al., 2016).

Even a rigorous longitudinal study cannot exclude *all* potential contributory factors (e.g., child abuse, subclinical mental illness, mild learning disabilities, and impoverished educational environment). However, the neuropsychological declines following cannabis use were present even after researchers controlled for factors like years of education, mental illness, and use of other substances. This finding is consistent with the view that early-onset and chronic drug use—at a developmental period when the brain is still shaping itself neurologically—can have deleterious and long-lasting effects on the brain.

Spotlight on mental health. Cannabis and mental health have also received a great deal of attention by researchers. Early and regular use of cannabis has been shown to increase the risk of developing a mental or behavioral disorder. Vulnerability factors are not currently clear but may include factors such as childhood trauma and genetics (Canadian Psychiatric Association's Research Committee, 2017). The strongest link is between cannabis use and psychotic illness, such as schizophrenia and delusional disorders (Miller, 2018). Cannabis use may also increase the risk of depression, suicidal ideation, bipolar disorder, panic disorder, and anxiety disorders (Volkow et al., 2014). Whereas it is not clear if cannabis use triggers the onset of the disorder, for youth who have already developed the disorder, it appears that continued cannabis use worsens long-term symptoms and life functioning. This was demonstrated by Large and colleagues (Large et al., 2011) in an analysis of several studies

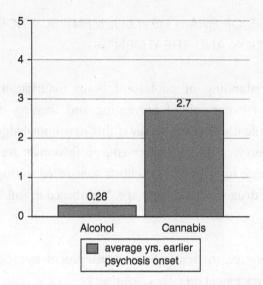

Figure 3.11 Average years earlier onset of psychosis based on history of substance use (Large et al., 2011).

that looked at the average age of onset of psychosis as a function of substance use or no substance use (see Figure 3.11). For alcohol, there was no difference in age of psychosis onset between those who used alcohol during youth and those who did not. But for early cannabis users, there was a significant difference: Those who used cannabis during their youth had their psychosis onset, on average, about 2.7 years earlier than youth who did use cannabis.

A prominent expert in the field, after a comprehensive review of the research literature on the possible link between cannabis use and mental illness, expressed this perspective: "The preponderance of evidence reviewed in this chapter substantiates not only a significant, causal role for cannabis in chronic psychotic syndromes but also a strong association with mood disorders and suicidal ideation. Thus, there can no longer be any doubt that the range of negative mental health impacts of this drug, too frequently dismissed as fear-mongering rhetoric, must be positioned at the front and center of international drug policy dialogue (Miller, 2018, p. 149).

IMPLICATIONS OF BRAIN DEVELOPMENT SCIENCE
ON PREVENTION AND TREATMENT

Can an understanding of adolescent brain maturation help service providers do a better job of preventing and treating drug abuse in teenagers? While it's too early to say if this new knowledge will dramatically impact prevention and treatment, professionals are beginning to mine this science to bolster their efforts toward educating youth about the dangers of drug use at an early age. Web-based examples include the following:

- https://drugfree.org/article/brain-development-teen-behavior/
  (*Brain Development and Teen Behavior*)
- https://teens.drugabuse.gov/ (*Teens: Drug Use and the Brain*)
- https://youtu.be/4S2qgEFEdKU (*Power of the Adolescent Brain*)

Here are five examples of prevention and treatment messages and strategies supported by brain development science.

1. Because many teenagers begin using drugs at a young age, coupled with concerns that such early use can impair the developing brain, the urgency for prevention is real. Even delaying the onset of drug use, especially if it is delayed until adulthood, helps protect the developing brain. Significant and perhaps lasting cognitive deficits can occur for teenagers who start drug use during adolescence, and especially those who are chronic and long-term users.

2. Creating age-appropriate health curriculum to educate youth about their developing brain is a priority. The emergence of developmental neuroscience provides new insights into how brain maturation influences how and why teenagers make critical and life-influencing decisions, including both positive, life-enhancing choices and possible unhealthy or risky ones that may promote a decision to use drugs. This perspective can be

harnessed to strengthen current drug prevention approaches by further encouraging youth to capitalize on the assets of the developing brain and to promote personal growth and healthy lifestyles.

3. This new science places importance on educating youth about the skill of using their "thinking breaks" when faced with having to make a decision to delay immediate gratification. Vulnerable conditions under which the teenager's self-control skills are particularly challenged should be highlighted (e.g., when with friends).

4. There is a need to educate parents about the developing teenage brain. Brain development science reinforces the importance of parents being actively involved in their teenager's life. Rather than the message "I need to know where you are and who you are with because I am not sure I can trust you," the more scientifically justified message is "I need to help you anticipate risky situations and how to deal with them." Indeed, there is a growing body of research that points to the impact of effective parenting on positive brain development (see Box 4 in Chapter 4).

5. What is being learned about brain maturation reinforces the current public policy of keeping the minimum legal age for alcohol at age 21 and the new federal regulation that the minimum age of smoking be moved up to age 21. This brain science evidence may not support the current trend in the United States to legalize cannabis for commercial sales.

MINI-REVIEW

- Adolescents go through significant brain development during the teenage years. This process likely contributes to increased risk taking and lapses in sound decision making but also supports learning and being open to new experiences. Adolescence is a developmental period replete with energy, trying new things, forging a sense of self and independence, heightened response to excitement and arousal, great interest in social information, and a willingness to learn.

- Whereas there are numerous open questions about the long-term effects of drug use, a growing research base disputes the view that drug use is a harmless activity for youth and points in direction that early-onset and frequent use of drugs may disrupt brain development. Several cognitive deficits have been linked to early use of alcohol or cannabis; the earlier age of onset of regular use, the worse the neurocognitive outcomes.
- The "brain under construction" of a teenager is vulnerable to the effects of stress, and in combination with biological risk, adolescence is period of onset of many mental illnesses. Also, the risk for addiction for all licit and illicit drugs is greatly increased when a person starts to use a drug during the teen years.
- Adults can help teenagers with their decision making. It is important that parents, teachers, and youth-serving professionals focus on the positive aspects of teenage risk behaviors.
- Given the trend in the United States to legalize cannabis for medical or recreational purposes, rigorously investigating the impact of cannabis on youth is a scientific priority in order to inform health policy decisions and prevention and treatment programs and practices.

DISCUSSION POINTS

1. Is there greater plasticity in adolescence than in other periods of development, or do we see a continuous decline of plasticity from childhood to adulthood? How do environmental influences such as cognitive training, social stress, or drug use affect brain development in humans?

2. During adolescence, executive function skills are not yet at adult levels, but often these skills are heavily taxed because of daily demands. Consider the following: Adolescents need to communicate effectively in multiple contexts; they need to manage their own school and after-school activities; abstract and complicated projects need to be completed.

3. What are some suggestions for helping teens to practice better self-regulation throughout the daily challenges they face?

4. What are the molecular mechanisms of plasticity in adolescence? Are they the same as in early childhood? What is the role of puberty in the onset of sensitive periods in adolescence? Is there variation in the timing and duration of sensitive periods within adolescence?

5. What is the role of individual differences in moderating the presence and onset of sensitive periods during this time of life? What are the effects of enrichment and training in adolescence as compared with other age groups? Conversely, what are the consequences of stress in humans across the life span? Can we harness adolescent brain plasticity for educational interventions?

6. Do cognitive training effects transfer to real-life measures such as academic performance? If so, what are the side effects of such interventions? What are the ethical implications of cognitive enhancement through training?

7. Discuss how brain maturation research may impact the debate in the United States to legalize the commercial sales of cannabis for adults.

Further Curiosity and Digging

Overviews of Adolescent Brain Development

Blakemore, S.-J. (2012). *The mysterious workings of the adolescent brain*. [Video]. TedGlobal.https://www.ted.com/talks/sarah_jayne_blakemore_the_mysterious_workings_of_the_adolescent_brain?language=en

Winters, K. C. (2012, April 19). *Teen brain video.wmv*. [Video]. YouTube. https://www.youtube.com/watch?v=Aiy2bPVfHg8

Intersection of Brain Development and Substance Use

Salmanzadeh, H., Ahmadi-Soleimani, S. M., Pachenari, N., Azadi, M., Halliwell, R. F., Rubino, T., & Azizi, H. (2020). Adolescent drug exposure: A review of evidence for the development of persistent changes in brain function. *Brain Research Bulletin, 16*, 105–117.

Winters, K. C. (2009). Adolescent brain development and alcohol abuse. Journal of Global Drug Policy and Practice, 3. http://www.globaldrugpolicy.org/

Children and Delaying Gratification

Igniter Video. (20029). *Marshmallow test*. [Video]. YouTube. https://www.youtube.com/watch?v=QX_oy9614HQ

Screen Time and Brain Development

Neophytou, E., Manwell, L. A., & Eikelboom, R. (2019). Effects of excessive screen time on neurodevelopment, learning, memory, mental health, and neurodegeneration: A scoping review. *International Journal of Mental Health and Addiction, 19*, 724–744. https://doi.org/10.1007/s11469-019-00182-2

REFERENCES

Albaugh, M. D., Ottino-Gonzalez, J., Sidwell, A., Lepage, C., Juliano, A., Owens, M. M., et al., for IMAGEN Consortium. (2021). Association of cannabis use during adolescence with neurodevelopment. *JAMA Psychiatry, 78*, 1031–1040.

American Psychiatric Association. (1994). *Diagnostic and statistical manual of mental disorders*, 4th ed., Washington, DC: American Psychiatric Association.

Andersen, S. L., & Teicher, M. H. (2008). Stress, sensitive periods and maturational events in adolescent depression. *Trends in Neurosciences, 31*, 183–191.

Baker, S. T., Lubman, D. I., Yücel, M., Allen, N. B., Whittle, S., Fulcher, B. D., Zalesky, A., & Fornito, A. (2015). Developmental changes in brain network hub connectivity in late adolescence. *Journal of Neuroscience, 35*, 9078–9087.

Bara, A., Ferland, J. M. N., Rompala, G., Szutorisz, H., & Hurd, Y. L. (2021). Cannabis and synaptic reprogramming of the developing brain. *Nature Reviews Neuroscience, 22*, 423–438.

Batalla, A., Bhattacharyya, S., Yücel, M., Fusar-Poli, P., Crippa, J. A., Nogué, S., Torrens, M., Pujol, J., Farré, M., & Martin-Santos, R. (2013). Structural and functional imaging studies in chronic cannabis users: A systematic review of adolescent and adult findings. *PloS ONE, 8*, e55821.

Brown, S. A., Tapert, S. F., Granholm, E., & Delis, D. C. (2000). Neurocognitive functioning of adolescents: Effects of protracted alcohol use. *Alcoholism: Clinical and Experimental Research, 24*, 164–171.

Canadian Psychiatric Association's Research Committee. (2017). *Implications of cannabis legalization on youth and young adults*. Canadian Psychiatric Association.

Carlson, S. M., Shoda, Y., Ayduk, O., Aber, L., Schaefer, C., Sethi, A., Wilson, N., Peake, P. K., & Mischel, W. (2018). Cohort effects in children's delay of gratification. *Developmental Psychology, 54*, 1395–1407.

Caspi, A., Sugden, K., Moffitt, T. E., Taylor, A., Craig, I. W., Harrington, H., McClay, J., Mill, J., Martin, J., Braithwaite, A., & Poulton, R. (2003). Influence of life stress on depression: Moderation by a polymorphism in the 5-HTT gene. *Science, 301*, 386–389.

Centifanti, L. C. M., Modecki, K. L., MacLellan, S., & Gowling, H. (2014). Driving under the influence of risky peers: An experimental study of adolescent risk taking. *Journal of Research on Adolescence, 26*, 207–222.

Chein, J., Albert, D., O'Brien, L., Uckert, K., & Steinberg, L. (2011). Peers increase adolescent risk taking by enhancing activity in the brain's reward circuitry. *Developmental Science, 14*, F1–F10.

Clark, D., & Winters, K. C. (2002). Measuring risks and outcomes in substance use disorders prevention research. *Journal of Consulting and Clinical Psychology, 70*, 1207–1223.

Cohen, G. L., & Prinstein, M. J. (2006). Peer contagion of aggression and health risk behavior among adolescent males: An experimental investigation of effects on public conduct and private attitudes. *Child Development, 77*, 967–983.

Crosnoe, R., Muller, C., & Frank, K. (2004). Peer context and the consequences of adolescent drinking. *Social Problems, 51*, 288–304.

Dahl, R. E. (2004). Adolescent brain development: A period of vulnerabilities and opportunities. Keynote address. *Annals of the New York Academy of Sciences, 1021*, 1–22.

Dahl, R. E., & Lewin, D. S. (2002). Pathways to adolescent health sleep regulation and behavior. *Journal of Adolescent Health, 31*, 175–184.

Davidson, R. J., & McEwen, B. S. (2012). Social influences on neuroplasticity: Stress and interventions to promote well-being. *Nature Neuroscience, 15*(5), 689–695.

Dishion, T. J., & Tipsord, J. M. (2011). Peer contagion in child and adolescent social and emotional development. *Annual Review of Psychology, 62*, 189–214.

Einon, D. F., & Morgan, M. J. (1977). A critical period for social isolation in the rat. *Developmental Psychobiology, 10*, 123–132.

Fuhrmann, D., Knoll, L. J., & Blakemore, S. J. (2015). Adolescence as a sensitive period of brain development. *Trends in Cognitive Sciences, 19*, 558–566.

Giedd, J. N. (2004). Structural magnetic resonance imaging of the adolescent brain. *The Annals of the New York Academy of Sciences, 1021*, 77–85.

Gogtay, N., Giedd, J. N., Lusk, L., Hayashi, K. M., Greenstein, D., Vaituzis, A. C., . . . Thompson, P. M. (2004). Dynamic mapping of human cortical development during childhood through early adulthood. *Proceedings of the National Academy of Sciences, 101*, 8174–8179.

Grant, B. F., Dawson, D. A., Stinson, F. S., Chou, S. P., Dufour, M. C., & Pickering, R. P. (2004). The 12-month prevalence and trends in DSM-IV alcohol abuse and dependence: United States, 1991–1992 and 2001–2002. *Drug and Alcohol Dependence, 74*, 223–234.

Greenough, W. T., Black, J. E., & Wallace, C. S. (1987). Experience and brain development. *Child Development, 58*, 539–559.

Institute of Medicine. (1991). *Why are animals used to study the brain?* The National Academies Press.

Jackson, N. J., Isen, J. D., Khoddam, R., Irons, D., Tuvblad, C., Iacono, W. G., McGue, M., Raine, A., & Baker, L. A. (2016). Impact of adolescent marijuana use on intelligence: Results from two longitudinal twin studies. *Proceedings of the National Academy of Sciences, USA*, *113*(5), E500–E508.

Johnston, L. D., O'Malley, P. M., Miech, R. A., Bachman, J. G., & Schulenberg, J. E. (2020). *Monitoring the Future national survey results on drug use: 1975–2019*. University of Michigan, Institute for Social Research.

Kaminer, Y., Zajac, K., & Winters, K. C. (2019). Assessment and treatment of internalizing disorders (depression, anxiety disorders and PTSD). In Y. Kaminer & K. C. Winters (Eds.), *Clinical manual of adolescent addictive disorders* (2nd ed., pp. 375–412). American Psychiatric Association.

Kaufmann, T., Alnæs, D., Doan, N. T., Brandt, C. L., Andreassen, O. A., & Westlye, L. T. (2017). Delayed stabilization and individualization in connectome development are related to psychiatric disorders. *Nature Neuroscience*, *20*, 513–515.

Kessler, R. C., Amminger, G. P., Aguilar-Gaxiola, S., Alonso, J., Lee, S., & Ustun, T. B. (2007). Age of onset of mental disorders: a review of recent literature. *Current Opinion in Psychiatry*, *20*, 359.

Kim-Cohen, J., Caspi, A., Moffitt, T. E., Harrington, H., Milne, B. J., & Poulton, R. (2003). Prior juvenile diagnoses in adults with mental disorder: developmental follow-back of a prospective-longitudinal cohort. *Archives of General Psychiatry*, *60*, 709–717.

Knoll, L. J., Magis-Weinberg, L., Speekenbrink, M., & Blakemore, S. J. (2015). Social influence on risk perception during adolescence. *Psychological Science*, *26*, 583–592.

Large, M., Sharma, S., Compton, M. T., Slade, T., & Nielssen, O. (2011). Cannabis use and earlier onset of psychosis: a systematic meta-analysis. *Archives of General Psychiatry*, *68*, 555–561.

Lisdahl, K. M., & Price, J. S. (2012). Increased marijuana use and gender predict poorer cognitive functioning in adolescents and emerging adults. *Journal of the International Neuropsychological Society*, *18*, 678–688.

Luby, J. L., Barch, D. M., Belden, A., Gaffrey, M. S., Tillman, R., Babb, C., Nishino, T., Suzuki, H., & Botteron, K. N. (2012). Maternal support in early childhood predicts larger hippocampal volumes at school age. *Proceedings of the National Academy of Sciences, USA*, *109*, 2854–2859.

Lutz, P. E., Tanti, A., Gasecka, A., Barnett-Burns, S., Kim, J. J., Zhou, Y., . . . Turecki, G. (2017). Association of a history of child abuse with impaired myelination in the anterior cingulate cortex: convergent epigenetic, transcriptional, and morphological evidence. *American Journal of Psychiatry*, *174*, 1185–1194.

Mahedy, L., Field, M., Gage, S., Hammerton, G., Heron, J., Hickman, M., & Munafò, M. R. (2018). Alcohol use in adolescence and later working memory: Findings from a large population-based birth cohort. *Alcohol and Alcoholism 53*, 251–258.

Martens, G. J. M., & van Loo, K. M. J. (2007). Genetic and environmental factors in complex neurodevelopmental disorders. *Current Genomics*, *8*, 429–444.

McEwen, B. S., & Gianaros, P. J. (2011). Stress- and allostasis-induced brain plasticity. *Annual Review of Medicine*, *62*, 431–445.

Meier, M. H., Caspi, A., Ambler, A., Harrington, H., Houts, R., Keefe, R. S. E., McDonald, K., Ward, A., Poulton, R., Moffitt, T. E. (2012). Persistent cannabis users show neuropsychological decline from childhood to midlife. *Proceedings of the National Academy of Sciences, USA, 109*, E2657–E2664.

Miller, C. L. (2018). The impact of marijuana on mental health. In K. Sabet & K. C. Winters (Eds.), *Contemporary health issues on marijuana* (pp. 122–164). Oxford University Press.

Moffitt, T. E., & Caspi, A. (2014). Bias in a protocol for a meta-analysis of 5-HTTLPR, stress, and depression. *BMC Psychiatry, 14*, 179–182.

National Epidemiological Survey of Alcohol and Other Conditions (NESARC) – Wave 1 (2001–2002), and Wave 2 (2004–2005). https://catalog.data.gov/dataset/natio nal-epidemiologic-survey-on-alcohol-and-related-conditions-nesarcwave-1-20012 002-and-

Nestler, E. J., & Malenka, R. C. (2004). The addicted brain. *Scientific American, 290*, 78–85.

Palmer, C. A., Oosterhoff, B., Bower, J. L., Kaplow, J. B., & Alfano, C. A. (2018). Associations among adolescent sleep problems, emotion regulation, and affective disorders: Findings from a nationally representative sample. *Journal of Psychiatric Research, 96*, 1–8.

Pascual-Leone, A., Amedi, A., Fregni, F., & Merabet, L. B. (2005). The plastic human brain cortex. *Annual Review of Neuroscience, 28*, 377–401.

Pattwell, S. S., Duhoux, S., Hartley, C. A., Johnson, D. C., Jing, D., Elliott, M. D., . . . & Soliman, F. (2012). Altered fear learning across development in both mouse and human. *Proceedings of the National Academy of Sciences, USA, 109*, 16318–16323.

Reyna, V. F., & Farley, F. (2006). Risk and rationality in adolescent decision making: Implications for theory, practice, and public policy. *Psychological Science in the Public Interest, 7*, 1–44.

Rubin, D. C., & Schulkind, M. D. (1997). The distribution of auto-biographical memories across the lifespan. *Memory and Cognition, 25*, 859–866.

Rudolph, M. D., Miranda-Domínguez, O., Cohen, A. O., Breiner, K., Steinberg, L., Bonnie, R. J., . . . & Richeson, J. A. (2017). At risk of being risky: The relationship between "brain age" under emotional states and risk preference. *Developmental Cognitive Neuroscience, 24*, 93–106.

Russotti, J., Warmingham, J. M., Duprey, E. B., Handley, E. D., Manly, J. T., Rogosch, F. A., & Cicchetti, D. (2021). Child maltreatment and the development of psychopathology: The role of developmental timing and chronicity. *Child Abuse & Neglect, 120*, 105215.

Schneider, M. (2013). Adolescence as a vulnerable period to alter rodent behavior. *Cell and Tissue Research, 354*, 99–106.

Schuster, R. M., Gilman, J., & Evins, A. E. (2018). Effects of adolescent cannabis use on brain structure and function: Current findings and recommendations for future research. In K. A. Sabet & K. C. Winters (Eds.), *Contemporary health issues on marijuana* (pp. 91–107). Oxford University Press.

Shin, S. H., Miller, D. P., & Teicher, M. H. (2013). Exposure to childhood neglect and physical abuse and developmental trajectories of heavy episodic drinking from early adolescence into young adulthood. *Drug and Alcohol Dependence, 127*, 31–38.

Simons-Morton, B., Lerner, N., & Singer, J. (2005). The observed effects of teenage passengers on the risky driving behavior of teenage drivers. *Accident Analysis & Prevention, 37,* 973–982.

Sirin, S. R., Ryce, P., Gupta, T., & Rogers-Sirin, L. (2013). The role of acculturative stress on mental health symptoms for immigrant adolescents: A longitudinal investigation. *Developmental Psychology, 49,* 736–738.

Spear, L. P. (2002). Alcohol's effects on adolescents. *Alcohol Health and Research World, 26,* 287–291.

Steinberg, L. (2004). Risk taking in adolescence: What changes, and why? *Annals of the New York Academy of Sciences, 1021,* 51–58.

Steinberg, L. (2008). A social neuroscience perspective on adolescent risk-taking. *Developmental Review, 28,* 78–106

Takizawa, R., Maughan, B., & Arseneault, L. (2014). Adult health outcomes of childhood bullying victimization: Evidence from a five-decade longitudinal British birth cohort. *American Journal of Psychiatry, 171,* 777–784.

Tapert, S. F., & Schweinsburg, A. D. (2005). The human adolescent brain and alcohol use disorders. *Recent Developments in Alcoholism, 17,* 177–197.

UNICEF. (2011). *The state of the world's children 2011: Adolescence—An age of opportunity.* UNICEF.

Ver Hoeve, E. S., Kelly, G., Luz, S., Ghanshani, S., & Bhatnagar, S. (2013). Short-term and long-term effects of repeated social defeat during adolescence or adulthood in female rats. *Neuroscience, 249,* 63–73.

Volkow, N. D., Baler, R. D., Compton, W. M., & Weiss, S. R. (2014). Adverse health effects of marijuana use. *New England Journal of Medicine, 370*(23), 2219–2227.

Volkow, N. D., Wang, G. J., Fowler, J. S., Tomasi, D., & Telang, F. (2011). Addiction: Beyond dopamine reward circuitry. *Proceedings of the National Academy of Sciences, USA, 108,* 15037–15042.

Winters, K. C., & Arria, A. (2011). Adolescent brain development and drugs. *The Prevention Researcher, 18,* 21–24.

Winters, K. C., & Lee, S. (2008). Likelihood of developing an alcohol and cannabis use disorder during youth: Association with recent use and age. *Drug and Alcohol Dependence, 92,* 239–247.

World Health Organization. (2014). *Health for the world's adolescents—A second chance in the second decade.* World Health Organization.

CO-OCCURING DISORDERS

Overview of Psychoactive Substances

CHAPTER OUTLINE

INTRODUCTION

Alcohol and other drugs (hereafter referred to as *drugs* or *substances*) have a long history. Marijuana was mentioned in the sacred Hindu texts (the Vedas). The Summerians around 3400 B.C.E. referred to the opium poppy, the source of opium, as the "plant of joy." Chinese immigrants in the 1800s introduced America to smoking opium. In the mid-1800s morphine was created from opium and was used as a powerful anesthetic for medical purposes. But morphine was found to be highly addictive and so a presumably safer drug was developed near the end of the 1800s from morphine—heroin. Heroin was thought to be safer; it was sold commercially and included in children's cough syrup. But heroin addiction soon escalated, resulting in restrictions and eventual status as an illegal drug. Alcohol production from all kinds of crops and from all corners of the world has taken place since practically the dawn of civilization. Some historians argue that the great transitions in human history, from the origin of farming to the origin of writing, have a possible link to alcohol (http://alcoholreviews. com/2017/02/17/our-9000-year-love-affair-with-booze/). The early history of tobacco places its discovery with the native peoples OF Mesoamerica and South America, and later it was introduced to Europe and the rest of the world. Following the Industrial Revolution, cigarettes became popularized in the United States as well as Europe.

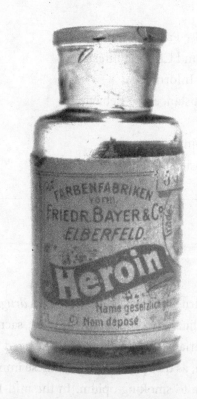

Use of drugs by *adolescents* in the United States continues to present a significant public health, despite the trend in recent years that declines in use for some drugs are observed 1 (National Institute on Drug Abuse, 2021), but the rates of use among adolescents are still a public health concern (Miech et al., 2019; National Institute on Drug Abuse, 2018). Often, drug use occurs in conjunction with other types of problems, including school difficulties, family disruption, risky sexual behavior, and delinquency (Khan et al., 2012).

Adolescence is a critical period for the first use of drugs. Fortunately, most adolescents who use drugs during the teen years do not experience serious health problems or develop a drug problem (technically termed a *substance use disorder [SUD]*, a concept that is the focus of Chapter 5). It is more common that youth who use drugs to do so at a level of chronicity and intensity that falls far short of meeting criteria for an SUD (Chung & Winters, 2018; Montana & Chung, 2019), and if problems occur, they often are subclinical in nature (e.g., a one-time argument with a parent after discovering the teenager has been drinking; feeling uneasy the day after a night of drinking).

When use of drugs begins during these teenage years, it is done so for reasons why all people begin to use drugs: to feel good, to feel better, to do better, or because other people are doing it (National Institute on Drug Abuse, 2018). Yet, use during the teenage years increases the likelihood of numerous negative health effects, including cognitive, physical, and psychosocial developmental factors. The following health-related and life-functioning areas are more likely to occur among or be reported by adolescents who use drugs than by non-drug users: failure to graduate from high school; engagement in unlawful behavior; reporting having a serious mental illness; affiliation with peers who also use drugs; victimization of sexual or physical abuse; and displaying more risk-taking tendencies (National Institute on Drug Abuse, 2018). And, as mentioned earlier, onset of drug use during adolescence increases the likelihood of developing an SUD (Volkow et al., 2014).

MAJOR DRUG USE PATTERNS AND TRENDS

Perhaps more is known about drug use trends among adolescents in the United States than in any other country. This is largely because two very large national surveys have been conducted annually for decades. The large and representative data sets produced from them provide a detailed view of the drug use habits of teenagers in the United States. One survey is the National Survey on Drug Use and Health (NSDUH). The NSDUH is sponsored by the Substance Abuse and Mental Health Services Administration (SAMHSA) of the U.S Department of Health and Human Services. It is conducted on a representative sample of the civilian, noninstitutionalized population 12 years of age and older in the United States (Center for Behavioral Health Statistics and Quality, 2015). A random sample of households across the United States is selected, then an interviewer visits the household and residents there are asked to participate by completing a face-to-face interview. Participation is voluntary and the information is confidential.

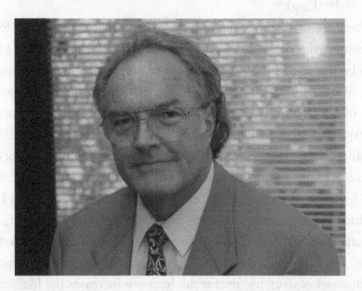

Lloyd Johnston, Ph.D., the pioneering epidemiologist and lead investigator for the MTF survey research.
Photo courtesy of Lloyd Johnston.

The other major survey is the Monitoring the Future (MTF) survey. MTF is an ongoing annual survey of 8th, 10th, and 12th graders among a representative sample of high schools, designed to study changes in the beliefs, values, attitudes, and behaviors of young people in the United

Table 4.1 Substance use patterns in 2021

2021 Trends in Substance Use
30-Day Prevalence in 12th Graders

Substance	Prevalence
Alcohol	26%
Cannabis	20%
Any Illicit Drug Other Than Cannabis	3%
Cigarettes	4%
Any Vaping	24%

Source: Retrieved from https://monitoringthefuture.org/data/21data.htm

States (Johnston et al., 2021). The survey began in 1975 with 12th-grade students only; starting in 1991 similar surveys of nationally representative samples of 8th and 10th graders have also been conducted annually. Each year's data collection of about 50,000 students takes place in approximately 420 public and private high schools and middle schools selected to provide an accurate representative cross section of students throughout the coterminous United States at each grade level. The MTF high school survey consists of the same set of questions over a period of years to understand how behaviors change over time. In addition to these annual surveys, beginning with the class of 1976, a randomly selected sample from each senior class has been followed up every other year after high school on a continuing basis. Data from the 2021 MTF survey of past 30-day use among 12th graders are shown in Table 4.1 (http://monitoringthefuture.org/data/21data.htm).

Based on our synthesis of survey findings from these two sources, we discuss next five general trends and patterns of drug use among adolescents in the United States.

1. Commonality of drugs used. The first major trend pertains to the *common drugs* used by adolescents. Throughout the history of surveying youth in the U.S., the drugs most commonly used at an overwhelming level are tobacco (primarily cigarettes), alcohol, and marijuana. Consider the data displayed in Figure 4.2 that illustrate this finding. Based on recent

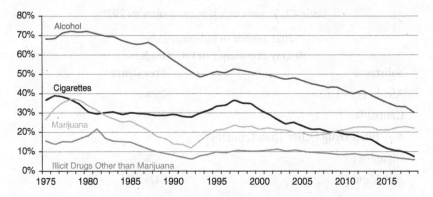

Figure 4.1 Past-month substance use by U.S. high school seniors: 1976–2018.
SOURCE: Miech, Richard A., Johnston, Lloyd D., Bachman, Jerald G., O'Malley, Patrick
M., and Schulenberg, John E. Monitoring the Future: A Continuing Study of American
Youth (12th-Grade Survey), 2018. Inter-university Consortium for Political and Social
Research [distributor], 2019-11-19. https://doi.org/10.3886/ICPSR37416.v1

MTF survey findings, the prevalence rates of prior 30-day use reported
by *12th-grade students* show trend lines for four drug classes (alcohol,
cigarettes, marijuana, and other illicit drugs) spanning from 1976 to 2018.
The data indicate that alcohol use is the most prevalent across the years,
with cigarette and cannabis use at lower rates. Other illicit drugs are used
at a much lower rate. This general pattern shown in Figure 4.1 is observed
across gender, race/ethnicity, geographic region, and grade (8th and 10th
grades). The most recent data from the MTF survey indicate that prevalence rates reported in 2021 show the same pattern (e.g., alcohol use is still
the most prevalent and other illicit drug use is very low) (http://monitori
ngthefuture.org/data/21data.htm).

The trend lines from Figure 4.1 indicate a downturn in use of most
drugs over the years by 12th graders. A more detailed look at this question is provided in Figure 4.2. Here the comparison is 2018 and 2019
rates based on the MTF data for all three age groups; vaping is included.
The bands in red indicate an increase from 2018; all of the increases are
either related to vaping and to marijuana use. Alcohol use shows a decline. The 2021 MTF data indicate one exception to these trends noted
above: marijuana use showed a decline compared to 2020.

2019 Monitoring the Future Survey
Key Findings: Percent Reporting Use of Selected Substances

	8th Grade	10th Grade	12th Grade		8th Grade	10th Grade	12th Grade
Vaping, Any				**Tobacco w/Hookah**			
Past Year	20.1	35.7	40.6	Past Year			5.6
Past Month	12.2	25.0	30.9	Past Month	1.3	2.4	4.0
Vaping, Nicotine				**Flavored Little Cigars**			
Past Year	16.5	30.7	35.3	Past Year	2.2	3.7	7.7
Past Month	9.6	19.9	25.5	Narcotics Other than			
Vaping, Marijuana				Heroin			
				Past Year			2.7
Past Year	7.0	19.4	20.8	Past Month			1.0
Past Month	3.9	12.6	14.0	**Marijuana**			
Vaping, Just Flavoring				Past Year	11.8	28.8	35.7
Past Year	14.7	20.8	20.3	Past Month	6.6	18.4	22.3
Past Month	7.7	10.5	10.7	Daily	1.3	4.8	6.4
Cigarettes				**Alcohol**			
Past Month	2.3	3.4	5.7	Past Month	7.9	18.4	29.3
Daily	0.8	1.3	2.4	Daily	0.2	0.6	1.7
½ Pack +/Day	0.2	0.5	0.9	Binge	3.8	8.5	14.4

Change from 2018 to 2019

■ Significant increase ■ Significant decrease

Figure 4.2 Substance use patterns comparing 2018 and 2019.
SOURCE: NIDA. 2019, December 18. Monitoring the Future Survey: High School and Youth Trends Drug Facts. https://www.drugabuse.gov/publications/drugfacts/monitoring-future-survey-high-school-youth-trends

The recent outbreak of EVALI is a public health problem related to vaping of nicotine or cannabis. EVALI is an acronym for "e-cigarette, or vaping, product use-associated lung injury." The first case of EVALI was officially reported in August, 2019, in an adult in Wisconsin. As of January 14, 2020, a total of 2,668 hospitalized EVALI cases had been reported to the Centers for Disease Control and Prevention (CDC) from all 50 states and the District of Columbia (Krishnasamy et al., 2020). Because the sharp increase in vaping by adolescents began much earlier than 2019, there is concern that the incidence of EVALI among youth will be surging.

It is important to consider adolescent trend data in the context that certain substances during some brief periods receive a lot of attention as the latest scourge among our youth (e.g., misuse of prescribed pain medication). Yet these occasional spikes in the use of other illicit drugs use do not exceed the prevalence rate of the three so-called common substances used by adolescents (alcohol, nicotine products, and marijuana).

There are concerns that recent trends in the United States to legalize marijuana for recreational or medical purposes may contribute to a rise in adolescent marijuana use. Marijuana is used at relatively high prevalence rates by adolescents in the United States; it is now used at higher rates than cigarettes (http://monitoringthefuture.org/data/21data.htm) (and as shown in Table 4.1, Figures 4.1, and 4.2). Some survey data indicate that marijuana use is on the rise among adolescents in states that have legalized it for recreational or medical purposes, although this complex question is not reliably occurring in all pro-marijuana states, and different sources of youth survey data do not reveal identical findings (see Carliner et al., 2017; Cerdá et al., 2020; Cottler & Okar, 2018; Lee et al., 2022; Smart & Pacula, 2019). Also, it is relevant to not lose sight that whereas it is common for youth to experiment with drugs during the teenage years, most do not develop a serious drug problem (Montana & Chung, 2019). More on this issue in Chapter 5.

One observation from Figure 4.2 is that daily marijuana use, defined as use on 20 or more occasions in the past 30 days by any method, significantly increased in 10th and 8th grade. In 10th grade it increased by 1.3 percentage points to 4.8%, which is the highest prevalence for this outcome ever measured by MTF since tracking began for this grade in 1991. In 8th grade, prevalence increased by 0.6 percentage points to 1.3%, which is the highest level ever tracked by the survey since tracking began for this grade in 1991 (it ties with the year 2011).

Sources: University of Michigan, Institute for Social Research. (2019). *National adolescent drug trends in 2019: Findings released. Marijuana vaping surges.* http://www.monitoringthefuture.org//pressreleases/19drugpr.pdf; https://nida.nih.gov/drug-topics/trends-statistics/infographics/monitoring-future-2019-survey-results-overall-findings

2. *Gateway pattern.* A second major theme of adolescent drug use is termed the *gateway pattern.* More than 40 years ago, Kandel and Faust

(1975) investigated adolescent involvement in drug use based on random and sequential sampling of students in New York State middle and high schools. Based on the survey responses from over 8,000 students, a common pattern emerged: students who smoked cigarettes and drank alcohol rapidly progressed to marijuana use within 5 to 6 months, but of those who had not initiated use of tobacco or alcohol, fewer than 10% had used marijuana. Also, the survey found that the majority of drug use progression to use other illicit drugs (e.g., amphetamines, cocaine) was much higher among marijuana users than non-marijuana users. This notion that there are gateway drugs has been reinforced by the findings from numerous other large national surveys of adolescents in the United States over the years (e.g., Moss et al., 2014).

The gateway effect of marijuana, if it exists, has at least two potential and quite different sources (MacCoun, 1998). One source may be the effect of marijuana itself. That is, trying marijuana leads the user to believe that other drugs are more pleasurable or less risky than previous expectations. A second possible source noted by MacCoun is the influence of peer groups. Marijuana involvement might contribute to affiliating more with peers who have pro-drug attitudes and behaviors and these social interactions lead to use of the harder drugs common to this peer group.

Yet, the gateway theory has its limits in *predicting* drug use at the individual level. For example, marijuana has often been viewed as a gateway drug. Whereas it's true that most amphetamine or heroin or barbiturate users once used marijuana, there is a greater proportion of youth who use marijuana and never escalate their drug use preference for so-called harder drugs. In this light, marijuana is a "limited gateway" drug.

3. *Collinearity of use.* We refer to the third major adolescent trend as the *collinearity of drug use.* This reflects that for the majority of teenagers who decide to use drugs, it is relatively more common for them to use all three of the major drugs of abuse by adolescents (tobacco, alcohol, and marijuana) than to use just one of them (DuPont et al., 2018). Thus, the common pattern is that the early onset of use of tobacco, alcohol,

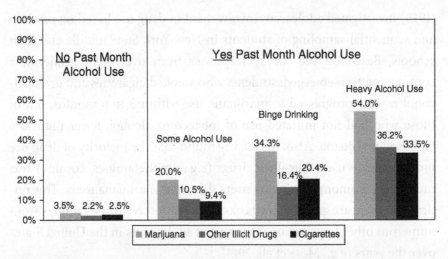

Figure 4.3 Past-month substance use among youth age 12–17 by past month alcohol use status, based on National Survey on Drug Use and Health (Dupont et al., 2018).
SOURCE: Drug use among youth: National survey data support a common liability of all drug use, by Robert L. DuPont, Beth Han, Corinne L. Shea, Bertha K. Madras, *Preventive Medicine*, Volume 113, August 2018, Pages 68–73.

marijuana, and their combined use is more common over the course of the teenage years than the initiation and use of just one or two of individual substances. Figure 4.3 shows this for alcohol; those youth who used any alcohol are far more likely to report also using cigarettes, marijuana, and other drugs than young people who have not used alcohol (Dupont et al., 2018). The same close association holds true when the question is based on the use in the past month of cigarettes and marijuana use. The decision to use a drug as a teenager most commonly involves eventually using more than a single drug. Of course, there are many individual and contextual factors that impact the specific sequence of the onset of use of these widely available drugs; most experts agree that the order is typically a tobacco product, followed by alcohol, and then marijuana (Montana & Chung, 2019). Sequence is most certainly affected by availability, social norms, and price. Nonetheless, the point of this third principle is that it further defines the "gateway" pattern: the initiation of a drug use rarely stops with initiation of a single drug type.

4. Abstaining from all drugs. Despite what might be perceived by the general public, there are some signs of a *downward trend in drug use* by adolescents in the United States over recent decades. As shown earlier in Figure 4.1, there is a general decline over the years in the prevalence rate of alcohol use, smoking cigarettes, and use of other illicit drugs (but not marijuana). The trend pattern for cannabis is less striking; its prevalence rate declined substantially from the late 1970s to early 2000, but the cannabis trend line has remained relatively flat since then (http://monitoringthefut ure.org/data/21data.htm).

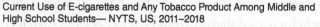

Current Use of E-cigarettes and Any Tobacco Product Among Middle and High School Students— NYTS, US, 2011–2018

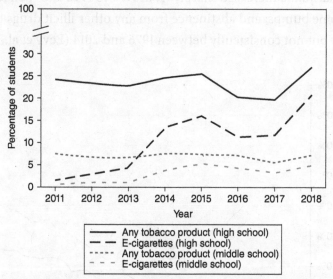

Source: Cullen KA, Ambrose BK, Gentzke AS, Apelberg BJ, Jamal A, King BA. *Notes from the Field*: Use of Electronic Cigarettes and Any Tobacco Product Among Middle and High School Students—United States, 2011–2018. MMWR Morb Mortal Wkly Rep 2018; 67:1276–1277.

The rise in the rate of abstinence from all substances by students in the United States may be slowed by the recent trend of vaping. A major finding from the 2018 Monitor the Future (MTF) survey data is the dramatic increase in vaping (shown as e-cigarettes in the graph) by adolescents. This trend is shown in the chart.

A trend related to the declining use of many substances is that the prevalence of *abstaining from all substances is on the rise.* A steadily growing percentage of American youth are refraining from any alcohol, tobacco, marijuana, and other drug use; many adolescents make it through high school drug free. A recent analysis of MTF survey data between 1975 and 2014 indicated that the percentage of high school students who did not use any alcohol, cigarettes, marijuana, or other drugs in their lifetimes increased from 2.9 to 26% (a five-fold increase), and that the percentage who abstained in the past month more than doubled to 52% (see Figure 4.4; Levy et al., 2018). The following abstinence trend lines for specific substances were observed by the authors: abstinence from alcohol use increased steadily over the past 38 years; abstinence from cigarettes increased dramatically over the past 20 years; abstinence from marijuana increased sharply from 1978 to 1992 and then leveled off with some bumps; and abstinence from any other illicit drugs increased slightly but not consistently between 1976 and 2014 (Levy et al., 2018). In

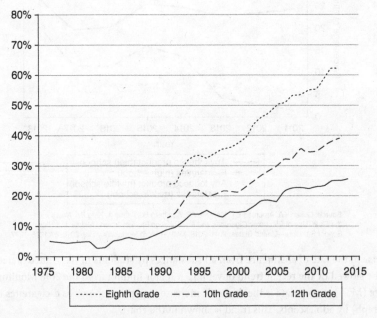

Figure 4.4 Abstaining from alcohol, marijuana and cigarettes lifetime, based on Monitoring the Future (MTF) data (Levy et al., 2018).
SOURCE: Levy, S., Campbell, M. C., Shea, C. L., & DuPont, R. L. (2018). Trends in abstaining from substance use in adolescents: 1975–2014. *Pediatrics, 142*, e20173498.

2014, students who identified as male, African American, or other race and those who reported greater religious commitment were significantly more likely to report lifetime abstinence. Students who lived in single-parent households, spent more evenings out, worked more hours during the school year, and reported lower grades and more truancy had lower abstinence rates.

5. *Drug use typically occurs in the presence of coexisting problems and disorders.* A sizeable proportion of teenagers who use drugs also suffer from *one or more co-occurring behavioral or psychological disorders.* As will be discussed in more detail in Chapter 5, many of these co-existing problems meet criteria for a formal "psychiatric" disorder. Psychosocial impairments that do not meet full *Diagnostic and Statistical Manual of Mental Disorders* (DSM) diagnoses of 29 well-defined disorders were identified as common among youth (Angold et al., 1999). Such coexisting problems likely influence the onset and course of a drug use habit. And the reverse is true—there is a bidirectional effect whereby drug use can aggravate a pre-existing condition or trigger a coexisting problem.

DRUGS' ACUTE AND CHRONIC EFFECTS

How Drugs Acutely Affect the Brain

Nearly all addictive drugs directly or indirectly target the brain's reward system by flooding this part of the brain with a neurotransmitter called *dopamine.* The reward system is the region of the brain that includes the amygdala, nucleus accumbens, and the hippocampus, and these regions regulate movement, emotion, cognition, motivation, and feelings of pleasure. All drugs of abuse, from nicotine to heroin, cause a particularly powerful surge of dopamine in the reward region. This dopamine release rewards our natural behaviors, produces the euphoric effects sought by people who use drugs, and teaches them to repeat the behavior (see Figure 4.5).

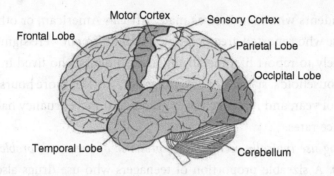

Figure 4.5 The key regions of the brain's reward center.
SOURCE: Figure 2 in Liu J, Sheng Y, and Liu H. (2019) Corticomuscular Coherence and Its Applications: A Review. *Front. Hum. Neurosci.* 13:100. doi:10.3389/fnhum.2019.00100. License: CC BY 4.0

Chronic Effects of Drug Use: Hijacking the Brain's Communication Network

Drugs have this powerful impact on users because they tap into the brain's communication system by disrupting the normal way neurotransmitters send, receive, and process information. Some drugs interfere with neuronal activity because the drug's chemical structure mimics the activity of normal neurotransmitter activity. This process "fools" the receiving part of a neuron to allow the drug to be attached and to activate it in abnormal ways. Examples of these "mimicking" drugs are marijuana and heroin. Other drugs, such as cocaine and amphetamine, cause an overamplification of neuronal activity because the drug prevents the normal amount of recycling of neurotransmitters, which produces excessive signaling of the neurons and ultimately disrupting the brain's normal communication network.

The bottom line is that drugs of abuse disrupt the normal amount and function of dopamine in the brain. A normal amount of dopamine is released when we eat food to satisfy hunger or when we engage in sex (Di Chiara & Imperato, 1988). Experts estimate that drugs can produce from 2 to 10 times the amount of dopamine compared to normally rewarding activities, either by virtue of the dopamine flooding the brain

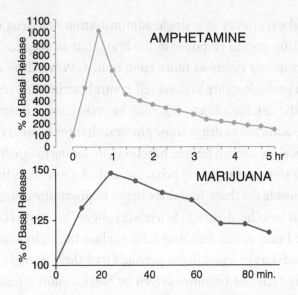

Figure 4.6 Changes in dopamine levels after administration of amphetamine and marijuana.

SOURCE: Graph adapted by NIDA from Tanda, G., Pontieri, F. E., & Di Chiara, G. (1997). Cannabinoid and heroin activation of mesolimbic dopamine transmission by a common µl opioid receptor mechanism. *Science, 276*(5321), 2048–2050.

almost immediately (when drugs are smoked or injected) or because the effects can last much longer than those produced by natural rewards (Di Chiara et al., 1997; Fiorino & Phillips, 1999). The former Director of the National Institute on Drug Abuse, C. Schuster, Ph.D., referred to this as the "wow" effect. The effect on dopamine elevations varies by drug; Figure 4.6 compares changes in dopamine after the administration of amphetamines and marijuana.

From initial use to addiction. The initial decision to take drugs is mostly voluntary. But our brains are wired to encourage the continuation of behavior that results in pleasure or reward. Thus, when the brain is exposed to a drug, our neural wiring signals pleasure and the brain "recognizes" that something important has occurred that needs to be remembered and will motivate us to repeat it. In this light, scientists characterize drug abuse as something we learn to do that is comparable to many other learned behaviors.

The initial experience of a single administration of a drug results in a noticeable drug reward response in the brain, but as drug use continues, the brain's response becomes more complicated. When drug use further continues, a person's ability to exert self-control can become seriously impaired and the risk for addiction greatly increases. Brain imaging studies from people addicted to drugs show physical changes in areas of the brain that are critical for various human functions, including judgment, decision making, learning, memory, and behavior control. Over time, the brain regions responsible for these functions begin to physically change, making certain behaviors "hard-wired." Scientists believe that these changes alter the way the brain works and may help explain the compulsive and destructive behaviors of an addicted person. Once these changes take place, drug-seeking behavior becomes driven by habit, almost a reflex, and the likelihood increases that the user may become a drug addict.

Consider the metaphor that taking a drug is like listening to music. The first time a drug is taken is like your brain listening to a favorite song at a pleasant volume. But continued drug use would be like the brain experiencing the song at a very loud volume. Similar to turning down the dial on the radio, the brain adjusts to the overwhelming surges in dopamine (and other neurotransmitters) by turning down the "drug volume" by producing less dopamine or by reducing the number of receptors that can receive signals. Whereas this adjustment provides a temporary correction for the brain, continued drug use and the repeated reductions in the brain's dopamine lead to abnormally low dopamine levels. With depressed levels of dopamine, the person's ability to experience any pleasure is reduced. This is why a person who abuses drugs will feel temporary spikes in dopamine (pleasure) but eventually feels flat, lifeless, and depressed and is unable to enjoy things that were previously pleasurable. You can appreciate how a vicious cycle can ensue: the person learns that taking drugs again and again will bring their dopamine function temporarily back up to normal. But doing so only makes the problem worse.

Brain changes due to prolonged drug use impact behavior. Chronic drug use influences the user's future behavior. The person will often need to take larger amounts of the drug to produce the familiar dopamine high—an effect known as *tolerance*. Drug addiction erodes a person's self-control and ability to make sound decisions, while producing intense impulses to take drugs. These intense feelings can drive a user to seek out and take drugs compulsively, ignore responsibilities, and channel their choices to ignore usual interests. Also, the brain's attempt to compensate for this change can cause impairment in thinking and learning.

The brain has memory of long-term drug use. Long-term drug abuse can trigger adaptations in the brain's memory systems. Conditioning is one example of this type of adaptation. Drug-related cues in a person's daily routine or environment can become associated with the person's prior drug experience and can trigger uncontrollable cravings whenever the person is exposed to these cues, even if the drug itself is not available (National Institute on Drug Abuse, 2018). This learned "brain reflex" is extremely robust; it can elicit cravings in a once addicted person for many years during abstinence.

Drug type and form of administration matter. The likelihood that the use of a drug will lead to continued use and, for some, addiction, is directly linked to the speed, intensity, and reliability with which the drug promotes dopamine release. The pharmacology of drugs varies with respect to dopamine potency; for example, methamphetamine is extremely potent and LSD is less so. Also, taking the same drug through different methods of administration can influence how likely it is to lead to addiction. Smoking a drug or injecting it intravenously, as opposed to swallowing it as a pill, for example, generally produces a faster, stronger dopamine signal and is more likely to lead to continued drug abuse. As discussed in detail in Chapter 5, the person's involvement with addictive drugs begins with "liking" it, and if use continues the experience can turn into "wanting" it.

Relative Harm of Different Drugs

Is there a science-based way to compare the relative addiction potential across drug categories? An interesting effort was attempted by Nutt and colleagues (Nutt et al., 2010). They viewed this question through the lens of comparing illicit and legal drugs on a nine-category matrix of harm. The authors used a sophisticated methodology by which the ratings were obtained from groups of experts regarding harms of drugs use. The experts rated each of 20 substances for their potential to contribute to a user's *physical harm, risk for developing a dependence,* and *harm to social functioning.* Figure 4.7 shows the mean rankings of each substance when all three "harm categories" are considered. Heroin was rated the most harmful; khat was rated the least harmful. It is of interest that the legal drugs alcohol and tobacco receive relative high harm rankings.

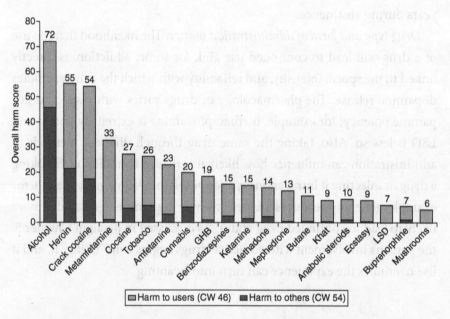

Figure 4.7 Drugs ordered by their overall harm scores, showing the separate contributions to the overall scores of harms to users and harm to others (Nutt et al., 2010).
SOURCE: Nutt, D. J., King, L. A., & Phillips, L. D. (2010). Drug harms in the UK: A multicriteria decision analysis. *The Lancet, 376,* 1558–1565.

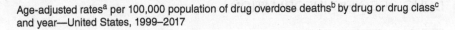

Age-adjusted rates[a] per 100,000 population of drug overdose deaths[b] by drug or drug class[c] and year—United States, 1999–2017

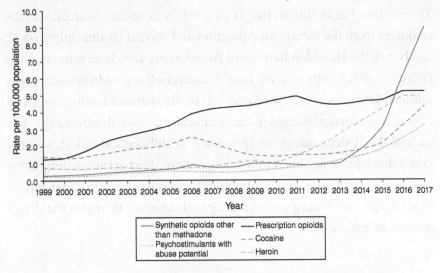

In the United States, the potential harm for certain substances has changed in recent years. The U.S. government does not track death rates for every drug, but the National Center for Health Statistics and the Centers for Disease Control and Prevention (CDC) collect information on many commonly used drugs. The CDC has a searchable database, Wonder, from which trends in drug-related fatalities are reported. Opioid deaths are by far the biggest problem when it comes to drug-related fatal overdoses.

Keep in mind that these rankings from the Nutt et al. study are based on the drug scene of the early 2000s, and as the drug culture changes, it is likely that a drug's harm status will also change.

Perceived harm for smoking may be trending in the direction that is concern from a public health perspective. Nationally representative data from the years 2016–2018 show that the prevalence of perceived great risk of cigarette smoking has continued to decline significantly (71.76% versus 72.77% in 2016 and 73.89% in 2006) (Pacek & McClernon, 2020).

DRUG-SPECIFIC INFORMATION

The information in this section is adapted from several sources: various resources from the Centre for Addiction and Mental Health (http://www. camh.ca/), the Hazelden Betty Ford Foundation's Teen Intervene resource (Winters, 2022; https://www.hazeldenbettyford.org/addiction/intervent ion/teen-intervene), and two sources from the National Institute on Drug Abuse (www.drugabuse.gov/parents-educators; www.drugfree.org). For each of the 17 drug categories (presented in alphabetical order), we provide a description and then information about short-term use, long-term use, signs of acute use, and legal status. There is one principal that applies to all drugs: combining use of a drug with another increases the drug's dangerous effects.

Alcohol

Categories and names of different types of alcohol include beer, wine, brew, booze, hooch, moonshine, vino, sauce, spirits.

Description. Alcohol is a depressant that reduces the activities of the central nervous system. Alcohol is created by the fermentation of grains, vegetables, and/or fruits.

Drinking to the point of getting drunk at least once is a common experience for adolescents. But excessive drinking is a particular problem for college students. About one-third of full-time undergraduate college students in the United States drink excessively, which includes heavy drinking and binge drinking (as defined by four or more drinks on a single occasion for females and five or more for males) (Lipari & JeanFrancois, 2016).

Short-term effects. Drinking alcohol is associated with several effects: greater relaxation; more sociability; and distorted thinking, decision-making, and reaction time. Alcohol's influence also disrupts one's coordination when engaged in physical and mental activity, can increase risk taking, and, for many, impair ability to control temper and anger. These effects of alcohol can be accentuated if drinking is combined with use of other drugs. When a person consumes a large amount of alcohol in a single occasion, it is called *binge drinking*. A *hangover* occurs when a person consumes a large amount of alcohol and feels ill several hours later or the next day. As discussed in Chapter 3, there is some evidence that adolescents are less sensitive to the short-term effects of alcohol than adults (Spear, 2002).

Long-term effects. The long-term health effects of using alcohol on a person who consumes alcohol heavily on a regular basis can be very deleterious. The chronic user is likely to suffer from numerous health problems, including cirrhosis of the liver, heart disease, high blood pressure, brain damage, nerve damage, and cancers of the gastrointestinal tract. At the extreme level, it can cause death. Other victims of the long-term effects of alcohol are unborn babies of pregnant women who drink. Prenatal exposure to alcohol can cause fetal alcohol syndrome (FAS) or fetal alcohol effects (FAE); symptoms of these disorders include facial abnormalities, growth deficiencies, learning disabilities, memory deficits, and hyperactivity and other behavioral disorders.

Some parents supply their adolescent children with alcohol in an attempt to educate them about the effects of alcohol and to protect them from heavy drinking and alcohol-related harms. The hope is that a drinking party under a watchful eye will not lead to problems. Alas, the research on parents supplying alcohol to an adolescent does not support this parenting policy as a harm reduction strategy (Mattick et al., 2018).

Signs of use. Drunken behavior includes impaired coordination and judgment, slurred speech, and the smell on a person's breath or clothing. Symptoms of a hangover include headache, stomach ache, low blood sugar, dehydration, and possibly an irritation of the lining of the digestive system.

Legal status. All states and the District of Columbia have a minimum drinking age of 21 years.

Caffeine

Description. Caffeine is a drug, albeit a relatively mild and low-harm one. Derived from many plants, including coffee, tea, cocoa, and some nuts, caffeine is likely the most widely used drug in the world. It is found in numerous popular foods and beverages like chocolate, coffee, tea, soft drinks, and energy drinks, the latter becoming increasingly popular.

Short-term effects. The short-term effects associated with caffeine intake are that it constricts the blood vessels and increases one's heart rate, blood pressure, production of gastric juices, and urine output. The caffeine user initially experiences an elevation in one's mood, with accompanying effects of reducing drowsiness and fatigue. Larger doses can cause irritability, restlessness, nervousness, and insomnia.

Long-term effects. If a person uses large doses of caffeine for an extended period, symptoms include irritability, restlessness, nervousness, muscle twitches, rapid and/or irregular heartbeat, inexhaustibility, agitation, and insomnia. The extent to which caffeine is addictive is a source of debate among experts. Caffeine use disorder is not a specified diagnosis in DSM-5, but it has been placed in the category of Conditions for Further Study (American Psychiatric Association, 2013). This category refers to conditions that appear to have some evidence of effects on psychological well-being but not enough of a research base to warrant their inclusion in the list of classifiable disorders.

Monitoring caffeine levels is difficult. It is common in low doses in many foods and beverages as a part of normal diets, and such low levels will not directly boost athlete performance. Caffeine is also metabolized at different rates by individuals, making it hard to determine from a blood test an athlete's recent caffeine intake (see https://nationalcoffee.blog/2018/02/12/can-olympic-athletes-have-caffeine/).

Signs of use. Caffeine users may appear jittery, hyperactive, talkative, and, for some, anxious. Withdrawal symptoms (e.g., headache, drowsiness) can occur when heavy users abstain.

Legal status. Caffeine is not a restricted drug. It is legal to purchase and consume with no age restrictions. However, for the period 1984–2004, Olympic athletes were restricted from its use, given that caffeine has been consistently shown to improve athletic performance.

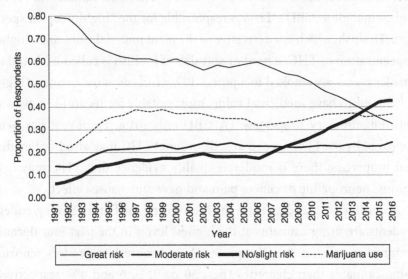

Perception of level of harm from using cannabis has been tracked by the Monitor the Future (MTF) survey. The figure below shows changes in perceptions of harm of any use of cannabis in the past year among U.S. 12th-grade students from 1991 to 2016. The trend line for "great risk" is on the general decline since 2006.

SOURCE: Risk is still relevant: Time-varying associations between perceived risk and marijuana use among US 12th grade students from 1991 to 2016, Yvonne M. Terry-McElrath, Patrick M. O'Malley, Megan E. Patrick, Richard A. Miech, *Addictive Behaviors*, Volume 74, November 2017, Pages 13–19.

Cannabis

Cannabis is referred to as marijuana, dope, THC, pot, hemp, weed, ganja, grass, reefer, Mary Jane, hashish, hash, hash oil, chronic, gangster, and boom.

Description. Cannabis is likely the most commonly used substance other than alcohol and nicotine products when considering all age groups in the United States. The drug's source is the cannabis plant, which appears as green, brown, or gray mixtures of dried, shredded leaves, stems, and seeds. Whereas the usual method of consumption is to smoke it in a pipe or water pipe ("bong"), or rolled up in cigarette or cigar papers, called "joints" or "blunts," there is increased popularity in marijuana edibles and inhaling cannabis via a vaporizer. The main pharmacologically active chemicals in cannabis are the cannabinoids Tetrahydrocannabinol (THC) and cannabidiol (CBD). THC is responsible for the "high" people experience. Hashish, which is a derivative of the plant material, contains a higher concentration of THC; a hard or soft slab of hashish is called hash and its smaller pieces are smoked in a pipe. CBD, which does not create a "high," is believed to have medicinal value, most notably for its anti-seizure and anti-inflammatory properties. (A CBD-only drug, Epidiolex, has been approved by the FDA for seizures disorders.) THC may also have medicinal properties; there is moderate-quality evidence that THC may help chronic neuropathic or cancer pain and have anti-nausea effects.

According to 2021 data from the Monitoring the Future Survey, college students are using cannabis at the highest levels in the past four decades (prior 12 months, 44%) (Knopf, 2021), and more 12th graders reported using cannabis than cigarettes (past 30 days, 20% and 4%, respectively (http://monitoringthefuture.org/data/21data.htm). Also, daily use of marijuana is still provocatively high: 1% 8th graders, 3% 10th graders, and 6% 12th graders (http://monitoringthefuture.org/data/21data.htm).

Short-term effects. There are numerous short-term behavioral effects of using marijuana. The person's pulse rate and blood pressure may rise. Many users feel elation and relaxation and are more talkative. Cognitive-related effects include short-term memory problems, difficulties with concentration, disorientated behavior, confusion, and the inability to think clearly. For some, using marijuana triggers symptoms of psychosis (paranoia, hallucinations), and there is compelling evidence that THC contributes to risk for developing psychosis (more on this issue in Chapter 7, *Externalizing Disorders*). Recent research indicates that marijuana secondhand smoke causes similar effects as tobacco secondhand smoke on the cardiovascular system.

These effects will vary based on the strength of the cannabis and the mode of delivery. Cannabis potency has been increasing over the past half century. During the 1960s, cannabis was typically about 1% to 5% THC by weight; many strains available today range from 15 to 25% THC by weight, with some strains much higher (www.learnaboutsam.org). When smoked, about 25% of the THC present in the plant material gets absorbed. However, when inhaling cannabis via a vaporizer, the user absorbs up to 33% of the THC. Both of these methods produce the effects quickly, with intoxication, on average, setting in within 2 minutes and lasting 2-4 hours. By contrast, when cannabis products are ingested orally, THC is absorbed inconsistently. Users typically experience the effects of THC about 2 to 4 hours after ingestion, and its effects may last for 6 to 8 hours.

Long-term effects. As with all psychoactive substances, one long-term effect of using marijuana is the possibility of developing a use disorder. (It is a myth that a person cannot become dependent on marijuana.) Other possible long-term effects include the following: loss of interest in formerly enjoyed activities; diminished intellectual performance (e.g., reduced IQ); a weakened immune system; chronic bronchitis or other lung-related ailments; and cardiovascular problems (e.g., blood pressure difficulties).

Signs of use. Most cannabis users exhibit talkativeness; difficulties with thinking, attention, judgment, and motor coordination; silliness or giddiness for no reason; red, bloodshot eyes; sleepiness; anxiety (for some); relaxation (for some); and thirst or hunger (called "the munchies").

U.S. public opinion on legalizing marijuana, 1969–2019

Do you think the use of marijuana should be made legal, or not? (%)

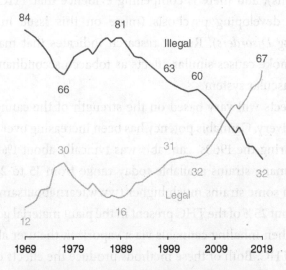

Note: No answer responses not shown. 2019 data from Pew Research Center's online American Trends Panel; prior data from telephone surveys. Data from 1969–1972 from Gallup: data from 1973–2008 from General Social Surveys.
Source: Survey of U.S. adults conducted Sept. 3–15. 2109.
PEW RESEARCH CENTER

Majorities of Millennials (those born between 1981 and 1997), Generation X (born between 1965 and 1980) and Baby Boomers (born between 1946 and 1964) say the use of cannabis should be legal. Members of the Silent Generation (born between 1928 and 1945) continue to be the least supportive of legalization (only 35% favor legalizing cannabis).
SOURCE: Two-thirds of Americans support marijuana legalization. BY ANDREW DANILLER, Pew Research Center, Washington, D.C. (NOVEMBER 14, 2019). https://www.pewresearch.org/fact-tank/2019/11/14/americans-support-marijuana-legalization/

Legal status. As of January 2022, the purchasing, selling, or possessing of marijuana is legal for adults age 21 or over in 19 U.S. states and the District of Columbia. An additional 18 states permit cannabis use for medicinal purposes. The trend to legalize marijuana for medicinal and recreational purposes that began in the 1990s has expanded. Also, some states have decriminalized cannabis laws related to possession (see https://marijuana. procon.org/view.resource.php?resourceID=006868).

There are credible reports by individuals suffering from a variety of intractable and often painful illnesses (e.g., cancer, AIDS wasting syndrome, etc.) and glaucoma that use of marijuana has uniquely beneficial effects on their conditions. Rigorous reviews of this science generally conclude among the more than 400 known elements and compounds within a typical marijuana plant that cannabidiol (CBD) and, to a lesser degree, tetrahydrocannabinol (THC) might have genuine medicinal effects for the treatment of pain and other ailments and conditions. As of this writing, one medication that contains 99% CBD and 1% THC, Epidiolex, has been approved by the U.S. Food and Drug Administration (FDA) to treat rare forms of childhood epilepsy. Also, Marinol and Syndros, synthetic forms of THC in pill form, are approved to treat or prevent nausea and vomiting caused by cancer medications and to increase the appetite of people with AIDS. Thus, it is reasonable to suggest that some compounds of the marijuana plant may possess medicinal properties.

The impact of legalizing cannabis in certain states has led researchers to examine if the trend in cannabis use is different in these states than in states without laws allowing for medical or recreational use of cannabis. There are numerous survey reports that have looked at this question (see *Further Curiosity and Digging* at the end of this chapter). It is the view of the present authors that the data represent relatively short time windows and thus are not conclusive. This important public health question will benefit from continued monitoring of trend data that spans extended time periods.

Nonetheless, nationwide calls for the legalization of the marijuana plant to treat medical conditions and ailments are premature. The scientific evidence to date is not sufficient for the marijuana plant to gain U.S. Food and Drug Administration (FDA) approval two main reasons (1): there have not been enough clinical trials showing that marijuana's benefits outweigh its health risks, and (2) to be considered a legitimate medicine, a substance must have well-defined and measurable ingredients that are consistent from one unit to the next (such as a pill or injection). This consistency allows doctors to determine the dose and frequency. Given that the marijuana plant contains hundreds of chemical compounds that might have different effects and that vary from plant to plant, its use as medicine is difficult to evaluate (Sabet et al., 2018).

Cocaine

Cocaine is known as crack, C, coke, flake, dust, blow, nose candy, rock, and white lines.

Description. Cocaine is a fine white powder that is processed from the leaves of the coca plant. The powder form is typically snorted, but it can also be injected. A derivative of cocaine, crack, is a cake-like substance made by mixing cocaine with baking powder or baking soda and water. This cake is cracked into small pieces about the size of a peanut, which are then then smoked (also called "freebasing").

Short-term effects. Cocaine is a powerful drug that activates the central nervous system, producing a brief "high" lasting about only 5 to 20 minutes. The user experiences a burst of energy, enhanced sense of alertness, and a decrease in appetite. For some, unpredictable and violent behavior, paranoia, and seizures may occur. One use of cocaine and/or crack cocaine can cause a stroke (due to an increase in one's hear rate and blood pressure) and a heart attack.

Long-term effects. For those who engage in repeated snorting of the drug, a long-term effect is the deterioration of the individual's nose tissues. Other long-term effects include developing a cocaine use disorder, paranoia, and medical conditions (for those who inject the drug). There is also a high risk of overdose.

Signs of use. A cocaine user will appear with pupils larger than normal and display mood swings and irritability, euphoria, and talkativeness.

Legal status. Possessing, purchasing, using, and selling cocaine are all illegal, with the one exception that it can be used in the United States as a topical anesthetic for some medical procedures (e.g., pain relief during rhinoplasty).

Ecstasy

Chemically, Ecstasy is MDMA, or methylenedioxymethamphetamine; it is called E, XTC, Adam, the love drug, designer drug. It is also called a "club drug" because of the use by those who attend nightclubs or parties called "raves."

Description. Ecstasy is a psychoactive drug with hallucinogenic and amphetamine-like effects. It is commonly taken orally in the form of a tablet or gelatin capsule, and the powder form can be snorted as well. There is no approved medical use for this drug at this time.

Short-term effects. The short-term effects from low to moderate doses include a mild intoxication, euphoria, and feelings of disinhibition and greater connectivity with others. Large doses of this drug increase the negative effects and may cause alterations in one's perceptions, thinking processes, and memory, and, in extreme instances, death due to a hazardous increase in the victims' body temperature. A fatal incident has occurred at raves as users overexert themselves while dancing all night long. Some reactions in certain people may be severe and unpredictable from only one use.

Long-term effects. There are several long-term effects of using Ecstasy: severe depression, irritability and paranoia; concentration difficulties; fatigue; weight loss; and damage to brain structures believed to cause permanent memory and learning disabilities. Some reactions in certain people may be severe and unpredictable from only one use.

Signs of use. Users may experience numerous physical and psychological effects, including sweating, increased heart rate and blood pressure, increased sensitivity to touch, nausea, convulsions, blurred vision, jaw pain (from grinding teeth), insomnia, anxiety, panic attacks, and paranoia.

Legal status. Ecstasy is illegal to purchase, sell, or consume in the United States.

GHB

GHB is the abbreviation for gamma hydroxybutyrate; it is also called "date-rape" drug, liquid Ecstasy, liquid X, easy lay, and "G."

Description. GHB is created in the human body naturally in small quantities and acts by depressing the central nervous system. In the liquid form, GHB looks and smells like water with a salty taste; it is also found in white powder or capsule form. GHB has been used to increase one's sensuality and physical responsiveness.

Short-term effects. The short-term effects of using GHB can include slower breathing and heart rate. The dosage is difficult, and it is very easy to overdose. Large quantities of GHB can cause nausea, vomiting, dizziness, amnesia, and vertigo, and extremely large does can reduce one's heart rate and place a person in a coma-like state. The heavy user has the risk of vomiting while sleeping and choking to death.

Long-term effects. The long-term effects of using GHB are unknown at this time, except that it can result in physical dependence for some (e.g., quitting suddenly can cause anxiety, insomnia, paranoia, and hallucinations).

Signs of use. Users exhibit sleepiness, nausea, vomiting, dizziness, amnesia, vertigo, and oversensitivity to touch.

Legal status. GHB is illegal to purchase, sell, or consume in the United States.

Ketamine is gaining attention as a promising treatment for cases of major depression that do not respond to traditional antidepressant medications. Because it is fast-acting, depressive symptoms can lift much sooner than is the case with other medications. Two types of ketamine are of interest. One is given as an infusion into the bloodstream (Racemic ketamine). The other is a Food and Drug Administration–approved drug that is given as a nasal spray (Spravato). Because ketamine is addictive, its use has to be weighed against the risks and benefits.

SOURCE: Walsh et al., 2021

Ketamine

Ketamine is known as "date-rape" drug, drug special, K, special K, vitamin K, baby food, kit kat, ketalar, ketaset, bump, cat Valium, jet, honey oil, super acid, purple, special la coke, and green.

Description. Ketamine is a fast-acting anesthetic and painkiller designed for use in veterinary medicine and in other special medical procedures. Generally, ketamine is found in liquid form but can also be in the form of a white pill or powder. The insidious use of this drug has involved the powder form sneaked into someone's drink in order to prevent the victim from fending off a sexual assault.

Short-term effects. The short-term effects of ketamine, which are experienced within 10 minutes of ingesting it, include lack of coordination, babbling, temporary amnesia, and a reduction of the heartbeat. High doses can result in unconsciousness and even death.

Long-term effects. Unknown.

Signs of use. Common signs are sleepiness, distraction, and confusion (e.g., perceptual distortions with regard to time).

Legal status. Ketamine is only legal for restricted and specialized medical purposes.

LSD

LSD is the abbreviation for lysergic acid diethylamide; it is also known as acid, blotter, dots, microdots, window pane, sugar cubes, and trips (the effect of using the drug is called "tripping").

Description. LSD is an odorless, clear or white, water-soluble material that has been synthesized from lysergic acid (found in rye fungus). LSD starts out as a crystal-like substance, and once it is crushed into powder, it is dissolved and diluted and then transferred to sheets of perforated paper (similar to quarter-inch postage stamps).

During the 1950s and early 1960s, research sponsored by the National Institute of Mental Health demonstrated potential for LSD and other psychedelic drugs to treat depression and the suffering associated with terminal illness. There is a growing base of recent evidence that has rekindled the potential benefits of LSD to treat some mental illnesses. The use of LSD and other psychedelics for therapeutic purpose faces regulatory and political challenges, but these challenges can be better addressed with well-designed studies. For more information on this topic, see *Further Curiosity and Digging* at the end of this chapter.

Short-term effects. A person who ingests LSD will begin to feel the effects within 30 to 90 minutes and its effects can last from 6 to 12 hours. The effects are highly unpredictable and may cause alterations in one's personality, emotions, mood, and sensory perceptions. Many users have experienced "bad trips," a nightmare-like state of anxiety, paranoia, and fear of insanity and/or death. For others, pleasant hallucination may occur.

Long-term effects. Some users of LSD have reported psychosis and other debilitating psychological effects that can last long after use of the drug. Flashbacks have also been reported by some long-term users. (A *flashback* is defined as continuous and recurring sensory distortions and hallucinations.) Experts do not agree if antipsychotic medications can help to reduce these LSD-induced symptoms.

Signs of use. A person's senses may become distorted and highly sensitive to colors, smells, lights, and sounds, and the person may appear to experience several emotions simultaneously or show an emotion that is out of context (e.g., laugh for no reason). Pupils can be dilated.

Legal status. Possessing, purchasing, using, and selling LSD are all illegal in the United States.

Methamphetamine and Other Amphetamines

These are known variously as meth, speed, crank, crystal, tweak, ice, glass, and uppers.

Two types of amphetamine, Adderall and Ritalin, are prescription medications used to treat attention-deficit/hyperactivity disorder (ADHD) in children and adults. Also, these psychostimulants are widely used for cognitive enhancement by people without ADHD. But research has shown little conclusive evidence for their effectiveness to boost brain power. It has been speculated that non-ADHD individuals experience the stimulant effects as more energy and misperceive this as improvements in attention and learning (Ilieva & Farah, 2013).

Description. In most cases, methamphetamine is found in the form of a pill or powder, which can be snorted, smoked, ingested orally, or injected. Due to the ignitable, corrosive, and toxic nature of the chemicals used to make this drug, there is a high risk of fires and toxic fumes from making the drug.

Short-term effects. Similar to cocaine, methamphetamine increases alertness and relieves fatigue. It arouses the central nervous system by giving the user an instant feeling of euphoria and creating a false sense of energy ("rush"). Physical effects can include an increase in heart rate and blood pressure; blurred vision; restlessness; and loss of coordination. After the initial euphoria abates, the user typically experiences a severe energy and emotional "crash." The drug carries with it a high risk of overdose.

Long-term effects. The long-term effects of using methamphetamine can include chronic fatigue, paranoia or delusional thoughts and thinking, and addiction. Whether it can cause permanent psychological damage is a matter of debate among experts. Other deleterious effects can include irreversible damage to blood vessels in the brain and risk of a heart attack and/or stroke.

Signs of use. Methamphetamine users can exhibit restlessness, nervousness, irritability, dizziness, dilated pupils, confusion, lack of appetite, increased sensitivity to sounds, paranoia, argumentativeness, and an increase in blood pressure and pulse rate. Users also suffer long periods without sleeping or eating.

Legal status. Possessing, purchasing, using, and selling methamphetamine are all illegal in the United States.

Nicotine

Varieties and names of nicotine include cigarettes, e-cigarettes, smokes, sticks, butts, Bogarts, bogies, chew, and snuff.

Description. The highly addictive drug, nicotine, follows alcohol in popularity of use around the globe. Nicotine is contained in the dried and crushed leaves of the tobacco plant. Tobacco can be smoked in pipes or cigarettes, chewed, or snorted in the powder form. E-cigarettes and other vaping devices heat a nicotine-based liquid to generate an aerosol, commonly called a "vapor," that the user inhales. The liquid solution often contains flavoring as well as a variety of other chemical components, which may or may not include nicotine. All of these forms of using nicotine are addictive.

Short-term effects. There are several short-term effects of using nicotine: an increase in brain activity and a feeling of enhanced attention; an increase in pulse and blood pressure; and suppression of appetite.

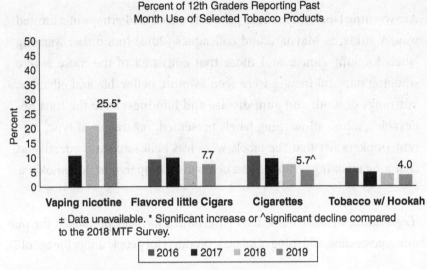

Percent of 12th Graders Reporting Past
Month Use of Selected Tobacco Products

± Data unavailable. * Significant increase or ^significant decline compared
to the 2018 MTF Survey.

■ 2016 ■ 2017 ■ 2018 ■ 2019

Source: University of Michigan, 2019 Monitoring the Future Study

Family smoking environment and family management have been shown to be associated with risk of adolescent smoking behaviors. The likelihood of adolescent daily smoking is greater when there is smoking among other family members. But a recent study showed that daily smoking can be reduced when parents engage in a high level of family management (Steeger et al., 2019). Protective parenting practices included effective monitoring of all risk behaviors, setting family rules, and appropriate application of consequences.

Long-term effects. The negative physical long-term effects of chronic, long-term use of nicotine are major. The smoker's blood vessels in the heart and brain will narrow or darken, causing shortness of breath, pneumonia, bronchitis, emphysema, and other lung-related ailments. Many different forms of cancer may develop. Women who smoke and take birth control pills have an elevated risk of developing blood clots or having a heart attack or stroke.

Signs of use. Nicotine users may display yellowish stain of fingers and teeth, decreased appetite, frequent coughing, and smoke smell on clothing and hair.

Are warning labels on tobacco products effective? Perhaps in a limited way. A study be Maynard and colleagues (2018) found that warning labels for lung cancer and those that consisted of the more severe smoking harmful images were seen as more believable and effective. Warnings of tooth and gum disease and blindness were the least believable. Across all warning labels presented, regardless of type, current smokers felt that the labels were less believable and effective at changing smoking attitudes and behaviors compared to nonsmokers.

Legal status. In 2020, the federal government formally prohibited the purchasing, possessing, and using of tobacco products for people under the age of 21.

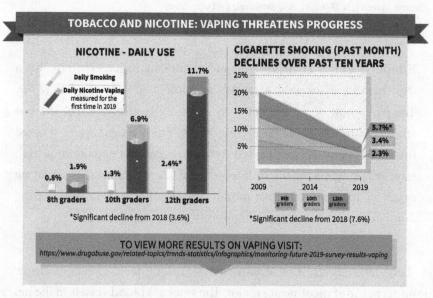

Trends in vaping and cigarette use are moving in opposite directions.
SOURCE: National Institute on Drug Abuse; National Institutes of Health; U.S. Department of Health and Human Services

Opioids

Heroin is known as junk, horse, smack, H, skag, shit, mud, black tar, and dope; methadone is known as meth; morphine: M, morph, and Miss Emma.

In October 2002, the Food and Drug Administration (FDA) approved Subutex® (buprenorphine hydrochloride) and Suboxone® tablets (buprenorphine hydrochloride and naloxone hydrochloride) for the treatment of opiate addiction. Naloxone (or Narcan), as a stand-alone medication, is an injection or nasal spray drug used to reverse the effects of an opioid overdose.

Description. Opioids include a broad range of natural, semisynthetic, and synthetic painkillers derived from the opium poppy. The most commonly used opioids include heroin and prescription painkillers such as morphine, codeine, methadone, hydrocodone (Vicodin), oxycodone (Percocet, OxyContin), fentanyl, and meperidine (Demerol). Buprenorphine is an opioid partial agonist, which means that it is an opioid and thus can produce typical opioid effects and side effects such as euphoria and respiratory depression. But as a partial agonist, its maximal effects are less than those of full agonists like heroin and methadone. All agonists, while still addictive, have therapeutic benefit to treat individuals with an opioid addiction (for detoxification, and for short- and long-term opioid replacement therapy).

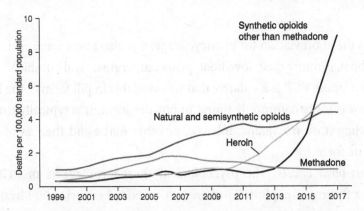

The statistics around opioid overdose deaths are staggering. The Center for Disease Control and Prevention (CDC) estimated that about 47,000 people died in 2017 of an overdose that involved a prescription or illicit opioid. It is estimated that over 75,000 people died in 2021 as a result of an opioid overdose. Shown are age-adjusted drug overdose death rates in the United States, by opioid category, 1999–2017.
SOURCE: Hedegaard H, Miniño AM, Warner M. Drug overdose deaths in the United States, 1999–2017. NCHS Data Brief, no 329. Hyattsville, MD: National Center for Health Statistics. 2018.

Short-term effects. Opioid use initially includes a pleasurable feeling or "rush," which is followed by the considerable slowing of one's thinking and reaction time. Other short-term effects include restlessness, nausea, vomiting, dry mouth, warm feelings in the body, heavy feelings of extremities, slower breath rate, constricted pupils, convulsions, lack of consciousness, cold skin that is moist and blue in color, and depression. Fatal overdose can occur with a single use.

Long-term effects. In addition to addiction and fatal overdose, the long-term effects of using opioids include infections and breathing problems, and infections for those using needles.

Signs of use. Signs include constricted pupils, loss of appetite, sniffles, watery eyes, cough, nausea, drowsiness, and restlessness. Injection users often have scars (or "tracks").

Legal status. Medical doctors can prescribe legal opiates for pain resulting from specific medical conditions. However, the use, purchase, or sale of legal opioids without a prescription is illegal in the United States. The same is the case for illegal opioids (e.g., heroin).

PCP

PCP is the abbreviation for phencyclidine; it is also known as angel, angel dust, boat, dummy dust, love boat, peace, supergrass, and zombie.

Description. PCP is a sedative that was available in pill form in the 1960s but now is more commonly found in powder form. It is typically used by sprinkling it on marijuana, tobacco, or other herbs and then smoked in cigarette form.

Short-term effects. The psychological short-term effects of PCP include a feeling of euphoria and an "out-of-body" experience. Physically, PCP can cause shallow, rapid breathing, an increase in heart rate, blood pressure, and body temperature, and nausea, blurred vision, and/or hallucinations. Higher doses can cause convulsions, coma, hyperthermia, violent episodes, and death.

Long-term effects. The long-term use of PCP can cause memory loss, depression, disorientation, and suicidal tendencies.

Signs of use. Users of PCP may exhibit multiple and dramatic behavioral changes, dizziness, nausea, and a lack of coordination.

Legal status. Possessing, purchasing, using, and selling PCP are all illegal in the United States.

Rohypnol

Rohypnol is also known as a "date-rape" drug, roofies, roachies, La Rocha, ruffies, ropes, pappas, ro-shays, robinal, the forget pill, pastas, and peanuts.

Description. Rohypnol is a benzodiazepine tablet that has sedative effects. Since 1999, these tablets have been adjusted to dissolve slower, make clear beverages blue, and make dark beverages murky so it is easier to detect. Yet this drug has been given underhandedly by men to women to make them unable to defend themselves from a sexual assault.

Short-term effects. The short-term effects of using Rohypnol include drowsiness, feelings of relaxation, dizziness, confusion, and discoordination. A user's inhibitions may be relaxed, and for some, the user appears to be intoxicated or drunk. When mixed with alcohol, the person may become unconscious or black out for several hours.

Long-term effects. Addiction to this drug is a long-term effect.

Signs of use. Slurred speech, confusion, physical weakness, severe drowsiness, and difficulty in walking are signs of a user.

Legal status. Rohypnol is illegal to purchase, sell, or consume in the United States.

Solvents and Aerosols/Inhalants

These are known as gas, glue, and sniff.

Description. Solvents and inhalants are found in many household products, including as gasoline, gas in aerosol cans, correction fluid, spray paint, air freshener, glues, and marking pens. The process of inhaling them is called "huffing."

Short-term effects. The short-term effects of inhaling these substances include lightheadedness, euphoria, loss of muscular coordination, nausea, and drooling.

Long-term effects. Some experts contend that permanent brain damage can occur from only one use, and this effect is greatly increased with long-term use. Other effects include fatigue, mental confusion, depression, irritability, hostility, and paranoia.

Signs of use. The user may reveal a sensitivity to light; have slurred speech, runny nose, and/or watery eyes; exhibit drowsiness and loss of muscle control; and develop sores on the nose and mouth.

Legal status. Possessing these types of solvents, aerosols, and inhalants is legal in the United States. However, a person must be 18 years old to purchase them in many states.

Steroids

Oral steroids include Anadrol, Oxandrin, Dianabol, Winstrol; injected forms include Deca-Durabolin, Durabolin, Depo-Testosterone, and Equipois.

Description. Anabolic steroids are synthetic compounds that are related to the male sex hormone testosterone. The street name for a steroid found in health food stores as a dietary supplement is Andro (dehydroepiandrosterone [DHEA]). Steroids, which come in either tablet or liquid forms, are taken orally or injected. Athletes and bodybuilders use them because they can facilitate skeletal muscle growth and are believed to enhance athletic performance. Research has found that steroid use can be highly addictive.

Short-term effects. Steroids contribute to an increase in body weight and muscular strength. Numerous physical side effects include damage to the liver, acne, cysts, oily hair and skin, disruption of the normal production of hormones, and even heart attacks. Psychologically, steroid use can trigger anger and aggressiveness. In males, steroids can cause a low sperm count, a reduction of the testes, hair loss, male breasts, and more; in females, steroids can lead to excessive body hair and loss of scalp hair, coarse skin, an enlarged clitoris, and a deepening of the voice. A danger among adolescent users is that steroids can signal bones to stop growing sooner than they should.

Long-term effects. Some of the short-term effects listed above are irreversible. Research has found that steroid use can be highly addictive.

Signs of use. Signs of irritability and aggression occur in some steroid users. For long-term users, significant physical changes may be noticeable.

Legal status. Most steroids require a prescription from a physician. But some steroids (e.g., Andro) can be found in health food stores, often sold as a dietary supplement.

Synthetic Cannabinoids

These agents are known as synthetic marijuana, K2, Spice, Skunk, Yucatan Fire, and Moon Rocks.

Description. Synthetic cannabinoids are man-made chemicals that are applied (sometimes sprayed) onto plant material and falsely marketed as a "legal" high. This dried, shredded plant material looks like marijuana. The chemicals used in the manufacturing of synthetic cannabinoids are constantly changing, and these contents are not regulated by the government. Dealers and users claim that synthetic cannabinoids are safe and that they produce effects similar to ingesting THC, the active ingredient in marijuana.

Short-term effects. These effects are often unpredictable and quite variable; they include elevated mood, relaxation (in some), agitation (in some), and altered perceptions such as hallucinations.

Long-term effects. Long-term users may experience severe agitation and anxiety, panic attacks, muscle tremors, suicidal thoughts, and psychotic symptoms.

Signs of use. User may have red or bloodshot eyes, fast pulse, pale skin, and nausea. There is potential for muscle spasms, panic attacks, and psychotic episodes.

Legal status. History tells us that individuals seek to stay ahead of legal restrictions and FDA regulatory oversight by manufacturing new addictive and dangerous substances. Policymakers have sought to address this problem by enacting more rigorous and wide-ranging legislation to prohibit the making and distribution of current and future synthetic drugs.

Synthetic Speed

Synthetic speed comes in the form of bath salts, jewelry cleaner, and plant food; it is known as Ivory Wave, Bloom, Cloud Nine, Lunar Wave, Vanilla Sky, White Lightning, and Scarface.

Description. This group of drugs, which contain synthetic chemicals related to cathinone, an amphetamine-like stimulant, produce effects that mimic amphetamines. Taken orally, snorted, or injected, it appears as a white or brown crystalline powder.

Short-term effects. In the short term, the user will have a euphoric, elevated mood, increased sociability and sex drive, confusion, headache, muscle tension, sweating, nausea, and dizziness.

Long-term effects. The long-term effects of the use of synthetic seed are significant. They include long-term depression, unpredictable behavior, paranoia, delusions, and suicidal thoughts.

Signs of usage. Users will show a reduced need for food and sleep, sweating, nausea, cold or blue fingers; if use occurs long term, signs include depression, paranoia, and unpredictable behavior.

Legal status. As with synthetic marijuana, policymakers have sought to address this problem with stronger legislation that would prohibit the making and distribution of these synthetic drugs.

MEASURING SUBSTANCE USE BEHAVIORS

Measuring substance use behaviors typically involves assessing the quantity, frequency, duration, and onset of use. These variables are typically included in screening and comprehensive tools. A *screening* process is often the first step when the task is to determine if an individual might have a behavioral problem, such as drug abuse, that might require more clinical services. The results from a screening inform the need for a *comprehensive assessment*, where an in-depth review of the extent and nature of problems, a diagnostic assessment, and a determination of need for treatment occurs. These two types of assessment procedures will be discussed in more detail in Chapter 5.

Measuring Use via Monitoring the Future

A useful guideline for measuring patterns of substance use is the method used by the MTF study, also known as the National High School Senior Survey (www.monitoringthefuture.org). This project is a long-term epidemiological study that surveys trends in and attitudes toward legal and illicit drug use among American adolescents and adults. The survey is conducted by researchers at the University of Michigan's Institute for Social Research and funded by research grants from the National Institutes of Health. Each year, a total of approximately 50,000 8th-, 10th-, and 12th-grade students are surveyed (12th graders since 1975, and 8th and 10th graders since 1991).

Items on the MTF questionnaire ask the respondent to report drug use frequency and duration across the main drug categories. For most drugs, they are asked to indicate "On how *many occasions* (if any) have you used (drug)" for three separate time periods ("in your lifetime?" "during the last 12 months?" "during the last 30 days?"). Each of the three questions is answered on the same scale: 0 times/1–2 times/3–5 times/6–9 times/10–19 times/20–39 times/40 or more occasions. Given the nature of cigarette use, the frequency of use is best scaled this way: "never," "once or twice," "occasionally but not regularly," "regularly in the past," and "regularly now." If quantity of use is desired, a suggested question and answer categories are the following: "How frequently have you smoked cigarettes during the past 30 days? "not at all," "less than one cigarette per day," "one to five cigarettes per day," and about one-half, one, one and one half, and two packs or more per day."

Getting intoxicated from alcohol, including binge drinking (typically defined as five or more drinks per occasion), are additional important variables to measure. We favor these additional MTF-based questions: "How many times (if any) have you been drunk over the past 2 weeks" and "How many times (if any) have you had five or more drinks in a row over the past 2 weeks." To assess extreme binge, now also called "high-intensity drinking," it can be measured with these similar questions: "How many times (if any) have you had 10 or more drinks in a row?" "How many times (if any) have you had 15 or more drinks in a row?"

There are considerations for drugs taken for therapeutic reasons, such as amphetamines, sedatives (barbiturates), tranquilizers, and pain medications (narcotics other than heroin), and for anabolic steroids. Respondents should be instructed to refer to use when it occurs "on your own—that is, without a doctor telling you to take the drug."

Timeline Follow-Back (TLFB)

TLFB (Sobell & Sobell, 1992) is a type of assisted interview used to collect detailed alcohol and other drug use information over a specified time period (sometimes up to a year). The traditional TLFB involves a structured interview with the use of a calendar to allow the respondent to indicate specific dates and events (e.g., birthdays, holidays, and vacations) and recording them on the calendar. These occasions enhance the respondent's recollection of their recent drug use. The interview then moves to a systematic overview of the person's drug use by reviewing each month, starting with the most recent and moving back each month for the specified time period. This method can yield extensive information about patterns, frequencies, and quantities of substance use behavior. Common variables from this method are number of drinking days, number of binge-drinking days, number of standard drinks (e.g., 12-oz. beer, 4-oz. wine, 1.25-oz. shot of distilled spirits) the person had each day, number drug use days, and number of times drugs were used each day. This method can be very useful in helping individuals examine their patterns of substance use and has demonstrated reliability and validity in individual and group settings and when self-administered via computer (Robinson et al., 2014; Sobell & Sobell, 2000). Figure 4.8 shows a sample of a TLFB interview completed for a prior month.

TLFB 2021

Name/ID#: _____   Date: _____

TIMELINE FOLLOWBACK CALENDAR: 2021

1 Standard Drink is Equal to

| One 12 oz can/bottle of beer | One 5 oz glass of regular (12%) wine | 1 ½ oz of hard liquor (e.g. rum, vodka, whiskey) | 1 mixed or straight drink with 1 ½ oz hard liquor |

Complete the Following

Start Date (Day 1): _____   End Date (yesterday): _____

MO   DY   YR   MO   DY   YR

2021	SUN	MON	TUES	WED	THURS	FRI	SAT
						1 New Year's	2
J A N	3	4	5	6	7	8	9
	10	11	12	13	14	15	16
	17	18 M. Luther King	19	20	21	22	23
	24	25	26	27	28	29	30
	31	1	2	3	4	5	6
F E B	7	8	9	10	11	12	13
	14 Valentine's Day	15 President's Day	16	17	18	19	20
	21	22	23	24	25	26	27
	28	1	2	3	4	5	6
M A R	7	8	9	10	11	12	13
	14	15	16	17 St.Patrick's Day	18	19	20
	21	22	23	24	25	26	27
	28	29	30	31	1 Passover	2 Good Friday	3
A P R	4 Easter	5	6	7	8	9	10
	11	12	13	14	15	16	17
	18	19	20	21	22	23	24
	25	26	27	28	29	30	1
M A Y	2	3	4	5	6	7	8
	9 Mother's Day	10	11	12	13	14	15
	16	17	18	19	20	21	22
	23	24 Memorial Day	25	26	27	28	29
	30	31					

1

Figure 4.8 Example of a TLFB Interview (Robinson et al., 2014).

TLFB 2021

2021	SUN	MON	TUES	WED	THURS	FRI	SAT
			1	2	3	4	5
J U N	6	7	8	9	10	11	12
	13	14	15	16	17	18	19
	20 Father's Day	21	22	23	24	25	26
	27	28	29	30	1	2	3
J U L	4 Independence Day	5	6	7	8	9	10
	11	12	13	14	15	16	17
	18	19	20	21	22	23	24
	25	26	27	28	29	30	31
A U G	1	2	3	4	5	6	7
	8	9	10	11	12	13	14
	15	16	17	18	19	20	21
	22	23	24	25	26	27	28
	29	30	31	1	2	3	4
S E P	5	6 Labor Day	7	8	9	10	11 Rosh Hashanah
	12	13	14	15	16	17	18
	19	20 Yom Kippur	21	22	23	24	25
	26	27	28	29	30	1	2
O C T	3	4	5	6	7	8	9
	10	11 Columbus Day	12	13	14	15	16
	17	18	19	20	21	22	23
	24	25	26	27	28	29	30
	31 Halloween	1	2 Election Day	3	4	5	6
N O V	7	8	9	10	11 Veterans' Day	12	13
	14	15	16	17	18	19	20
	21	22	23	24	25 Thanksgiving	26	27
	28	29	30	1	2	3	4 Hanukkah
D E C	5	6	7	8	9	10	11
	12	13	14	15	16	17	18
	19	20	21	22	23	24	25 Christmas
	26	27	28	29	30	31	

© Sobell, L. C. & Sobell, M. B., 2008

2

Figure 4.8 Continued

Drug Use Onset

There are clinical implications based on when a person begins to use drugs; the earlier the onset of drug use, the greater the likelihood the person will develop a substance use problem (a topic we will discuss in more detail in the next chapter). Thus, assessing when a teenager begins to use drugs is highly recommended. We suggest that for each drug that the respondent has indicated lifetime use at least once the following question: "At what age did you first use (drug)?" Some experts recommend replacing "age" with "school grade" because grade can be an easier reference point for youth.

MINI-REVIEW

- Initiation to substance use peaks at a time when the developing brain may be particularly vulnerable to the neurotoxic effects of heavy substance use, highlighting the importance of efforts to prevent substance use.
- In recent years, the gender gap in rates of substance involvement has narrowed, with females catching up to or surpassing males in rates of use for certain substances, such as tobacco.
- Cannabis use continues to be a drug that is used at relatively high rates, although its rate of use among adolescents has remained relatively stable over recent years, whereas the rates of use of other so-called "hard drugs" (e.g., opioids, cocaine) are declining.
- Vaping of nicotine and of cannabis is a new trend among adolescents, contributing to health concerns.
- Several psychometrically sound assessment tools exist to maser patterns of substance use by adolescents.

DISCUSSION POINTS

1. Discuss the pros and cons of adults hosting a drinking party for underage youth. What laws exist about adult hosting? Do you have any experience of attending a drinking party that was hosted by parents? How did it go?
2. Imagine you are developing a high school prevention program that focuses on cannabis. What themes would you emphasize?

What misperceptions or myths about cannabis would you
   address?
3. Does use of e-cigarettes help a person quit from using regular
   cigarettes? This question is debated among the experts. Do you
   have any personal experience about this? Do you know of any
   friends who switched from regular smoking and now vape? How
   is it going for them?
4. A related discussion question: How healthy or unhealthy is
   vaping? Discuss these two perspectives: 1. Vaping may be
   safer than smoking. (Is it linked to a reduced risk of lung
   and other cancers? Does it help many quit regular smoking?)
   versus 2. Vaping may be a gateway to regular smoking and is
   not healthy.
5. Imagine you are the Drug Czar of the U.S. What policies and
   practices would you prioritize to address the opioid crisis?

FURTHER CURIOSITY AND DIGGING

Dopamine: More information on how dopamine is involved in healthy brain function
and its role in the development of substance use disorder is provided below.

Drug Abuse, Dopamine, and the Brain's Reward System

Butler Center for Research. (2015). *Why do people use alcohol and drugs even after suffering consequences?* https://www.hazeldenbettyford.org/education/bcr/addiction-
research/drug-abuse-brain-ru-915

**Cannabis: Issues Pertaining to Its Legalization as Medicine and for Commercial Sales
to Adults**

Smart Approaches to Marijuana. (n.d.) *Home page.* www.learnaboutsam.org

Cannabis: Impact of Its Legalization on Adolescent Cannabis Use

Carliner, H., Brown, Q. L., Sarvet, A. L., & Hasin, D. S. (2017). Cannabis use, attitudes,
and legal status in the US: A review. *Preventive Medicine, 104*, 13–23.

Substance Use Trend from the National Survey on Drug Use and Health

Substance Use and Mental Health Services Administration. (2022). *Key substance use
and mental indicators in the United States: Results from the National Survey on Drug
Use and Health (NSDUH).* https://www.samhsa.gov/data/.

Electronic Cigarettes, General Information

Breland, A., Soule, E., Lopez, A., Ramôa, C., El-Hellani, A., & Eissenberg, T. (2017). Electronic cigarettes: What are they and what do they do? *Annals of the New York Academy of Sciences, 1394,* 5–30.

Centers for Disease Prevention and Control. (2020). *Outbreak of lung injury associated with the use of e-cigarette, or vaping, products.* https://www.cdc.gov/tobacco/basic_information/e-cigarettes/severe-lung-disease.html

Cerdá, M., Mauro, C., Hamilton, A., Levy, N. S., Santaella-Tenorio, J., Hasin, D., . . . Martins, S. S. (2020). Association between recreational marijuana legalization in the United States and changes in marijuana use and cannabis use disorder from 2008 to 2016. *JAMA Psychiatry, 77,* 165–171.

Dai, H., & Leventhal, A. M. (2019). Association of electronic cigarette vaping and subsequent smoking relapse among former smokers. *Drug and Alcohol Dependence, 199,* 10–17.

Hajek, P., Phillips-Waller, A., Przulj, D., Pesola, F., Myers Smith, K., Bisal, N., Li, J., Parrott, S., Saseini, P., . . . Hayden, J. (2019). A randomized trial of e-cigarettes versus nicotine-replacement therapy. *New England Journal of Medicine, 380,* 629–637. https://www.nejm.org/doi/full/10.1056/NEJMoa1808779?query=TOC

Weaver, S. R., Huang, J., Pechacek, T. F., Heath, J. W., Ashley, D. L., & Eriksen, M. P. (2018). Are electronic nicotine delivery systems helping cigarette smokers quit? Evidence from a prospective cohort study of US adult smokers, 2015–2016. *PLoS One, 13,* e0198047.

Overview of the Effectiveness of Smoking Cessation Interventions

A Report from the Surgeon General, Executive Summary: http://www.surgeongeneral.gov/

Potential of Psychedelics to Treat Mental Illness

Byock, I. (2018). Taking psychedelics seriously. *Journal of Palliative Medicine, 21,* 417–421.

Potential for Cannabis to Treat Chronic Pain

Bhaskar, A., Bell, A., Boivin, M., Briques, W., Brown, M., Clarke, H., . . . Moulin, D. E. (2021). Consensus recommendations on dosing and administration of medical cannabis to treat chronic pain: Results of a modified Delphi process. *Journal of Cannabis Research, 3,* 1–12.

REFERENCES

American Psychiatric Association. (2013). *Diagnostic and statistical manual of mental disorders* (5th ed.). American Psychiatric Association.

Angold, A., Costello, E. J., & Erkanli, A. (1999). Comorbidity. *The Journal of Child Psychology and Psychiatry and Allied Disciplines, 40,* 57–87.

Carliner, H., Brown, Q. L., Sarvet, A. L., & Hasin, D. S. (2017). Cannabis use, attitudes, and legal status in the US: a review. *Preventive Medicine, 104,* 13–23.

Center for Behavioral Health Statistics and Quality. (2015). *Behavioral health trends in the United States: Results from the 2014 National Survey on Drug Use and Health* (HHS Publication No. SMA 15-4927, NSDUH Series H-50). https://www.samhsa.gov/data/sites/default/files/NSDUH-FRR1-2014/NSDUH-FRR1-2014.pdf

Chung, T., & Winters, K. C. (2018). Clinical characteristics of cannabis use disorder. In K. A. Sabet & K. C. Winters (Eds.), *Contemporary health issues on marijuana* (pp. 71–88). Oxford University Press.

Cottler, L., & Okafor, C. (2018). Recent epidemiological trends in marijuana use. In. K. A. Sabet & K. C. Winters (Eds.), *Contemporary health issues on marijuana* (pp. 14–38). Oxford University Press.

Di Chiara, G., & Imperato, A. (1988). Drugs abused by humans preferentially increase synaptic dopamine concentrations in the mesolimbic system of freely moving rats. *Proceedings of the National Academy of Sciences, USA, 85*, 5274–5278.

Di Chiara, G., Tanda, G., Cadoni, C., Acquas, E., Bassareo, V., & Carboni, E. (1997). Homologies and differences in the action of drugs of abuse and a conventional re-inforcer (food) on dopamine transmission: An interpretive framework of the mechanism of drug dependence. *Advances in Pharmacology, 42*, 983–987.

DuPont, R. L., Han, B., Shea, C. L., & Madras, B. K. (2018). Drug use among youth: National survey data support a common liability of all drug use. *Preventive Medicine, 113*, 68–73.

Fiorino, D. F., & Phillips, A. G. (1999). Facilitation of sexual behavior and enhanced dopamine efflux in the nucleus accumbens of male rats after D-amphetamine-induced behavioral sensitization. *Journal of Neuroscience, 19*, 456–463.

Ilieva, I. P., & Farah, M. J. (2013). Enhancement stimulants: Perceived motivational and cognitive advantages. *Frontiers in Neuroscience, 7*, 198. doi:10.3389/fnins.2013.00198

Johnston, L. D., Miech, R. A., O'Malley, P. M., Bachman, J. G., Schulenberg, J. E., & Patrick, M. E. (2021). *Monitoring the Future national survey results on drug use, 1975–2021: Overview, key findings on adolescent drug use*. Institute for Social Research, University of Michigan.

Kandel, D., & Faust, R. (1975). Sequence and stages in patterns of adolescent drug use. *Archives of General Psychiatry, 32*, 923–932.

Khan, M. R., Berger, A. T., Wells, B. E., & Cleland, C. M. (2012). Longitudinal associations between adolescent alcohol use and adulthood sexual risk behavior and sexually transmitted infection in the United States: Assessment of differences by race. *American Journal of Public Health, 102*, 867–876.

Knopf, A. (2021). College students use marijuana at highest level since 1980s: MTF. *Alcoholism & Drug Abuse Weekly, 33*, 1–3.

Krishnasamy, V. P., Hallowell, B. D., Ko, J. Y., et al. (2020). Update: Characteristics of a nationwide outbreak of e-cigarette, or vaping, product use—associated lung injury—United States, August 2019–January 2020. *MMWR Morbidity and Mortality Weekly Reports, 69*, 90–94. http://dx.doi.org/10.15585/mmwr.mm6903e2

Lee, M. H., Kim-Godwin, Y. S., & Hur, H. (2022). Adolescents' marijuana use following recreational marijuana legalization in Alaska and Hawaii. *Asia Pacific Journal of Public Health, 34*, 65–71.

Levy, S., Campbell, M. C., Shea, C. L., & DuPont, R. L. (2018). Trends in abstaining from substance use in adolescents: 1975–2014. *Pediatrics, 142*, e20173498.

Lipari, R., & Jean-Francois, B. (May 26, 2016). A day in the life of college students aged 18 to 22: Substance use facts. The CBHSQ Short Report, Substance Abuse and Mental Health Services Administration (SAMHSA). https://www.samhsa.gov/data/sites/default/files/report_2361/ShortReport-2361.html

MacCoun, R. (1998). In what sense (if any) is marijuana a gateway drug. FAS Drug Policy Analysis Bulletin, 4, 3–5.

Mattick, R. P., Clare, P. J., Aiken, A., Wadolowski, M., Hutchinson, D., Najman, J., . . . Vogl, L. (2018). Association of parental supply of alcohol with adolescent drinking, alcohol-related harms, and alcohol use disorder symptoms: A prospective cohort study. The Lancet Public Health, 3, e64–e71.

Maynard, O. M., Gove, H., Skinner, A. L., & Munafò, M. R. (2018). Severity and susceptibility: Measuring the perceived effectiveness and believability of tobacco health warnings. BMC Public Health, 18, 468. https://doi.org/10.1186/s12889-018-5385-x

Miech, R., Johnston, L., O'Malley, P., Bachman, J., Schulenberg, J., & Patrick, M. (2019). Monitoring the Future national survey results on drug use, 1975–2018: Volume I, secondary school students. Institute for Social Research, University of Michigan.

Montana, G., & Chung, T. (2019). Diagnosis, epidemiology and course of youth substance use and use disorders. In Y. Kaminer & K. C. Winters (Eds.), Clinical manual of adolescent addictive disorders (2nd ed., pp. 3–24). American Psychiatric Association.

Moss, H. B., Chen, C. M., & Yi, H. Y. (2014). Early adolescent patterns of alcohol, cigarettes, and marijuana polysubstance use and young adult substance use outcomes in a nationally representative ample. Drug and Alcohol Dependence, 136, 51–62.

National Institute on Drug Abuse. (2018). Drugs, brain, and behavior: The science of addiction. https://www.drugabuse.gov/publications/drugsbrains-behavior-science-addiction

National Institute on Drug Abuse. (2021). Monitoring the Future 2021 survey results. https://www.drugabuse.gov/drug-topics/related-topics/trends-statistics/infographics/monitoring-future-2021-survey-results

Nutt, D. J., King, L. A., & Phillips, L. D. (2010). Drug harms in the UK: A multicriteria decision analysis. The Lancet, 376, 1558–1565.

Pacek, L. R., & McClernon, F. J. (2020). Risk perceptions regarding cigarette smoking in the United States continue to decline. Drug and Alcohol Dependence, 209, 107887. https://doi.org/10.1016/j.drugalcdep.2020.107887

Robinson, S. M., Sobell, L. C., Sobell, M. B., & Leo, G. I. (2014). Reliability of the timeline follow-back for cocaine, cannabis, and cigarette use. Psychology of Addictive Behaviors, 28, 154–162.

Sabet, K. A., Atkinson, D., & Sabet, S. M. (2018). What is the evidence of marijuana as medicine? In K. A. Sabet & K. C. Winters (Eds.), Contemporary health issues on marijuana (pp. 256–294). Oxford University Press.

Smart, R., & Pacula, R. L. (2019). Early evidence of the impact of cannabis legalization on cannabis use, cannabis use disorder, and the use of other substances: Findings from state policy evaluations. The American Journal of Drug and Alcohol Abuse, 45, 644–663.

Sobell, L. C., & Sobell, M. B. (1992). Timeline follow-back: A technique for assessing self-reported ethanol consumption. In J. Allen & R. Z. Litten (Eds.), *Measuring alcohol consumption: Psychosocial and biological methods* (pp. 41–72). Humana Press.

Sobell, L. C., & Sobell, M. B. (2000). Alcohol timeline follow-back (TLFB). In American Psychiatric Association, *Handbook of psychiatric measures* (pp. 477–479). American Psychiatric Association.

Spear, L. P. (2002). Alcohol's effects on adolescents. *Alcohol Health and Research World*, *26*, 287–291.

Steeger, C. M., Epstein, M., Hill, K. G., Kristman-Valente, A. N., Bailey, J. A., Lee, J. O., & Kosterman, R. (2019). Time-varying effects of family smoking and family management on adolescent daily smoking: The moderating roles of behavioral disinhibition and anxiety. *Drug and Alcohol Dependence*, *204*, 107572. https://doi.org/10.1016/j.drugalcdep.2019.107572

Volkow, N. D., Baler, R. D., Compton, W. M., & Weiss, S. R. (2014). Adverse health effects of marijuana use. *New England Journal of Medicine*, *370*, 2219–2227.

Walsh, Z., Mollaahmetoglu, O. M., Rootman, J., Golsof, S., Keeler, J., Marsh, B., . . . Morgan, C. J. (2021). Ketamine for the treatment of mental health and substance use disorders: comprehensive systematic review. *BJPsych Open*, *8*(1). https://www.ncbi.nlm.nih.gov/pmc/articles/PMC8715255/

Winters, K. C. (2022). *Teen Intervene as a Screening, Brief intervention and Referral to Treatment (SBIRT) Program*, 4th edition. Center City, MN: Hazelden Betty Ford Foundation.

Substance Use Disorders

INTRODUCTION

In this chapter we discuss many perspectives that pertain to the construct known as addiction, or the equivalent but more commonly used term in the research literature, a *substance use disorder (SUD)*. An SUD is defined by the American Psychiatric Association's *Diagnostic and Statistical Manual of Mental Disorders, Fifth Edition* (DSM-5; American Psychiatric Association, 2013). Like other categorical disorders described in DSM-5, an SUD is a diagnostic category indicating that a person is experiencing a certain number of clinically significant symptoms.

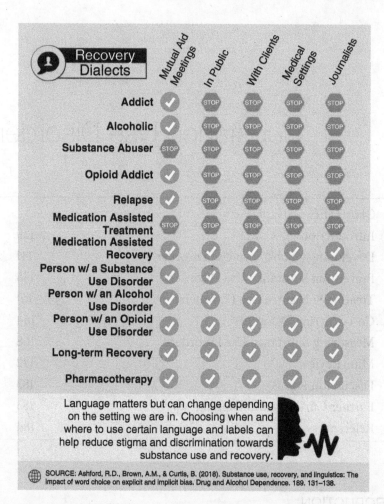

Recovery Dialects	Mutual Aid Meetings	In Public	With Clients	Medical Settings	Journalists
Addict	✓	STOP	STOP	STOP	STOP
Alcoholic	✓	STOP	STOP	STOP	STOP
Substance Abuser	STOP	STOP	STOP	STOP	STOP
Opioid Addict	✓	STOP	STOP	STOP	STOP
Relapse	✓	STOP	STOP	STOP	STOP
Medication Assisted Treatment	STOP	STOP	STOP	STOP	STOP
Medication Assisted Recovery	✓	✓	✓	✓	✓
Person w/ a Substance Use Disorder	✓	✓	✓	✓	✓
Person w/ an Alcohol Use Disorder	✓	✓	✓	✓	✓
Person w/ an Opioid Use Disorder	✓	✓	✓	✓	✓
Long-term Recovery	✓	✓	✓	✓	✓
Pharmacotherapy	✓	✓	✓	✓	✓

Language matters but can change depending on the setting we are in. Choosing when and where to use certain language and labels can help reduce stigma and discrimination towards substance use and recovery.

SOURCE: Ashford, R.D., Brown, A.M., & Curtis, B. (2018). Substance use, recovery, and linguistics: The impact of word choice on explicit and implicit bias. Drug and Alcohol Dependence. 189. 131–138.

The term *addiction* is controversial, and there is a school of thought that it creates a negative bias and distracts from the reality that having a serious drug problem is a legitimate behavioral disorder. Researchers at the University of Pennsylvania studied how people responded to several addiction-related terms. Terms such as *addict*, *alcoholic*, and *substance abuser* elicited the strongest negative biases. The alternative term, a *person with a substance use disorder*, was associated with less negative implicit bias (Ashford et al., 2018). The authors argue that a wider adoption of less biased terms, including by public officials and the media, could help reduce the stigma that stops some people from seeking help. Listed here is a summary of the acceptability of terms given a setting or context (Ashford et al., 2018).

SOURCE: Substance use, recovery, and linguistics: The impact of word choice on explicit and implicit bias, Robert D. Ashford, Austin M. Brown, Brenda Curtis, *Drug and Alcohol Dependence*, Volume 189, 1 August 2018, Pages 131–138.

Most Americans know someone (including a teenager) with a current or history of an SUD, and many know someone who has lost or nearly lost a family member or friend as a consequence of drug abuse. Yet, at the same time, few other medical conditions are surrounded by as much shame and misunderstanding as SUDs. Fortunately, the myths of addiction have been replaced by the science of addiction. We now have a more complete and research-informed view that developing an SUD during adolescence is a complex phenomenon involving biology, developmental psychology, and the environment.

Since 1971, when President Nixon declared a war on drugs, it is estimated that over $1 trillion has been spent on fighting this war in America. How to end drug abuse has been a long-standing topic of debate among politicians, law enforcement, and drug abuse researchers. It is the authors' viewpoint that it will take more than interdiction (control) policies and that the best hope is the widespread application of effective prevention programs.

But addiction can gravely affect a young person who is not a user. When parents and adults abuse drugs or avoid intervening when a family member has a problem, too often the young people in the family suffer the brunt of the impacts all around them. Crime and violence, abuse and neglect—these are downstream effects that land most harshly and directly on children in families and communities who have no voice and can't adequately defend themselves from the onslaught and the economic and emotional toll it brings through the door.

DEVELOPING A SUBSTANCE USE DISORDER

As we discussed in Chapter 4, drugs of abuse can have a powerful influence on the user. Some individuals, including adolescents, repeatedly use illegal drugs or misuse legal drugs to seek pleasure, alleviate stress, or avoid reality. An SUD might occur when a person cannot control the impulse to use drugs even when there are negative consequences. Such compulsive use causes clinically and functionally significant impairment, such as health problems, disability, and failure to meet major responsibilities at work, school, or home. And as we have discussed earlier, these behavioral changes are also accompanied by changes in brain functioning, especially in the brain's natural inhibition and reward centers.

Definition

Although drug use involvement may be optimally represented by a continuum of severity in use and problems, an SUD is operationally defined by a list of 11 criteria, of which no single symptom is necessary or sufficient, but at least 2 are needed to define the presence of a diagnosis. The DSM-5 (American Psychiatric Association, 2013) no longer uses the terms *substance abuse* and *substance dependence*. These terms were viewed as an unreliable distinction; rather, DSM-5 has mild, moderate, or severe distinctions which indicate the level of severity. Each level is determined by how many of the 11 diagnostic symptoms are present. A feature of the DSM-5 is that none of the criteria directly refer to onset, quantity, and frequency variables. This is not to say that these variables are not important to assess. Indeed, consumption history does produce important information, particularly when data are compared with regularly updated norms of use. But any DSM-based symptom can occur regardless of level of use.

The DSM-5 criteria for an SUD have changes that are relevant to adolescents and supported by research and clinical observation: the elimination of the abuse and dependence categories, the elimination of the "legal problems" symptom, and the addition of the symptom pertaining to craving and a strong desire to use. But some of the criteria are problematic when applied to adolescents. For example, the two physiological symptoms, tolerance and withdrawal, are not highly relevant to young people who are going through neurodevelopmental changes and are not yet chronic users. Furthermore, the meaning of some symptoms for adolescents, who are relatively inexperienced with the effects of drugs, may lead to higher rates of false-positive endorsements (Winters et al., 2011).

The diagnosis of an SUD is based on significant behavioral and physiological impairment associated with drug use. SUDs are diagnosed when, during a 12-month period, a person displays 2 or more symptoms out of a set of 11 symptoms pertaining to inability to control one's use, health problems, social impairment, tolerance, withdrawal, and failure to fulfill major responsibilities at home, school, or work. Individuals would be assigned a diagnosis based on how many symptom criteria the individual met: no disorder (0–1), mild (2–3), moderate (4–5), or severe (6 or more).

Descriptors of the SUD criteria, based on DSM-5. Provided below are descriptors of the 11 DSM-5 criteria for an SUD (American Psychiatric Association, 2013).

1. Taking the substance in larger amounts or for longer time than you had intended to
2. Wanting to cut down or stop using the substance but efforts are unsuccessful
3. Spending a great deal of time obtaining, using, or recovering from use of the substance
4. Strong cravings and urges to use the substance
5. Disruptions in personal obligations and responsibilities at work, home, or school because of substance use

6. Continuing to use, even in the face of problems the use is causing in interpersonal relationships
7. Giving up or avoiding social, occupational, or recreational activities once important to you because of substance use
8. Continuing to use substances even when doing so is dangerous
9. Continuing to use despite doing so exacerbates physical or psychological problems
10. (Tolerance) Needing more of the substance to get the effect you want
11. (Withdrawal) Development of withdrawal symptoms after prolonged non-use, which can be relieved by taking more of the substance

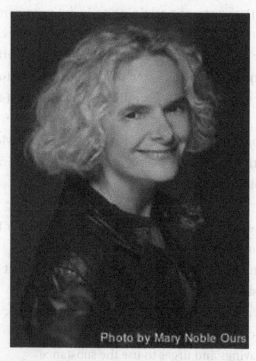

Photo by Mary Noble Ours

Nora Volkow, M.D., the Director of the National Institute on Drug Abuse since 2003, has led the institute's research on the science of addiction.
Photo courtesy of Mary Noble Ours.

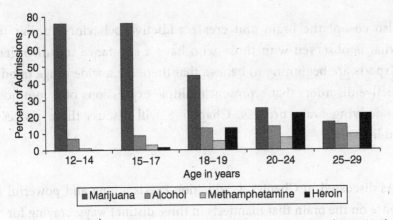

Figure 5.1 Treatment admissions by primary drug for youth age groups (2002–2012). SOURCE: SAHMSA, Treatment Episode Data Set 2002–2012.

From "Wow Effect" to Wanting

People do not intentionally get addicted, but many fall peril to its devastating effects. National data in the U.S. indicate that nearly 23 million Americans—almost 1 in 10—are addicted to at least one substance (https://drugfree.org/learn/drug-and-alcohol-news/new-data-show-millions-of-americans-with-alcohol-and-drug-addiction-could-benefit-from-health-care-reform/). More than two-thirds of them are addicted to alcohol, and other drugs with high addiction prevalence rates are nicotine, marijuana, opioids, and cocaine.

What about adolescents? It is estimated that approximately 4–6% will develop an SUD at some point during their teenage years (Montana & Chung, 2019; Winters & Lee, 2008). And the two drugs that most commonly cause an SUD for youth are marijuana and alcohol. These two drugs are the primary drug of abuse for teenagers who seek treatment for an SUD (see Figure 5.1).

Addiction is not limited to substance-based features. Neuroimaging technologies and more recent research have shown that certain pleasurable activities, such as gambling, shopping, and sex, can also co-opt the brain and create addictive behaviors similar to what is observed with those who have a substance use disorder. Experts are beginning to believe that there are a wide range of addictive disorders that represent multiple expressions of a common underlying brain process. Chapter 8 will discuss these process addictions.

As discussed in Chapter 4, addiction exerts a long and powerful influence on the brain that manifests in three distinct ways: craving for the object of addiction, loss of control over its use, and continuing involvement with it despite adverse consequences. It is considered a brain disease because drugs change the brain; the drugs change the brain's structure and how it works. These brain changes can be long-lasting and can lead to many harmful, often self-destructive, behaviors. Whereas overcoming addiction is possible, the process is often long, slow, and complicated. Repeated cycles of abstinence and relapse are common. And there are indications that this addiction process occurs with a greater likelihood when drug use begins during adolescence. Figure 5.2 shows this trend

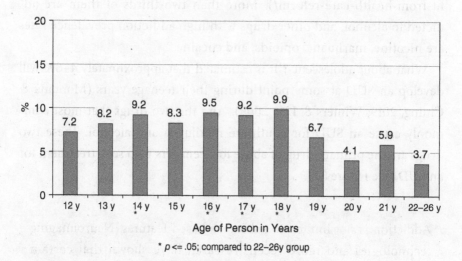

Figure 5.2 Percentages of past-year alcohol use disorder among those with a recent onset (prior 2 years) of alcohol use ($N = 4074$) (Winters & Lee, 2008).

with respect to early alcohol use and rate of subsequent alcohol use disorder (Winters & Lee, 2008).

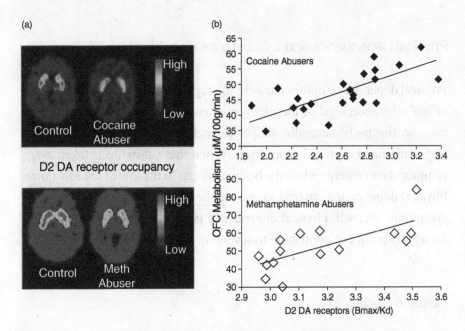

Brain images showing decreased glucose metabolism, which indicates reduced activity, in the orbitofrontal cortex (OFC) in a control subject (a) and a cocaine-addicted subject (b).

SOURCE: Imaging dopamine's role in drug abuse and addiction, by N.D. Volkow, J.S. Fowler, G.J. Wang, R. Baler, F. Telang, *Neuropharmacology*, Volume 56, Supplement 1, 2009, Pages 3–8.

The recognition that addiction is a chronic disorder that changes both brain structure and function was discovered over decades of research. Historically, it was thought that people who developed addictions were somehow morally flawed or had a deficit in willpower. In this moralistic light, addiction's source was viewed as a character weakness. Treating addiction typically involved punishment or encouraging the person to muster the will to break the habit. In the late 1950s, the 12-Step movement gained momentum as it provided the individual with a framework for leading a life of sobriety (see Chapter 13). Contemporary treatment strategies to address adolescents with a substance use disorder typically use multiple strategies, as we will discuss in upcoming chapters.

Physical Dependence and a Substance Use Disorder

Physical dependence may occur with the regular (daily or almost daily) use of any substance, legal or illegal, even when taken as prescribed. It occurs because the body naturally adapts to regular exposure to a substance (e.g., caffeine or a prescription drug). When that substance is taken away, symptoms can emerge while the body readjusts to the loss of the substance. Physical dependence can lead to craving the drug to relieve the withdrawal symptoms. By itself, physical dependence is not sufficient to meet criteria for a SUD but it can contribute to several of the disorder's criteria.

Costs to Society

As reported by a recent Surgeon Surgeon's report (U.S. Department of Health and Human Services, 2016), drug addiction is a major public health challenge that is taking an enormous toll on individuals, families, and society. This impact occurs by virtue of drug-related crime and violence, abuse and neglect of children, and the increased costs of health care. It is estimated that the yearly economic impact of substance misuse is $249 billion for alcohol misuse and $193 billion for illicit drug use (Sacks et al., 2015).

One perspective on the social and health costs of excessive alcohol use is to compare costs to revenues generated from alcohol taxes. Sacks and colleagues (Sacks et al., 2015) estimated that the economic costs of excessive alcohol consumption to governments (in 2010 dollars) are almost 7 times greater, and total economic costs are about 16 times greater, than the revenue generated by alcohol taxes (in 2011 dollars).

Costs to Adolescents

Adolescence is a critical period both for experimenting with drugs and the development of SUDs. Critical neural circuits are still actively forming, particularly those regions of the brain that govern impulse control, seeking new sensations, and peer influences. These parts of the brain may steer a teenager to a decision to use drugs. Thus, the adolescent brain is particularly susceptible to being affected by legal and illicit drugs in a lasting way, and this makes the development of an SUD much more likely. Even when drug involvement falls short of the compulsive use that causes addiction, drug use during adolescence can interfere with meeting crucial social and developmental milestones and also compromise cognitive development. For example, heavy marijuana use that starts during adolescence and extends for many years has been linked to a loss of several IQ points; this loss might not be regained even if the user later quits in adulthood (Meier et al., 2012). The dangers of abusing pain medication and synthetic drugs (e.g., "Spice") is underappreciated by many adolescents; and even scientists still do not know much about how abusing these drugs may affect the developing brain.

Whereas most teens do not escalate from trying drugs to developing an SUD, which is good news, even experimenting with drugs can be a risk to one's health. Drug use can be part of a pattern of risky behavior, including driving while intoxicated, or other hazardous, unsupervised activities. Repeated drug use can aggravate a pre-existing mental disorder (to be addressed in depth later in this chapter) and contribute to other serious social and health risks, including the following:

- School failure
- Problems with family and other relationships
- Loss of interest in normal healthy activities
- Impaired memory
- Increased risk of contracting an infectious disease (such as HIV or hepatitis C) because of unsafe, risky sexual behavior or sharing contaminated injection equipment
- The very real risk of overdose death

A more precise estimate of the type and extent of problems that accompany adolescent drug abuse is provided in Figure 5.3 (Dennis, Clark, & Huang, et al., 2014). Based on a survey from a large community-based sample of adolescents, it is evident that a strong relationship exists between severity of substance use and the number of coexisting problems. The number of 24 problems covering SUD diagnosis, mental health diagnoses, and problems pertaining to health, school, work, and the legal system go up with the number of SUD symptoms. At the severe end, those youth who reported six or more SUD symptoms were nearly nine times more likely to have three or more problems compared to those with no SUD symptoms.

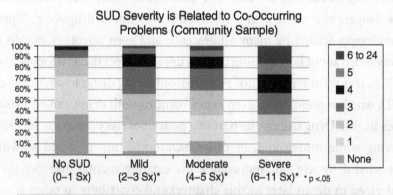

Figure 5.3 The number of co-occurring problems as a function of the number of substance use disorder (SUD) symptoms (Dennis et al., 2014).
SOURCE: Dennis, M. L., Clark, H. W., & Huang, L. N. (2014). The need and opportunity to expand substance use disorder treatment in school-based settings. *Advances in School Mental Health Promotion, 7,* 75-87. © The Clifford Beers Foundation, reprinted by permission of Informa UK Limited, trading as Taylor & Francis Group, www.tandfonline.com on behalf of The Clifford Beers Foundation.

SUD Patterns Among Adolescents

The most common SUDs among adolescents parallel the substances most frequently used by adolescents—alcohol, cannabis, and tobacco (Montana & Chung, 2019). Also, the occurrence of poly-SUDs involving the combination of more than one of the three aforementioned substances is frequently observed (Winters, Botzet, & Lee, 2018). An adolescent who suffers from multiple SUDs compared to having a single SUD is likely to experience more severe problems in multiple areas of functioning (e.g., home, school, in relationships with peers) linked to their substance involvement.

From 2002 to 2014, the prevalence rate of meeting diagnostic criteria for any SUD among adolescents *who had used any substance* decreased from 27.0% to 19.2% (Han et al., 2017). That is a significant decrease of about 30% across this time period.

Another way of looking at trends in SUD is to examine how prevalence rates of SUDs vary as a function of age. The most recent survey of a representative sample of U.S. residents indicates that the prevalence of SUD varies as a function of age group; SUD rates peak during young adulthood (in the age range of 18 to 25 years). Here are data from the 2019 National Survey on Drug Use and Health (rates are based on all respondents per group): The prevalence of any SUD during the prior year among 12- to 17-year-olds was 4.5%, among 18- to 25-year-olds was 14.1%, and among adults age 26 and older was 6.7% (for all age groups, alcohol and marijuana diagnoses were the most common ones) (Substance Abuse and Mental Health Services Administration, 2020). Table 5.1 shows these data across recent years (2015–2018).

Table 5.1 SUBSTANCE USE DISORDER IN THE PAST YEAR BY AGE GROUPS (SUBSTANCE ABUSE AND MENTAL HEALTH SERVICES ADMINISTRATION, 2020)

Age (years)	2015	2016	2017	2018	2019
12 or older	7.8	7.5	7.2	7.4	7.4
12 to 17	5.0	4.3	4.0	3.7	4.5
18 to 25	15.3	15.1	14.8	15.0	14.1
26 or older	6.9	6.6	6.4	6.6	6.7

Transitioning to a Substance Use Disorder

Adolescence is likely a developmental period when the transition from initial use of a substance to developing an SUD may occur within a time frame that is much shorter than what is observed among adults. For any individual, an addiction consists of a vicious cycle of chronic, compulsive drug use leading a person to realign their priorities, followed by the alteration of key brain areas necessary for judgment and self-control, which further reduces the individual's ability to control or stop their drug use. Repeated drug use compromises the very parts of the brain that account for resisting use or for the ability to say "no."

Some adolescents develop an SUD within 2 or 3 years of first use of that substance (Substance Abuse and Mental Health Services Administration, 2021). This pattern for alcohol is displayed in Figure 5.2; the data indicate that the earlier the initiation of alcohol use during the teenage years, the higher the rate of a rate DSM-IV alcohol use disorder (Winters & Lee, 2008). The study by Winters and Lee also found a similar pattern for cannabis use and transitioning to a cannabis use disorder (see Figure 5.4). These data emphasize the importance of early detection and intervention for substance-related problems.

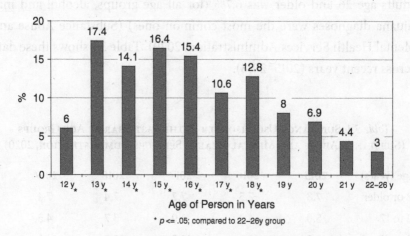

Figure 5.4 Percentages of past-year DSM-IV cannabis use disorder among those with a recent onset (prior 2 years; n = 2176) of cannabis use (Winters & Lee, 2008).

Mild-to-Moderate Drug Involvement

Many adolescents who use substances will develop a mild-to-moderate level of severity in terms of negative consequences and symptomology and do not progress to a severe-end disorder. In fact, a larger percentage of adolescents who use substances will not develop a serious SUD compared to the percentage that will likely develop a mild-to-moderate problem. Figure 5.5 shows an estimate of the percentage of adolescents aged 12–17 who fall into three mutually exclusive groups: dependence (red), mild–moderate (yellow), and non-problem (green). The data are based on a national sample collected in 2004 (Substance Abuse and Mental Health Services Administration, 2005). These groups were defined on the basis of youths' reports of current substance use and presence of DSM-IV substance abuse or dependence disorder symptoms (DSM-IV criteria included the distinction of abuse and dependence). As the data in the figure show, 5.2% of adolescents met the definition of a DSM-IV-defined substance dependence disorder for at least one substance; an additional 24.7% met the criteria for a mild–moderate substance problem (which included either meeting the definition of an abuse disorder for at least one substance, reporting binge or heavy drinking pattern, or reporting use of an illicit substance); and an additional 70.1% were in the group of non-problem by virtue of reporting only light drinking or reporting no use of any substances.

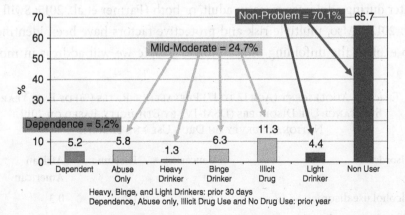

Figure 5.5 Rates of mutually exclusive drug-abusing groups, ages 12–18 years (Substance Abuse and Mental Health Services Administration, 2005).

Differences in SUD Prevalence by Gender and Ethnicity

The 2019 National Survey on Drug Use and Health (NSDUH; Substance Abuse and Mental Health Services Administration, 2020) indicates slightly higher rates of past-year SUD (DSM-IV) by female adolescents than for males (12- to 17-year-olds) (5.0% for females and 4.0% for males), although adolescent females and males reported the same rate of past-year nicotine dependence (Substance Abuse and Mental Health Services Administration, 2020). The 2019 survey indicated both similarities and differences in terms of ethnicity: Caucasian, Hispanic, and African American youth had comparable rates of past-year any illicit drug use disorder; African American youth had the lowest rate of past-year alcohol use disorder; and Caucasian youth had the highest rate of past-year nicotine dependence (cigarettes; see Table 5.2) (Substance Abuse and Mental Health Services Administration, 2020).

SUD Symptom Development and Course

The speed and specifics pertaining to the onset and maintenance of SUD symptoms for adolescents, despite individual differences, follow a fairly reliable profile. Longitudinal studies indicate that regular and heavy use of any drug will increase the likelihood that the person will develop an SUD later during adolescence, as an adult, or both (Farmer et al., 2015; Swift et al. 2012). Also, multiple risk and protective factors have been identified to explain the unfolding of symptoms, a topic we will address in more

Table 5.2 ADOLESCENT (AGE 12 TO 17) PREVALENCE RATES (%) OF PAST YEAR SUBSTANCE USE DISORDERS (DSM-IV) BY ETHNICITY, BASED ON 2019 NATIONAL SURVEY ON DRUG USE AND HEALTH

Disorder	Caucasian	Hispanic	African American
Alcohol use disorder	2.2	1.7	0.3
Illicit drug use disorder	3.5	4.2	3.5
Nicotine dependence (cigarettes)	1.1	0.6	0.3

detail later in this chapter. But the bottom line is that the symptom pro-file for adolescent heavy and regular drinkers tends to be the following: alcohol-related interpersonal problems tend to emerge first and within the first 2 years of regular drinking; this is followed by other alcohol-related consequences and symptoms of an alcohol use disorder; and for some withdrawal generally emerges last (Wagner & Anthony, 2002). The symptom pattern for adolescent cannabis users tends to look like this: signs of impaired control over cannabis use, such as using more than intended, commonly emerge within the first year of regular (typically daily) use; and then cannabis-related physical or psychological problems occur within subsequent years (Chung & Winters, 2018; Rosenberg & Anthony, 2001). Finally, there are data regarding symptom development for adolescent regular cigarette smokers: the first symptoms to emerge are typically related to strong cravings for nicotine that typically emerge within the first year of occasional smoking; this is followed by a pattern of regular (often daily) smoking (DiFranza et al., 2002). Some experts believe that the early emergence of symptoms indicating impaired control over use for cannabis and nicotine may reflect greater addiction liability for these substances relative to alcohol. This issue will continue to be examined given its public health significance and as the legalization landscape changes.

There is considerable controversy as to whether the prevalence of a cannabis use disorder among adolescents is on the rise in recent years due to current pro-marijuana trends in the United States. Creda and colleagues (Creda et al., 2019) examined this issue by comparing cannabis use disorder (CUD) rates before and after states approved recreational marijuana laws (RML). The data below show rates of past-year CUD among past-year users of cannabis. Increases in CUD rates after RML occurred in all three age groups.

PREVALENCE OF PAST YEAR CANNABIS USE DISORDER AMONG RECENT CANNABIS USERS BEFORE AND AFTER RECREATIONAL MARIJUANA LAWS (RML)

Age Group (years)	Before RML (%)	After RML (%)
12–17	22.8	27.2
18–25	16.6	15.7
≥26	9.1	10.4

Based on research with the prior diagnostic system, the DSM-IV SUD symptoms that are most often endorsed by adolescents include tolerance and using more or longer than intended, whereas the least frequently reported is withdrawal (Chung & Martin, 2005). There is some empirical support that early in the development of an SUD, the most common initial symptoms are substance-related interpersonal problems and impairment in meeting major role obligations (e.g., at school or work) due to substance use (Chung & Martin, 2005).

What Causes a Substance Use Disorder?

There are several reasons adolescents use drugs, including peer influences, an attempt to deal with personal or emotional problems, and an interest in pursuing novel experiences. As noted in Chapter 3, the adolescent brain is developing in a way that promotes the seeking of new experiences and to take risks; the regions of the brain responsible for processing feelings of pleasure, important drivers of drug use, are the first to mature during childhood. Parts linked to decision making and controlling of emotions mature later during adolescence. Also, adolescence is a time when drug use might be a vehicle for the teenager to forge a social identity. In this light, experimenting with drugs is driven by normal developmental processes.

Underlying reasons to use are the numerous factors that influence whether an adolescent tries drugs and then is at risk for developing an SUD. This body of knowledge is framed in the literature as risk and protective factors; risk factors contribute to the likelihood to use drugs and protective factors promote the non-use of drugs. Major factors identified by experts include the following (Sussman et al., 2008):

- Availability of drugs within the neighborhood, community, and school
- Peer drug use
- Drug use by family members
- Being victimized by violence or physical or emotional abuse in the family

- Family history of mental illness or drug use
- Personality traits like poor impulse control or a high need for excitement
- Attitudes that drug use is normative and that drugs are harmless
- Seeking emotional relief or pleasure
- Early use of drugs
- Genetic vulnerability
- Mental health conditions such as depression, anxiety, or attention-deficit/hyperactivity disorder (ADHD) (more on the contributing role of coexisting mental illness and SUD later in this chapter).

As we noted earlier in this chapter (and highlighted in Figures 5.2 and 5.4), drug use at an early age is a noteworthy predictor of development of a subsequent SUD. The majority of those who have an SUD at some time in their life started using before age 18. For example: data collected in the 2012 national household survey indicated that nearly 13% of those with an SUD began using marijuana by the time they were age 14 (Substance Abuse and Mental Health Services Administration, 2013).

The figure below further demonstrates this principle by showing that the risk increases for eventually developing an alcohol use or cannabis use disorder as a function of the younger the age of onset of use.

It is relevant to ask if some risk and protective factors are more influential than others. The simple answer is that, in general, no. Of course, for any given teenager, there may be a salient factor that distinguishes their risk profile. Consider an adolescent whose biological parents both have a history of addiction; this person's genetic vulnerability is much higher than that of an adolescent with biological parents having no addiction history. But the basic principle is that not all young people are equally at risk for developing an addiction, and one's "risk index" is based on the number of risk factors associated with that person. To counter risk factors, such protective factors as nurturing parents or a healthy school environment might lessen the risk of an SUD. Consider these two examples. An adolescent who begins using drugs early during youth, has friends who are drug users, has a parent with a history of addiction, and finds it difficult to control impulses is at a very high risk to develop an SUD. By

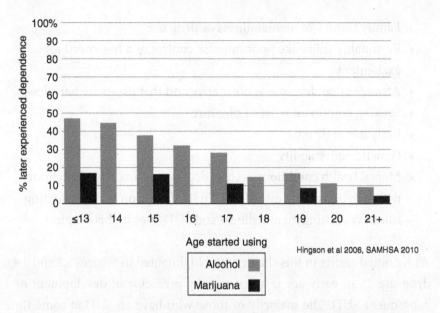

Hingson et al 2006, SAMHSA 2010

As we have noted earlier in this chapter (and highlighted in Figures 5.2 and 5.4), drug use at an early age is a noteworthy predictor of development of a subsequent SUD. The majority of those who have an SUD at some time in their life started using before age 18. For example: data collected in the 2012 National Household Survey indicated that nearly 13% of those with a substance use disorder began using marijuana by the time they were age 14 (Substance Abuse and Mental Health Services Administration, 2013). The figure further demonstrates this principle by showing that the risk increases for eventually developing an alcohol use or cannabis use disorder as a function of the younger the age of onset of use.

contrast, an adolescent who is using drugs but has no other risk factors and has parents who are very supportive and exhibit effective monitoring behaviors would be at a much lower risk to develop an SUD.

PREVENTING SUBSTANCE USE DISORDERS

Adolescence is a crucial time for preventing drug abuse, a view supported by several lines of evidence already discussed in this book: early use of drugs increases a person's chances of developing addiction; the developing brain is particularly vulnerable to the effects of drugs; and the life functioning of an adolescent with an SUD is significantly impaired. Thus, there is great health significance in preventing young people from experimenting with drugs.

It is logical that prevention programs are typically implemented in schools. When youth advance from elementary through middle school, they face new and challenging social and academic situations. Often during this period, children are exposed to cigarettes and alcohol for the first time. When they enter high school, adolescents might encounter greater availability of drugs (typically marijuana) and social activities where drugs are used.

Do prevention programs work? This issue has been extensively researched for over 25 years and the authors' answer to this question is "yes." But there are two conditions to this answer. Effective programs require that (1) the content is developmentally appropriate, and (2) rigorous research has documented that the program produces positive results. Researchers have developed a diverse range of evidence-based programs and practices that significantly reduce early use of drugs. The typical strategy of a prevention program is to shape the balance between underlying factors that cause drug and substance use disorder by reducing risk factors and increasing protective factors. One key factor is to educate youth about the potential harm of drugs. This variable has shown to be related to drug use—when the perception of harm of taking drugs is greater, there tends to be less drug use (Scheier et al., 2019).

Key Principles of Effective Prevention

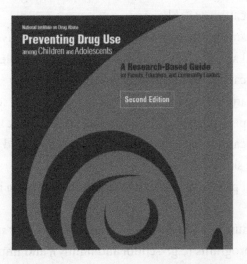

SOURCE: Robertson, E. B., David, S. L., & Rao, S. A. (2003). *Preventing drug use among children and adolescents: A research-based guide for parents, educators, and community leaders* (2nd ed.). Rockville: MD: National Institute on Drug Abuse.

A group of prominent research-based programs are described in the National Institute on Drug Abuse's (NIDA's) *Preventing Drug Use among Children and Adolescents: A Research-Based Guide for Parents, Educators, and Community Leaders* (Robertson et al., 2003). Major themes from this publication are that evidence-based prevention interventions are cost-effective and that programs exist for use in schools or in communities. This publication also identifies key elements of effective prevention programs and practices, which we list below.

1. All forms of drugs are addressed.
2. Prevention is an ongoing effort with repeated programming over time to reinforce earlier goals and develop new skills.
3. Identify risk and protective factors relevant to the local community.
4. Modifiable protective factors are enhanced and modified risk factors are reduced or reversed.
5. The content and delivery of the program are tailored to address the target population's developmental status, race/ethnicity, and other local factors.
6. For family programs: Family bonding, parenting skills, and communication are enhanced.
7. For programs in the elementary school years: Focus on behavioral self-control, emotional awareness, problem solving, communication, and academic readiness.
8. For programs in the middle, junior high, and high school years: Focus on peer relations, study habits and academic support, communication, self-efficacy and assertiveness, and drug resistance skills.
9. For school programs: Teacher training in classroom management is critical.
10. For community programs: Seek to combine two or more effective programs (e.g., school and family), and implement consistent messages across settings.

TREATING SUBSTANCE USE DISORDERS

Principles of treatment for adolescents with an SUD are summarized in the NIDA publication *Principles of Adolescent Substance Use Disorder Treatment: A Research-Based Guide* (National Institute on Drug Abuse, 2014).

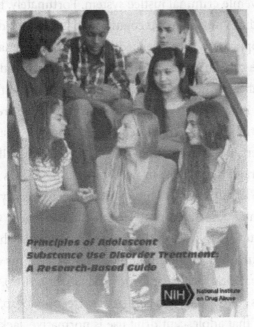

Principles of treatment for adolescents with a SUD are summarized in this NIDA Publication (National Institute on Drug Abuse, 2004)
SOURCE: National Institute on Drug Abuse. (2014). *Principles of adolescent substance use disorder treatment: A research-based guide*. NIH Publication Number 14-7953. Rockville, MD: National Institute on Drug Abuse.

SUD is a treatable disorder. Research shows that comprehensive assessment, addressing mental conditions that may coexist with an SUD, having staff trained in adolescent treatments, and using strategies that combine behavioral and family therapies provide, on average, the best outcomes when treating adolescents with an SUD (National Institute on Drug Abuse, 2014; Tanner-Smith et al., 2013; Winters, Botzet, Stinchfield, et al., 2018). Treatment approaches must be tailored to address each patient's drug use patterns and drug-related medical, psychiatric, and social problems

(National Institute on Drug Abuse, 2014). In subsequent chapters, we discuss a wide range of SUD treatment strategies and approaches.

Historically, treating adolescents who have a drug problem reflected society's view that drug abuse was a sign of moral weakness or a willful rejection of societal norms, and these problems were typically addressed through the juvenile criminal justice system. Fortunately, health care systems in recent times now reflect recognition that treating adolescent SUDs requires the application of evidenced-based behavior change strategies. Yet it is still the case that the same level of attention to adolescent SUDs is not comparable to the level that other behavioral health concerns affecting similar numbers of youth receive. Drug abuse treatment in the United States still remains largely segregated from the rest of health care services (Winters, Botzet, Stinchfield, et al., 2018), and available treatment serves only a fraction of those in need of treatment. It is estimated that only about 10% of adolescents with an SUD receive any type of specialty treatment (Center for Behavioral Health Statistics and Quality, 2016). Further, estimates are that fewer than half of individuals who have both an SUD and a mental health condition receive treatment for either disorder (Center for Behavioral Health Statistics and Quality, 2016).

Many factors contribute to an adolescent "treatment gap," including parental attitudes that adolescent drug use is normative, lack of motivation to change by adolescents, fear of family shame, the inability to access or afford care, and lack of screening for drug abuse in youth-serving health care settings (Winters, Botzet, Stinchfield, et al., 2018). It can be expected that the majority of adolescents who are abusing drugs do not recognize the dangers of their behavior and simply believe they do not have a problem or need treatment. These attitudes may be also held by many parents after discovering their son or daughter is using.

Post-Treatment Course of Substance Use Disorder

Adolescents treated for SUD generally show reductions in drug use compared to pretreatment levels, along with concurrent improvements in psychosocial functioning over short- and longer-term follow-up (Chung & Maisto, 2006). However, there is considerable variability in the course of adolescents' post-treatment substance involvement. Studies of *short-term post-treatment clinical course* (i.e., ≤18-month follow-up) have identified multiple prototypical paths or trajectories of drug use that include these types: stable low levels of use, stable high levels of use, increasing pattern of use, and decreasing pattern of use (e.g., Chung et al., 2005; Waldron et al., 2005). These trajectory types have been identified for both alcohol and cannabis use following treatment (Waldron et al., 2005). When trajectory types were examined for level and type of drug-related problems, one study examined alcohol symptoms (Chung et al., 2005). The symptoms most often reported over 1-year follow-up were interpersonal problems linked to alcohol use and impaired control over alcohol use (Chung et al. 2005).

Most studies of *longer-term post-treatment clinical course* in treated adolescents have examined changes in level of substance use following treatment (e.g., Winters et al., 2008), and some studies have documented post-treatment changes in SUD symptoms (e.g., Chung et al., 2008). Comparable trajectory types have been identified across these studies, despite differences in substance examined (e.g., alcohol, cannabis, other illicit drugs), how drug use severity was defined (e.g., frequency of use, substance-related problems), and regional differences in study location. The long-term trajectory types were the following: stable abstinence, infrequent use, slow improvers (gradually decreasing substance involvement), and persistent high-level drug using. Generally, this group of studies showed that proportionally most youth were classified as either infrequent users or slow improvers, and the smallest proportions were the two "endpoint" groups—stable abstinence and persistent high-level drug using.

The extent and nature of long-term cross-drug patterns have also been examined. Chung and colleagues (Chung et al., 2008) found a moderate level of cross-drug concordance in post-treatment pattern of change. To make this point another way: It was rare for a youth to reveal a trajectory type for one drug and a distinctly different trajectory for a different drug.

This finding of cross-drug similarity in post-treatment patterns of change suggests that drug substitution effects are not prevalent among youth, and that treatment has widespread, positive effects in reducing poly-drug use.

CO-OCCURRING DISORDERS

Any psychiatric disorder among adolescents is relatively common. The prominent Great Smoky Mountain Study (GSMS) examined longitudinally the DSM-IV diagnosis of 1,420 adolescents between 9 and 13 years of age in the community annually until the age of 16 years. At least one psychiatric disorder was met by 36.7% of respondents (Costello et al., 2003). Social anxiety, panic, depression and substance use disorders increased in prevalence over time, while disorders such as ADHD decreased (Costello et al., 2003). *Co-occurring* (or co-existing) disorders (CODs) refers to two or more behavioral or psychiatric conditions that may occur simultaneously or sequentially in a person. Co-occurring conditions might affect the timing of SUD onset, its severity, and trajectory (National Institute on Drug Abuse, 2014; Substance Abuse and Mental Health Services Administration, 2021). A review of community-based studies indicates that a majority (~60%) of adolescents with an SUD had a COD (Armstrong & Costello, 2002). Among adolescents in substance use treatment, more than half are estimated to have a co-occurring mental illness (Chan et al., 2008). Thus, COD is the rule rather than the exception. Some studies of adolescents with SUD have found that females were more likely to exhibit internalizing (e.g., depression, anxiety) symptoms and trauma syndromes than are males (e.g., Kaminer & Bukstein, 2008). But Angold and colleagues found that both sexes showed more similarities than differences in terms of the course of early substance use and its future risk for CODs (Angold, Costello, & Erkanli, 1999). Little is known about ethnic differences in SUD and co-occurring psychiatric conditions. The pattern of CODs among adolescents with an SUD in terms of the number and type of conditions present is quite heterogeneous. Nonetheless, there are conditions that are commonly associated with adolescent SUD: conduct

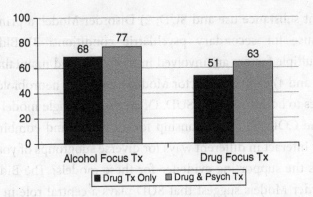

Figure 5.6 Drug treatment outcome improves in the presence of treatment for co-occurring disorders (Sterling & Weisner, 2005).

problems, mood disorders (e.g., depression, ADHD, physical trauma, and sexual trauma; Armstrong & Costello, 2002).

Adolescent drug treatment programs that formally address coexisting disorders are still relatively rare, but recognition is growing that the multiple problems that typically accompany an SUD need to be assessed and treated (National Institute on Drug Abuse, 2014) and that when CODs are addressed, substance use outcomes are enhanced (Substance Abuse and Mental Health Services Administration, 2021). Sterling and Weisner (2005) compared the rates of abstinence at 6 months post-treatment in a sample of youth with an SUD that received only drug treatment (dark blue bars) versus a sample with an SUD that received both drug and COD treatment (light blue bars) (see Figure 5.6). The abstinence rates are better for the SUD youth that received both drug and COD treatment. (Subsequent chapters in this volume address co-occurring internalizing disorders [Chapter 6] and externalizing disorders [Chapter 7].)

Explanations for Co-Occurring Disorders

The nature of the relationship between COD and SUD during adolescence is complex. Research points to these four explanatory models: 1) Self-Medication Model: early-onset psychiatric symptoms contribute to subsequent substance use and SUD; 2) Disorder Model: a primary SUD is the cause for secondary psychiatric conditions; 3) Bidirectional Model: multiple factors are involved in triggering and maintaining COD and SUD; and 4) Common Factor Model: a common neurobiological risk contributes to both COD and SUD. Of course, no single model may fully explain the COD–SUD relationship for all youth, and combinations of them may interact in different ways for diverse subgroups of youth.

What is the supporting evidence for these models? The Bidirectional and Disorder Models suggest that SUD plays a central role in the onset and course of COD, but epidemiological data do not support them. In an Epidemiological Catchment Area study conducted with community samples of 18–30 years old, in three out of four cases the psychiatric disorder *preceded* the substance use (Christie et al., 1988). These data actually support the Self-Medication Model, which is likely the most popular one among professionals. The Common Factor Model has received support from recent genetic studies, which show shared or overlapping genetic involvement among some psychiatric disorders and SUD (Groenman et al., 2017). One example is the relative salience of behavioral and emotional components of psychological dysregulation that are observed in a range of psychiatric disorders and SUD, and this dysregulation has been shown to be highly heritable (Tarter & Horner, 2016).

Diagnostic Issues

The stability or change of diagnostic status among adolescents with COD/SUD has not been systematically examined, which limits our understanding of how co-occurring conditions affects their trajectories of relapse and recovery. The amount and direction of change typically varies across disorders and much of the shift occurs between subthreshold and threshold status (Costello et al., 2003). Complicating matters is that youths with SUD often have psychosocial impairments that do not meet full DSM diagnoses; Angold and colleagues conducted a large epidemiological study and found significant psychosocial impairments were common among youth that did not meet full DSM diagnoses (Angold, Costello, Farmer, et al., 1999).

These subclinical problems may go undetected and untreated, and such impairments may impact the recovery/relapse trajectory of SUD. Consider an example in which a girl with a history of learning problems is being treated for an SUD and this important coexisting condition goes undetected. Her ability to maximally benefit from the program may be compromised unless adjustments are made with written materials and assignments that requite reading and writing skills. Also, her aftercare plan would want to include attention to this problem in order to support recovery.

Another diagnostic issue pertains to the temporal sequencing for the onset and course of specific disorders. Little is known about factors associated with the persistence (i.e., length of the index episode) of CODs over time among adolescents. Identifying the temporal sequence of multiple disorders requires implementing a detailed historical diagnostic interview that pinpoints the onset and progression of separate disorders. A rough gauge of the onset of a specific disorder is when the first clinical-level symptom or cluster of symptoms are experienced by the individual, and an approximation of a COD's course can be assessed by then asking when these symptoms reached their peak in terms of negatively affecting the adolescent's functioning (e.g., impairment in school functioning, disturbances in sleep).

Treatment Issues

Adolescents with COD present many treatment challenges. Youth with COD and SUD, compared to youth with just SUD, are associated with greater overall impairment in level of functioning and poorer recovery (Priester et al., 2016). Regarding the latter issue, trajectories of relapse and recovery from SUD are likely influenced by fluctuations in symptom severity of the COD and access to quality aftercare services for youth with COD.

As noted above, there is a growing trend in adolescent health to integrate treatment services for COD and SUD, and integration likely improves outcome (as we showed in Figure 5.6). But barriers to widespread integration in the service delivery arena include the persistent historical trend to separate drug treatment and mental health services, and the limited number of clinicians and researchers with expertise in assessing and treating COD. Piecemeal unidimensional treatments targeting just SUD or just one COD when many are present will not optimize treatment outcome. There is a growing clinical consensus that the future of adolescent treatment will require the coordination of treatment protocols for both SUD and COD. Indeed, a major impetus for this book is to provide an educational vehicle for upgrading such coordinated clinical services.

MEASURING SUBSTANCE USE DISORDERS

Developmental Issues

Many developmental factors influence the measurement of SUD among adolescents. As we have noted earlier, adolescents who use substances can develop a drug problem within a relatively short period of time, and many contextual factors are adolescent specific (e.g., living with parents; powerful influence from peers). Another consideration is the rapid biological growth during adolescence, a factor that impacts the measurement of tolerance to alcohol. A teenager who shows "overt" tolerance by drinking twice as much to get the same effect compared to use level when they started to drink may be interpreted differently than when an adult shows the same pattern. The teenager's physical growth can be quite significant during a short period of time, and this alone can account for tolerance to the effects of drinking.

Another example is this symptom for an alcohol use disorder: "spending much time trying to obtain alcohol or getting over its effects." An adolescent might endorse this item due to difficulties in acquiring alcohol because they are a minor, not because the person is showing a compulsive drinking pattern, which is the intended meaning of this symptom (Harford et al., 2005). Thus, SUD symptoms might manifest differently in adolescent and adults, which reinforces the need to adapt assessment tools and the constructs and criteria they address to optimize the overall accuracy of SUD diagnoses in adolescents. Thus, the assessment process with adolescents requires careful and developmentally suitable construction of the questions, and sufficient symptom queries and probing when interviews are conducted, about the presence or absence of symptoms, to ensure valid measuring of the phenomenon being queried.

Optimizing Accurate Measurement

There are several steps that can improve the accuracy of measuring SUD symptoms.

1. Brief descriptions should be provided to the adolescent to ensure a common understanding of constructs being queried. For example, one symptom of an SUD is "failed attempt to cut down on use." An accompanying description for this item could be this: "Are there any instances in which you thought about or tried to cut back or stop using but you did not or could not?"

2. Recall may be facilitated by providing a contextual example of how the symptom may occur in relation to the adolescent's own experiences or specific situation. With respect to the symptom noted above, here is an example: "Was there a time recently when you were at a party and you told yourself that you were going to limit how much you drank but you did not?"

3. Probes can be used to reduce a person saying that they have a problem or symptom when in fact it is not present (referred to as a "false positive"). For example, clarification for the possible presence of the symptom "much time spent obtaining alcohol" would require probing if this is present as a reflection of a compulsive pattern of use (the intended meaning of the

criterion) or of difficulties obtaining alcohol due to minor status (possible false positive).

4. Some SUD criteria are complex and need to be split into separate questions. One example is the criterion "using more or longer than intended." The possible manifestations of "using more than intended" and "using longer than intended" should be assessed with separate questions.

Following is a sample of assessment items to measure an adolescent's recent substance use history.

1. During the prior 12 months, how often (if at all) have you used the following drugs? Choose one option for each drug:

1 = Not at all
2 = Less than monthly
3 = About monthly
4 = About weekly or daily
    A. Alcohol (including beer, wine, liquor)
    B. Marijuana (grass, pot) or hash
    C. Tobacco or nicotine products (cigarettes, vaping, chew)

5. The specifics of drug use behavior (e.g., frequency, quantity, duration) are not directly related to determining diagnostic criteria for individual SUD symptoms. But it advisable to review the adolescent's drug use history prior to measuring SUD criteria, and for drugs that have been used at least five or more times in their lifetime, to assess the SUD criteria for that drug.

The measurement process also benefits from various approaches and strategies that optimize a detailed and accurate self-report from an adolescent during a clinical assessment. Self-report is a hallmark of clinical assessment, given its convenience, comprehensiveness, and low cost. Plus, the individual is the most knowledgeable reporter. The most common self-report formats of measurement tools are self-administered questionnaires and interviews; other types include the timeline follow-back (TLFB; see Figure 4.9 in Chapter 4) and computer-assisted interviews. Research on the concordance of self-report questionnaires, interview, TLFB, and computer-based formats suggests that, for the most part, the various formats yield similar levels of disclosure (Winters et al., 2014). Provided in a subsequent section are examples of these different types of measurement tools.

Though commonly used, the overall accuracy of the self-report method for assessing adolescent drug use and related problems is still debated. Underreporting of the quantity and type of drug use on self-report measures by adolescents can occur. Youth may also see the self-report assessment as an opportunity to "cry for help" or exaggerate their responses. Other variables that can influence the accuracy of assessment include cognitive factors (e.g., comprehension, recall), perceived lack of confidentiality, lack of trust in the provider, and fear of reprisal (Brener et al., 2003). Despite possible limitations, the validity of self-report for adolescent drug use has been supported by several lines of evidence: Only a small percentage of youth endorse improbable questions; adolescent self-reports agree with corroborating sources of information, such as archival records and, for the most part, urinalyses; and the percentage of elevations on scales intended to detect compromised self-report (e.g., "faking-good" and "faking-bad" scales) is relatively low (Maisto et al., 1995).

A counselor has a duty to warn when the following are present:

- A client or patient expresses specific and immediate threat.
- The threat entails serious bodily injury or death.
- The threat includes an identifiable or easily identifiable person.
- The counselor believes that the client has the ability to carry out the threat imminently.

How can the validity (accuracy) of self-report be optimized? Several keys to this are provided below.

1. Describe the confidentiality protections that the teenager is entitled to. For example, an adolescent can disclose illegal drug

use without that information being disclosed to law enforcement. Of course, mandated reporters are required to report instances of victimization of abuse and suicidality.

Time Window for Detecting Drugs from Urinalysis

Substance	Detection Period
Alcohol	7–12 hours
Short-acting barbiturates	24 hours
Long-acting barbiturates	3 weeks
Amphetamines	48 hours
Heroin	48 hours
Cocaine metabolites	2–4 days
Cannabis	3 days to 30 days (depends on use pattern)

Source: Sissons, B. (2018, October 18). *Approximate drug detection time in the urine* [table]. *Medical News Today*. https://www.medicalnewstoday.com/articles/323378#how-to-prepare-for-a-urine-test

2. Establish good rapport with the client by being nonjudgmental, expressing empathy, avoiding argumentation, and using other motivational interviewing techniques (a topic that is the focus of Chapter 11).

3. Corroborate self-report with other sources, such as archival records, report from parents, clinical observation, and use of bioassay techniques (e.g., urine test).

4. Use measurement tools that were developed specifically for and normed on adolescents. As we discuss in a subsequent section, there are numerous developmentally appropriate tools available for use in clinical settings.

5. For self-administered questionnaires, ensure that the tool's reading level is appropriate to the adolescent's reading ability. It is common for self-administered tools to have a fourth-grade reading level and yet some youth cannot read at this

level. Naturally, a tool that is difficult for a teenager to read can contribute to inaccurate responses.

6. Given that many youth suspected of having an SUD have attention problems, a computer-assisted format can be beneficial and the assessment process should not be burdensomely long.

Distinguishing Screening and Comprehensives Assessment

Screening is the first step in identifying whether a youth may be involved with drugs. Screening results should be used to determine the need for a comprehensive assessment, rather than used to directly determine treatment need. The comprehensive assessment is used to explore the extent and nature of the drug involvement, consequential problems, and treatment needs.

Screening. A good screening tool is brief, easy to use, and accurate. Typical screening questions for adolescents pertain to recent drug use quantity and frequency (e.g., "How often did you use the following drugs in the past 6 months?"), the presence of adverse consequences of use (e.g., "Has your drug use led to problems with your parents?"), and situations in which drug use is common (e.g., "Describe typical situations when you use."). A universal screening for SUD and related substance use problems can be ideal; if a screening tool is routinely administered "to all teens that walk through the door," teens might be less likely to feel singled out and more likely to provide honest responses.

Provided below is a well-known screening tool, the CRAFFT + N Interview (www.crafft.org). This interview leads off with four questions about drug use during the past 12 months (Part A), and then is followed by six items pertaining to problems associated with drug use (Part B). Two or more "yes" responses on the problem severity items (questions 5–10) is considered a "red flag" score and suggests a need for a comprehensive assessment. (Not shown here is Part C, which consists of seven questions about use of nicotine products, and the scoring interpretation rules.)

The CRAFFT+N Interview

To be verbally administered by the clinician

Begin: *"I'm going to ask you a few questions that I ask all my patients. Please be honest. I will keep your answers confidential."*

Part A
During the PAST 12 MONTHS, on how many days did you:

1. Drink more than a few sips of beer, wine, or any drink containing **alcohol**? Say "0" if none.

   # of days

2. Use any **marijuana** (cannabis, weed, oil, wax, or hash by smoking, vaping, dabbing, or in edibles) or **"synthetic marijuana"** (like "K2," "Spice")? Say "0" if none.

   # of days

3. Use **anything else to get high** (like other illegal drugs, pills, prescription or over-the-counter medications, and things that you sniff, huff, vape, or inject)? Say "0" if none.

   # of days

4. Use a **vaping device* containing nicotine or flavors,** or use any **tobacco products†**? Say "0" if none.
   *Such as e-cigs, mods, pod devices like JUUL, disposable vapes like Puff Bar, vape pens, or e-hookahs. †Cigarettes, cigards, cigarillos, hookahs, chewing tobacco, snuff, snus, dissolvables, or nicotine pouches.

   # of days

If the patient answered...

"0" for all questions in Part A	"1" or more for Q. 1,2, or 3	"1" or more for Q. 4
↓	↓	↓
Ask 1st question only in Part B below, then STOP	Ask all 6 questions in Part B below	Ask all 10 questions in Part C on next page

Part B   Circle one

C Have you ever ridden in a **CAR** driven by someone (including yourself) who was "high" or had been using alcohol or drugs?   No   Yes

R Do you ever use alcohol or drugs to **RELAX,** feel better about yourself, or fit in?   No   Yes

A Do you ever use alcohol or drugs to while you are by yourself, or **ALONE**?   No   Yes

F Do you ever **FORGET** things you did while using alcohol or drugs?   No   Yes

F Do your **FAMILY** or **FRIENDS** ever tell you that you should cut down on your drinking or drug use?   No   Yes

T Have you ever gotten into **TROUBLE** while you were using alcohol or drugs?   No   Yes

Two or more YES answers in Part B suggests a serious problem that needs further assessment. See Page 3 for further instructions. ⟶

Following are sample items from the Alcohol Use Disorder section of the *Adolescent Diagnostic Interview* (Winters & Henly, 1993).

During the past 12 months. . . .

1. Has your use of alcohol caused you to miss school or work more than once or twice?
2. Have you gone to work or school while drunk from drinking alcohol?
3. Has your use of alcohol upset any of your friends to the point where they argued with you or no longer speak to you?

Comprehensive assessment. If the screening suggests a possible drug use problem, a more comprehensive assessment can determine details of drug use history, consequences, whether criteria are met for an SUD, what other behavioral and mental co-occurring problems may exist, and what level or type of treatment might be needed. This assessment, which should include at least a detailed clinical interview and the use of at least one standardized questionnaire, might also involve several sources. A common type of comprehensive assessment tool is the structured interview. Such interviews mean that the items are to be read verbatim, following a decision-tree format, and responses consist of a few predefined options. Areas of inquiry include the following: age of onset and progression of use for specific substances; the type, frequency, and variability of drugs used recently and historically; circumstances or settings in which substances were used; use patterns of peers; environmental factors that are triggers of use; symptoms of SUD for each substance recently used; other negative consequences of use that are not part of SUD criteria (e.g., problems in school or with family linked to drug use); and problem recognition and readiness for treatment.

See Box 7 for a set of items from the Adolescent Diagnostic Interview, a standardized interview for use with adolescents suspected of problems associated with drug use (Winters & Henly, 1993).

Differences. There are distinct differences between screening and comprehensive assessment in terms of length of time conducting the assessment and clinical goals, as shown in Figure 5.7.

Length	Clinical purpose
Screening	Few minutes	Further assessment?
Assessment	1+ hours	Treatment indicated?

Figure 5.7 Comparison of screening and comprehensive assessment.

Assessing coexisting disorders. As we have noted above, there is general consensus that certain psychiatric or behavioral disorders are the most frequent among youth with an SUD (Kaminer & Winters, 2019). The formal psychiatric disorders and related problems that have the greatest coexistence with adolescent SUD are the following:

- Attention deficit hyperactivity disorder
- Conduct disorder
- Oppositional defiant disorder
- Depressive disorders
- Anxiety disorders
- Post-traumatic stress disorder
- Learning disorders
- Eating disorders
- Other problems (e.g., suicidality, learning problems, eating disorders)

Parents as an Assessment Source

Whereas parents are usually willing to provide a report about their adolescent, it is not likely that they can provide detailed reports about the types, frequency, and quantity of drug use by their child (Winters et al., 2000). Often, parents and other caregivers are unaware if their adolescent has initiated substance use, and symptoms of use during the early stages of use can be short-lived and might be concealed from parents. Yet some of the early behavioral signs of drug use that might be detected include withdrawal from previously enjoyed activities (e.g., quitting a hobby), an increase in academic problems (e.g., rapid drop in grades, skipping school), a change in social behavior (e.g., isolating oneself, changing peer group), and trouble with the law (e.g., charged with possession) (Bukstein, 2005).

With respect to mental health, parents typically provide more detailed and accurate information for the so-called "externalizing" disorders (e.g., ADHD; conduct disorder), which manifest by highly observable behaviors, compared to "internalizing" disorders (e.g., depressive disorders), symptoms of which can often go undetected by another person. Diagnostic interviews that focus on formal criteria for psychiatric disorders typically have both parent and youth versions. Prominent examples include the *Diagnostic Interview for Children and Adolescents* (DICA) (Reich et al., 1992) and the *Diagnostic Interview Schedule for Children* (DISC) (Shaffer et al., 1996). These interviews cover recent and lifetime psychiatric symptoms and other content areas of functioning (e.g., social and school functioning).

Family influences. The importance of including parents in the assessment process is further heighted given they are a valuable source of information pertaining to a wide range of family-related variables. Family influences encompass several factors, including familial genetic risk and parenting practices. Children whose parents have a history of an SUD are at increased risk for the development of an SUD (McGue, 1999). Also, parental antisocial behavior history is relevant in offspring SUD liability. The importance of parenting factors cannot be understated; increased drug use among adolescents is associated with families that lack closeness or affection, lack effective discipline, lack supervision, have excessive or weak parental control, and have inconsistent parenting (LaBrie & Cail, 2011). There is converging evidence that incorporates both types of family influences with respect to alcohol abuse. The evidence is such that the initiation of alcohol use during adolescence is significantly influenced by parental monitoring factors, yet after alcohol use is initiated, youth with genetic risk factors are more likely to maintain alcohol use and an alcohol use disorder (Rose et al., 2001).

The Clinical Interview

The importance of the initial clinical assessment interview with the adolescent dictates that we discuss it in some detail. Seven key issues that will promote a therapeutic initial interview with a teenager are highlighted below.

1. Decide up-front who will be present for the initial interview. In most instances, it is preferable to briefly begin with the teenager and the parent to orient both to the procedure and to obtain signatures on any administrative forms; then follow with the adolescent alone and end the first interview with the adolescent and the parent to review next steps.

2. It is advisable to situate oneself out from behind the desk. Maintain as much eye contact as possible and avoid too much note taking during the interview.

Examples of opening interview questions:

1. What circumstances led you to come and see me today?
2. What do you understand as the reasons why you are here today?
3. It is helpful that I get to know you a little better. How do you like to spend your free time? What is school like for you? Describe your friends.

3. Spend the first part of the interview building rapport by using motivational interviewing techniques (an interviewing style that is the focus of Chapter 11). Begin with small talk and nonthreatening openers. Also, focus early in the interview on the present situation; withhold historical issues until later in the interview. The comprehensive interviews cited below provide good examples of opening interview questions.

4. Acknowledge that you are aware that the current situation may be difficult for the adolescent. But level with the adolescent that your job is to help to assess the situation and to work with them to determine a course of action.

5. Act as the teenager's advocate as much as possible; highlight positive behaviors; when offering criticism, criticize the activity, not the person.

6. Acknowledge that using drugs has functional value and is serving some purpose for the individual (e.g., drugs might have social and psychological benefits for the user). Acknowledgment does not mean you are approving drug use.

7. Be aware of your own biases and "resentments" so they don't interfere with your judgment. Avoid pontificating, lecturing, and admonishing.

Selecting Assessment Tools

Choosing screening and comprehensive assessment tools depends on the setting in which it will be used, its purpose, and the suitability of the tool with respect to the youth's demographics and the staffing resources that can support the task. Also important is to select an instrument associated with favorable psychometric properties of reliability and validity for the relevant population it was designed to assess. A reliable instrument means that it measures the construct of interest with consistency (e.g., the person's score would be similar if the same test were taken within a short period of time, such as 1 week). A valid tool means that it accurately measures the construct it is intended to measure (e.g., a person's score on the measure accurately reflects the real-world manifestation of that construct). An instrument should not be used if there is no published research to describe the degree of its reliability or validity when administered to adolescents.

Other desirable features when selecting instruments include the following (Winters, Botzet, & Lee, 2018): (1) normative scores are provided according to gender, various ages, and various ethnic backgrounds; (2) the reading level is not too high (e.g., fourth-grade reading level or lower is desirable when assessing adolescents); (3) wording of interview and questionnaire items are suitable for youth of diverse ethnic, cultural, and linguistic backgrounds; (4) the length of administration is congruent with the type of instrument (e.g., screening tools typically have about a 15-minute administration time; most comprehensive tools take at least 60 minute to administer); (5) if not a public domain tool, the cost is not prohibitive (e.g., some instruments might cost several dollars per case through purchase of the materials or contracts with commercial computer-based assessment systems); and (6) the expertise of existing personnel administering and interpreting the instrument is adequate to meet the requirements of the instrument (e.g., little training may be needed to administer a standardized questionnaire, but formal training may be needed to interpret the results).

Existing Instruments and Tools

A recent online catalogue, the PhenX Toolkit (https://www.phenxtoolkit.org/), describes a compendium of rigorously vetted and public-domain measures for a broad range of research domains, including drug use, underlying factors that trigger and maintain drug use, diagnostic symptoms, and co-occurring problems.

There are dozens of screening and comprehensive assessment instruments that measure aspects of adolescent drug abuse, mental health, and related issues (e.g., treatment readiness, personality traits). Table 5.3 provides brief descriptions of select screening and comprehensive instruments for assessing adolescent substance abuse and coexisting problems. We

Table 5.3 SELECT SCREENING AND COMPREHENSIVE ASSESSMENT TOOLS

Screening Tools

Instrument	Format	Administration Time (minutes)	Scoring Time (minutes)	Fee for Use	Source
CRAFFT+N 2.1	10 items	5	2	No	http://www.projectcork.org/clinical_tools/pdf/CRAFFT.pdf
GAIN-SS	20 items	10	2	No	http://gaincc.org/instruments/
PESQ	40 items	10	5	Yes	http://lib.adai.washington.edu/instruments

Comprehensive Tools

Instrument	Settings in Which Studied	Format	Administration Time (minutes)	Computer Scoring	Source
GAIN	Clinic, drug treatment, juvenile detention	Semi-structured interview	75–100	Yes	http://gaincc.org/instruments/
T-ASI	Clinic, drug treatment, juvenile detention	Semi-structured interview	25–45	No	kaminer@psychiatry.uchc.edu
PEI	Clinic, drug treatment, juvenile detention	Self-report	45–60	Yes	http://lib.adai.washington.edu/instruments

included tools associated with favorable psychometric data and that have been published in the peer-reviewed literature.

MINI-REVIEW

- Addiction occurs when repeated use of drugs changes how a person's brain functions over time. The transition from voluntary to compulsive drug use reflects changes in the brain's natural inhibition and reward centers that keep a person from exerting control over the impulse to use drugs even when there are negative consequences—the defining characteristic of addiction.

- Some people are more vulnerable to drug addiction than others, due to a range of possible risk factors. Stressful early life experiences, such as being abused or suffering other forms of trauma, are one important risk factor. Adolescents with a history of physical and/or sexual abuse are more likely to be diagnosed with substance use disorders. Many other risk factors, including genetic vulnerability, prenatal exposure to alcohol or other drugs, lack of parental supervision or monitoring, and association with drug-using peers, also play an important role.

- On average, adolescents tend to show a reduction in use following treatment, but post-treatment course is variable. Aftercare helps to maintain treatment gains, and more than one episode of treatment may be needed for some adolescents with more severe substance involvement.

- Accurately identifying those adolescents in need of drug-related services has been aided by over two decades of assessment research. Service providers and researchers have a range of adolescent screening and comprehensive assessment tools from which to choose. Developmentally informed assessment and intervention involve querying substance-related problems that are relevant to the adolescent's developmental stage and environmental context, and also assessing coexisting mental or behavioral problems.

DISCUSSION POINTS

1. Some experts have argued that "addiction does not discriminate. It can affect anyone." What are the arguments for and against this statement?

2. Cigarette taxation, warning labels, and smoke-free workplace laws have contributed to the reduction of use of tobacco products by youth (although the latest vaping trend is a current challenge). Discuss how these documented impacts of tobacco control interventions offer insights into interventions that might be adopted to combat other forms of substance abuse. Discuss what strategies might be fruitful if enacted.

3. From 2002 to 2014, the prevalence rate of meeting diagnostic criteria for any substance use disorder among adolescents who had used any substance decreased from 27.0% to 19.2% (Han et al., 2017). That is a significant decrease of about 30% across this time period. Why might this reduction have occurred? But this trend has not been maintained in recent years. Why might this be the case?

4. You are a counselor for a 17-year-old teenage girl who discloses that she is not practicing safe sex. Discuss the issues about whether or not this information should be disclosed to the parent.

5. Imagine you are the director of a local, community-based drug abuse prevention program. What steps and initiatives can you take to optimize the sustainability of your program?

6. How might adolescent brain development affect insight, motivation, and other factors related to an adolescent's willingness to engage in drug treatment?

FURTHER CURIOSITY AND DIGGING

Overview of the Science of Addiction

Learn.Genetics. (n.d.). *The science of addiction: Genetics and the brain.* University of Utah. https://learn.genetics.utah.edu/content/addiction/

Volkow, N. (2015). *The science of addiction.* [Video]. YouTube. https://acnp.org/videos/nora-volkow-the-science-of-addiction/

A Personal View of the Devastating Impact of Addiction

Sheff, D. (2008). *Beautiful boy: A father's journey through his son's addiction.* Houghton Mifflin.

The DSM-5 and Relevance to Adolescents

Winters, K. C., Martin, C. S., & Chung, T. (2011). Commentary on O'Brien: Substance use disorders in DSM-5 when applied to adolescents. *Addiction, 106,* 882–884.

The Health and Social Costs of Nicotine Addiction

Ekpu, V. U., & Brown, A. K. (2015). The economic impact of smoking and of reducing smoking prevalence: Review of evidence. *Tobacco Use Insights, 8,* TUI-S15628.

REFERENCES

American Psychiatric Association. (2013). *Diagnostic and statistical manual of mental disorders* (5th ed.). American Psychiatric Association.

Angold, A., Costello, E. J., & Erkanli, A. (1999). Comorbidity. *Journal of Child Psychology and Psychiatry and Allied Disciplines, 40*(1), 57–87.

Angold, A., Costello, E. J., Farmer, E. M., Burns, B. J., & Erkanli, A. (1999). Impaired but undiagnosed. *Journal of the American Academy of Child & Adolescent Psychiatry, 38,* 129–137.

Armstrong, T. D., & Costello, E. J. (2002). Community studies on adolescent substance use, abuse, or dependence and psychiatric comorbidity. *Journal of Consulting and Clinical Psychology, 70,* 1224–1239.

Brener, N. D., Billy, J. O., & Grady, W. R. (2003). Assessment of factors affecting the validity of self-reported health-risk behavior among adolescents: Evidence from the scientific literature. *Journal of Adolescent Health, 33,* 436–457.

Bukstein, O. G. (2005). Practice parameter for the assessment and treatment of children and adolescents with substance use disorders. *Journal of the American Academy of Child & Adolescent Psychiatry, 44,* 609–621.

Center for Behavioral Health Statistics and Quality. (2016). *Results from the 2015 National Survey on Drug Use and Health: Detailed tables.* Substance Abuse and Mental Health Services Administration.

Chan, Y. F., Dennis, M. L., & Funk, R. R. (2008). Prevalence and comorbidity of major internalizing and externalizing problems among adolescents and adults presenting to substance abuse treatment. *Journal of Substance Abuse Treatment, 34,* 14–24.

Christie, K. A., Burke, J. D., Regier, D. A., Rae, D. S., Boyd, J. H., & Locke, B. Z. (1988). Epidemiologic evidence for early onset of mental disorders and higher risk of drug abuse in young adults. *American Journal of Psychiatry, 145,* 971–975.

Chung, T., & Maisto, S. A. (2006). Relapse to alcohol and other drug use in treated adolescents: Review and reconsideration of relapse as a change point in clinical course. *Clinical Psychology Review, 26*, 149–161.

Chung T., Maisto, S. A., Cornelius, J. R., Martin, C. S., & Jackson, K. M. (2005). Joint trajectory analysis of treated adolescents' alcohol use and symptoms over 1-year. *Addictive Behavior, 30*, 1690–1701.

Chung, T., & Martin, C. S. (2005). What were they thinking?: Adolescents' interpretations of DSM-IV alcohol dependence symptom queries and implications for diagnostic validity. *Drug and Alcohol Dependence, 80*, 191–200.

Chung, T., Martin, C. S., & Clark, D. (2008). Concurrent change in alcohol and drug problems in treated adolescents over 3 years. *Journal of Studies on Alcohol, 69*. 420–429.

Chung, T., & Winters, K. C. (2018). Clinical characteristics of cannabis use disorder. In K. A. Sabet & K. C. Winters (Eds.), *Contemporary health issues on marijuana* (pp. 71–88). Oxford University Press.

Costello, E. J., Mustillo, S., Erkanli, A., Keeler, G., & Angold, A. (2003). Prevalence and development of psychiatric disorders in childhood and adolescence. *Archives of General Psychiatry, 60*, 837–844.

Dennis, M. L., Clark, H. W., & Huang, L. N. (2014). The need and opportunity to expand substance use disorder treatment in school-based settings. *Advances in School Mental Health Promotion, 7*, 75–87.

DiFranza, J. R., Savageau, J. A., Fletcher, K., Ockene, J. K., Rigotti, N. A., McNeill, A. D., Coleman, M., & Wood, C. (2002). Measuring the loss of autonomy over nicotine use in adolescents: The DANDY (Development and Assessment of Nicotine Dependence in Youths) Study. *Archives of Pediatrics & Adolescent Medicine, 156*, 397–403.

Farmer, R. F., Kosty, D. B., Seeley, J. R., Duncan, S. C., Lynskey, M. T., Rohde, P., . . . Lewinsohn, P. M. (2015). Natural course of cannabis use disorders. *Psychological Medicine, 45*, 63–72.

Groenman, A. P., Janssen, T. W. P., & Oosterlaan, J. (2017). Childhood psychiatric disorders as risk factor for subsequent substance abuse: A meta-analysis. *Journal of the American Academy of Child and Adolescent Psychiatry, 56*, 556–569.

Han, B., Compton, W. M., Blanco, C., & DuPont, R. L. (2017). National trends in substance use and use disorders among youth. *Journal of the American Academy of Child & Adolescent Psychiatry, 56*, 747–754.

Harford, T. C., Grant, B. F., Yi, H. Y., & Chen, C. M. (2005). Patterns of DSM-IV alcohol abuse and dependence criteria among adolescents and adults: Results from the 2001 National Household Survey on Drug Abuse. *Alcoholism: Clinical and Experimental Research, 29*, 810–828.

Kaminer, Y., & Bukstein, O. G. (2008). *Adolescent substance abuse: Psychiatric comorbidity and high-risk behaviors.* Taylor & Francis.

Kaminer, Y., & Winters, K. C. (Eds.) (2019). *Clinical manual of adolescent addictive disorders* (2nd ed.). American Psychiatric Association.

LaBrie, J. W., & Cail, J. (2011). Parental interaction with college students: The moderating effect of parental contact on the influence of perceived peer norms on drinking during the transition to college. *Journal of College Student Development, 52*, 610–621.

Maisto, S. A., Connors, G. J., & Allen, J. P. (1995). Contrasting self-report screens for alcohol problems: A review. *Alcoholism: Clinical and Experimental Research, 19,* 1510–1516.

McGue, M. (1999). Behavioral genetics models of alcoholism and drinking. In K. E. Leonard & H. T. Blane (Eds.), *Psychological theories of drinking and alcoholism* (2nd ed., pp. 372–421). Guilford.

Meier, M. H., Caspi, A., Ambler, A., Harrington, H., Houts, R., Keefe, R. S., . . . Moffitt, T. E. (2012). Persistent cannabis users show neuropsychological decline from childhood to midlife. *Proceedings of the National Academy of Sciences, USA, 109*(40), E2657–E2664.

Montana, G., & Chung, T. (2019). Diagnosis, epidemiology, and course of youth substance use and use disorders. In Y. Kaminer & K. C. Winters (Eds.), *Clinical manual of adolescent addictive disorders* (2nd ed., pp. 3–24). American Psychiatric Association.

National Institute on Drug Abuse. (2014). *Principles of adolescent substance use disorder treatment: A research-based guide.* NIH Publication Number 14-7953. National Institute on Drug Abuse.

Priester, M. A., Browne, T., Iachini, A., Clone, S., DeHart, D., & Seay, K. D. (2016). Treatment access barriers and disparities among individuals with co-occurring mental health and substance use disorders: An integrative literature review. *Journal of Substance Abuse Treatment, 61,* 47–59.

Reich, W., Shayla, J. J., & Taibelson, C. (1992). *The Diagnostic Interview for Children and Adolescents-Revised* (DICA-R). Washington University.

Robertson, E. B., David, S. L., & Rao, S. A. (2003). *Preventing drug use among children and adolescents: A research-based guide for parents, educators, and community leaders* (2nd ed.). National Institute on Drug Abuse.

Rose, R. J., Dick, D. M., Viken, R. J., Pulkkinen, L., & Kaprio, J. (2001). Drinking or abstaining at age 14? A genetic epidemiological study. *Alcoholism: Clinical and Experimental Research, 25,* 1594–1604.

Rosenberg, M. F., & Anthony, J. C. (2001). Early clinical manifestations of cannabis dependence in a community sample. *Drug and Alcohol Dependence, 64,* 123–131.

Sacks, J. J., Gonzales, K. R., Bouchery, E. E., Tomedi, L. E., & Brewer, R. D. (2015). 2010 national and state costs of excessive alcohol consumption. *American Journal of Preventive Medicine, 49,* e73–e79.

Scheier, L. S., Catalano, R., & Winters, K. C. (2019). Prevention of substance use and use disorders: Risk and protective factors, programs and implementation. In Y. Kaminer & K. C. Winters (Eds.), *Clinical manual of adolescent addictive disorders* (2nd ed., pp. 25–50). American Psychiatric Association.

Shaffer, D., Fisher, P., Dulcan, M. K., Davies, M., Piacentini, J., Schwab-Stone, M. E., . . . Canino, G. (1996). The NIMH Diagnostic Interview Schedule for Children Version 2.3 (DISC-2.3): Description, acceptability, prevalence rates, and performance in the MECA study. *Journal of the American Academy of Child & Adolescent Psychiatry, 35,* 865–877.

Sterling, S., & Weisner, C. (2005). Chemical dependency and psychiatric services for adolescents in private managed care: Implications for outcomes. *Alcoholism: Clinical and Experimental Research, 29,* 801–809.

Substance Abuse and Mental Health Services Administration. (2005). *Results from the 2004 National Survey on Drug Use and Health: Mental health findings*. Center for Behavioral Health Statistics and Quality, Substance Abuse and Mental Health Services Administration.

Substance Abuse and Mental Health Services Administration. (2013). *Results from the 2012 National Survey on Drug Use and Health: Summary of national findings*. NSDUH Series H-46, HHS Publication No. (SMA) 13-4795. Substance Abuse and Mental Health Services Administration.

Substance Abuse and Mental Health Services Administration. (2020). *Results from the 2019 National Survey on Drug Use and Health: Detailed tables*. Substance Abuse and Mental Health Services Administration. https://www.samhsa.gov/data

Substance Abuse and Mental Health Services Administration. (2021). *Treatment considerations for youth and young Adults with serious emotional disturbances/serious mental illnesses and co-occurring substance use*. Publication No. PEP20-06-02-001. National Mental Health and Substance Use Policy Laboratory, Substance Abuse and Mental Health Services Administration.

Sussman, S., Skara, S., & Ames, S. L. (2008). Substance abuse among adolescents. *Substance Use & Misuse, 43*, 1802–1828.

Swift, W., Coffey, C., Degenhardt, L., Carlin, J. B., Romaniuk, H., & Patton, G. C. (2012). Cannabis and progression to other substance use in young adults: Findings from a 13-year prospective population-based study. *Journal of Epidemiology and Community Health, 66*, e26–e26.

Tanner-Smith, E. E., Wilson, S. J., & Lipsey, M. W. (2013). The comparative effectiveness of outpatient treatment for adolescent substance abuse: A meta-analysis. *Journal of Substance Abuse Treatment, 44*, 145–158.

Tarter, R. E., & Horner, M. S. (2016). Developmental pathways to substance use disorder and co-occurring psychiatric disorders in adolescents. In Y. Kaminer (Ed.), *Youth substance abuse and co-occurring disorders* (pp. 1–22). American Psychiatric Association Publishing.

U.S. Department of Health and Human Services. (2016). *Surgeon General's report on alcohol, drugs, and health: Executive summary*. https://addiction.surgeongeneral.gov/executive-summary

Wagner, F. A., & Anthony, J. C. (2002). From first drug use to drug dependence: Developmental periods of risk for dependence upon marijuana, cocaine, and alcohol. *Neuropsychopharmacology, 26*, 479–488.

Waldron, H. B., Turner, C. W., & Ozechowski, T. J. (2005). Profiles of drug use behavior change for adolescents in treatment. *Addictive Behaviors, 30*, 1775–1796.

Winters, K. C., Anderson, N., Bengston, P., Stinchfield, R. D., & Latimer, W. W. (2000). Development of a parent questionnaire for use in assessing adolescent drug abuse. *Journal of Psychoactive Drugs, 32*, 3–13.

Winters, K. C., Botzet, A. M., & Lee, S. (2018). Assessing adolescent substance use problems and other areas of functioning: State of the art. In P. Monti, S. Colby, & T. O'Leary (Eds.), *Adolescents, alcohol and substance use: Reaching teens through brief intervention* (2nd ed., pp. 83–107). The Guilford Press.

Winters, K. C., Botzet, A. M., Stinchfield, R., Gonzalez, R., Finch, A., Piehler, T., Ausherbauer, K., Chalmers, K., & Hemze, A. (2018). Adolescent substance abuse treatment: A review of evidence-based research. In C. Leukefeld, T. Gullotta, & M. Staton Tindall (Eds.), *Adolescent substance abuse: Evidence-based approaches to prevention and treatment* (2nd ed., pp. 141–171). Springer Science+Business Media.

Winters, K. C., Fahnhorst, T., Botzet, A. M., Nicholson, A., & Stinchfield, R. D. (2014). Assessing adolescent substance use. In R. Reis, D. Fiellin, S. Miller, & R. Saitz (Eds.), *The ASAM principles of addiction medicine* (5th ed., pp. 1609–1626). Wolters Kluwer.

Winters, K. C., & Henly, G. A. (1993). *Adolescent Diagnostic Interview schedule and manual*. Western Psychological Services.

Winters, K. C., & Lee, S. (2008). Likelihood of developing an alcohol and cannabis use disorder during youth: Association with recent use and age. *Drug and Alcohol Dependence, 92*, 239–247.

Winters, K. C., Martin, C. S., & Chung, T. (2011). Commentary on O'Brien: Substance use disorders in DSM-5 when applied to adolescents. *Addiction, 106*, 882–884.

Winters, K. C., Stinchfield, R., Latimer, W. W., & Stone, A. (2008). Internalizing and externalizing behaviors and their association with the treatment of adolescents with substance use disorder. *Journal of Substance Abuse Treatment, 35*, 269–278.

Internalizing and Related Disorders

CHAPTER OUTLINE

INTRODUCTION

The next two chapters discuss the two largest domains of disorders that coexist with adolescent substance use disorder (SUD)—internalizing and externalizing disorders. Both of these domains consist of several subgroups. For each we will review the epidemiology, clinical characteristics, and treatment and will provide case examples. As discussed in the Introduction, adolescents diagnosed with an SUD also commonly suffer from one or more co-occurring behavioral or mental disorders. As numerous survey studies indicate, it is the rule rather than the exception for a co-occurring disorder; approximately 70–80% of adolescents receiving treatment for an SUD have at least one coexisting disorder (Kaminer & Winters, 2019). And the presence of a coexisting disorder typically negatively impacts the course and treatment outcomes of SUD. In general, comorbid disorders are associated with more severe substance use and SUD symptoms, more substance-related problems, and poorer treatment outcome (Kaminer & Winters, 2019). Also as we noted in the Introduction, the coexisting disorders of depression, attention-deficit/hyperactivity disorder (ADHD), oppositional defiant disorder, and conduct disorder appear to be reliably linked to adolescent SUDs with less of a link between anxiety disorders and SUDs (Groenman et al., 2017).

In this chapter we address *internalizing disorders* and their main disorder subgroups—depression, anxiety, and post-traumatic stress disorder (PTSD). Internalizing disorders share the feature of emotional distress to the point of contributing to functioning problems. We will also briefly discuss bipolar disorder and autism, disorders that have some features common to the core internalizing disorders.

EMOTION

Underlying all internalizing disorders is emotion. Emotions reflect our relations with our surroundings, including people, and serve as an adaptive tool to deal with life's challenges (Miu et al., 2019). Adolescents in particular respond emotionally to both positive opportunities and negative events, and when emotions are extreme, they may dominant one's decision making. We described in Chapter 3 how brain development during adolescence contributes to high emotionality, which in turn may lead to regrettable decisions. The state of one's emotions will impact our mood, social functioning, cognitive functioning, and overall health.

Ways that high emotionality may affect an adolescent's decision making:

1. Seeing multiple options
2. Predicting outcome of an action
3. Appreciating consequences
4. Considering differential weight of options
5. Considering risk of situation
6. Controlling self-control

The consequences of emotions can be adaptive or maladaptive. Germaine to our chapter is the issue that poor regulation of emotions can contribute to developing an internalizing disorder. Indeed, the disorders discussed in their chapter are often noted as "emotional difficulties" associated with experiencing a lot of stress, whereas ameliorating underlying emotional distress is a key to treating internalizing disorders. This latter point will become apparent when treatment approaches for internal disorders are discussed.

INTERSECTION OF INTERNALIZING DISORDERS AND SUBSTANCE USE DISORDER

Symptoms of internalizing disorders (e.g., anxiety, depression) have been found to predict SUDs in adolescents. For example, the Oregon Adolescent Depression Project found that anxiety and depressive disorders at baseline (adolescence) were associated with significantly greater odds of abusing cannabis and alcohol at the early adulthood follow-up after controlling for relevant variables (e.g., gender, depression, conduct disorder) (e.g., Buckner et al., 2008). Similar findings were found in a large longitudinal study of a New Zealand cohort (Goodwin et al., 2004). These and other studies provide support for the model that substance use is a way for the adolescent to cope with internalizing issues. However, the effects of substances on internalizing symptoms are complex, and these symptoms may emerge as or be exacerbated by substance use (Kushner et al., 2000).

An adolescent's age and the type and severity of the substance use are important considerations. Thus, the directionality of the internalizing problems and substance use connection is not clearly one direction.

Some experts have argued that internalizing disorders may be a "protective factor" for using substances. What features or depression, anxiety, and PTSD may provide a protection again using? Possible answers:

1. Internalizing disorders are associated with elevated behavioral inhibition and behavioral inhibition may counteract reward seeking associated with negative consequences.
2. Individuals with internalizing disorders are less likely to affiliate with deviant peers; these persons may experience cannabis to be less reinforcing.
3. Substance use may lead to the worsening of internalizing symptoms thus making continued use less likely.

DEPRESSION

Prevalence

One of the most common mental and behavioral disorders among adolescents in the United States is depression. According to a report from the Blue Cross Blue Shield Association (2018), which examined health claims for treatment from over millions of commercially insured Americans, those who met an official diagnosis of a major depressive disorder (MDD) has appreciably risen since 2013. Based on results from the National Survey on Drug Use and Health, rates of major depression in adolescents have increased by 47% for boys and 65% for girls, and among millennials (born 2000 or later) this rate is also rising—up by 47% (McCance-Katz, 2019). Also trending is that its onset is moving to an earlier age. In the mid-1990s only 8.3% of adolescents met criteria for a current (within a prior year) MDD (described below) (McCance-Katz, 2019). Yet in 2016 this figure was 12.8%. And the coexistence with substance use was significant: Among those suffering from depression, nearly a third of those reported using at least one substance (only 13% were substance users among those adolescents without an MDD) (McCance-Katz, 2019). The COVID-19 pandemic and the resulting lockdown and in-school prohibitions have been cited as contributing to higher rates of depression and suicidal ideation among adolescents (Hollenstein et al., 2021).

Characteristics

An MDD is a period of at least 2 weeks of low mood that is present in most situations. Symptoms include low self-esteem, loss of interest in normally enjoyable activities, and problems with sleep, energy, and concentration. Early warning signs are likely to include many features that can be mistaken for normal adolescent behavior: irritability, fatigue, changes in sleep patterns, changes in eating patterns, social withdrawal, and anger.

An adolescent with MDD finds it difficult or impossible to do normal daily activities, such as studying, sleeping, and eating, and they typically lose interest in social activities. Without treatment, MDD episodes can last for long periods of time; those who have had one episode are at high risk of having another.

The diagnostic criteria for MDD in the DSM-5 are very similar to the criteria in the DSM's previous edition, DSM-IV. But there is one important difference: DSM-5 now allows a diagnosis of MDD if depressive symptoms persist for longer than 2 months after the loss of a loved one. Also required are a marked functional impairment, chronic preoccupation with worthlessness, and suicidal ideation.

DSM-5 diagnostic criteria for depression. The official criteria from the American Psychiatric Association for MDD, published in their most recent publication of diagnostic criteria for mental disorders (DSM-5; American Psychiatric Association, 2013), are provided below. To receive a diagnosis of MDD, the adolescent must be experiencing five or more symptoms among the eight during the same 2-week period, at least one of the symptoms needs to be either depressed mood (symptom #1) or loss of interest or pleasure (symptom #2), and these symptoms must contribute to significant distress or impairment in social, occupational, or other important areas of functioning for the person. Also, the symptoms must also not be a result of a medical condition or substance use.

1. Depressed mood most of the day, nearly every day
2. Markedly diminished interest or pleasure in all, or almost all, activities most of the day, nearly every day
3. Significant weight loss when not dieting or weight gain, or decrease or increase in appetite nearly every day
4. A slowing down of thought and a reduction of physical movement (observable by others, not merely subjective feelings of restlessness or being slowed down)
5. Fatigue or loss of energy nearly every day
6. Feelings of worthlessness or excessive or inappropriate guilt nearly every day
7. Diminished ability to think or concentrate, or indecisiveness, nearly every day
8. Recurrent thoughts of death, recurrent suicidal ideation without a specific plan, or a suicide attempt or a specific plan for committing suicide

Other Features

Individuals with MDD are at elevated risk to commit suicide, which is one reason this disorder is associated with high mortality. Also, depressed individuals may experience anxiety and excessive worry over physical health and may show irritability and brooding. The revised

DSM-5, DSM-5-TR, will include options for the counselor to specifically document the presence or history of suicidal behavior and nonsuicidal self-injury, the later defined as intentional self-inflicted damage to one's body that is likely to induce bleeding, bruising, or pain but absent of suicidal intent.

Subthreshold depression. Many adolescents have significant depressive symptoms but do not meet strict DSM-5 criteria for MDD. It has been estimated that 5–29% of adolescents have significant depressive symptoms without meeting diagnostic criteria for MDD (Carrellas et al., 2017). These individuals have significant psychosocial impairment and elevated rates of psychiatric comorbidities and SUD, and many will suffer from subsequent episodes of MDD (Hill et al., 2014). Thus, adolescents with less than five symptoms of depression can benefit from treatment to address their clinically significant depressed mood.

Some experts have warned that the rate of adolescents who have seriously considered committing suicide is increasing at an alarming rate. Suicide was the 10th most common cause of death among Americans of all ages in 2017, it was the second leading cause of death among young Americans in the United States who are ages 15 to 24 (Curtin & Heron, 2019). In the home state of the authors—Minnesota—a recent statewide student health survey indicated that 13% of 11th graders reported seriously considering suicide.

SOURCE: https://www.mprnews.org/story/2019/10/17/survey-finds-mn-students-feel-less-safe-less-healthy

Despite decades of research on correlates and risk factors for adolescent suicide, little is known about why suicidal ideation and behavior frequently emerge in adolescence and how to predict, and ultimately prevent, suicidal behavior among youths.

A recent scholarly review of the literature on this topic concluded that adolescent suicide is a failure of biological responses to acute distress that is unusual and severe and exceeds the adolescent's perceived capacity to cope (Miller & Prinstein, 2019). Due to variability in biological responses to stress, youth vary in the extent to which they experience adaptive or nonadaptive biological responses (e.g., autonomic nervous system), as manifested by differences in stress thresholds, during these critical stress situations. The authors suggest the need for more education of youth about the nature of stress and coping strategies.

Sadness Differs from Depression

There is a difference between depression and sadness, but the difference can be difficult to distinguish. The most prominent distinction is in terms of severity. Sadness is a normal emotional reaction that most individuals will experience as a result of some disappointment (e.g., the end of a relationship) or loss (e.g., death of a loved one). This type of sadness usually leads to feeling down in the dumps for a day or two, but the person is still able to find joy or enjoyment from daily experiences, such as having a favorite meal or talking with a friend. But for those suffering from MDD, the sadness does not have to be triggered by an event and it is very severe and lasting, and other symptoms occur (e.g., problems sleeping, physical symptoms, impairment with every day functioning).

Sadness can stem from experiencing a significant life event. Common ones faced by adolescents are the following (Low et al., 2012):

1. Romantic breakup
2. Family disruption (divorce/separation or new family)
3. Relationship with father
4. Relationship with mother

5. Relationship with siblings
6. Relationship with friends
7. Health problem
8. Weight
9. School work

Treatment of depressive disorders with psychotherapeutic strategies, whether individual or group format, can be effective treatments for MDD. A common approach is the use of cognitive behavioral therapy (CBT) that restructures depressive cognitions (e.g., "I will not feel better") and supports skills to cope with depression (e.g., confronting the urge to be socially isolated) (Hawke et al., 2008).

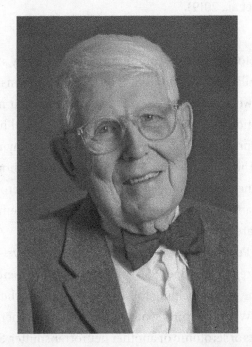

Aaron Beck, M.D. (born 1921) is regarded as the father of cognitive-based therapy for depression.
Photo courtesy of Beck Institute for Cognitive Behavior Therapy, www.beckinstitute.org.

Group therapy has many advantages when treating teenagers: They can connect with other adolescents who understand their struggles; strategies for dealing with depression are shared; and support networks beyond their immediate families and close friends can be created.

Severe cases of MDD may need medication. A physician needs to determine whether medication is necessary and carefully evaluate the teenager during the course of medication treatment. Selective serotonin reuptake inhibitors (SSRIs) are antidepressant medications that have been shown to be effective for adolescents diagnosed with MDD. Yet antidepressant medication does come with risks. In 2004, the U.S. Food and Drug Administration issued a warning about SSRI medications for children and adolescent in that they may increase the risk of suicidal thoughts or behavior in some adolescents. There is also the concern that introducing SSRIs while the adolescent brain is developing can hinder healthy brain maturation (Kaminer et al., 2019).

Selective serotonin reuptake inhibitors (SSRIs) work by affecting brain chemicals called *neurotransmitters*. These neurotransmitters send messages between brain cells, also called *neurons*. Their messages help regulate emotion and therefore directly impact mental health. To understand the process better, let's break down the acronym.

Selective: The word *selective* indicates that SSRIs primarily increase levels of the neurotransmitter known as *serotonin*. Serotonin is only one of the many neurotransmitters in the brain. Dopamine and norepinephrine are two of the other brain chemicals.

Serotonin: People with depression often have low levels of serotonin in areas that regulate mood. SSRIs increase levels of serotonin in the brain, with the goal of helping these areas to function better.

Reuptake: When neurons send signals to one another, they release small amounts of serotonin or another neurotransmitter. Subsequently, they take back the neurotransmitter they released in order to use it to send another signal. This process is called *reuptake*.

Inhibitor: SSRIs for anxiety and depression block the reuptake of serotonin in the brain. Therefore, more serotonin is available to regulate mood.

Adolescents with *combined depression and SUD* have higher rates of perceived service needs, receive more treatment services than non-comorbid adolescents, and pose more challenges when it comes to treatment (Kaminer et al., 2019). Treating both depression and SUD likely optimizes the outcomes for both problem areas, whereas treatments for SUD alone or depression alone do not adequately address the need of all youth with co-occurring depression and SUD (Curry et al., 2012; Rohde et al., 2018). Hersh and colleagues conducted a comprehensive review of 11 studies that investigated the influence of co-occurring depression on SUD treatment outcome. The findings were varied. The relationship between depression and substance abuse treatment outcome across the studies did not show a consistent pattern, suggesting that depression does not have a simple relationship with substance-related treatment outcomes (Hersh et al., 2014). Maximizing the effects of treatment may be achieved by combining medication (e.g., an antidepressant such as Prozac) and behavioral treatment in an integrative model (Riggs et al., 2007).

Adolescents who show a relatively quick response to treatment for depression tend to maintain their positive response more so than those who take longer to respond. Known as *rapid responders,* youth who show this treatment effect can achieve positive treatment outcomes that are considerably better than the minimal effects typically achieved by those judged as nonresponders. One study found that approximately 40% of adolescents aged 13–21 years with SUD and co-occurring depression showed a rapid clinical response 4 weeks after onset of treatment (Kaminer et al., 2008).

Case Illustration of Depression

Jimmy; age: 14; ethnicity: Caucasian; gender: male; sexual orientation: heterosexual; family situation: biological mother; step-father; collage-age brother (not at home); 11-year-old sister; school: mainstream middle high school

Jimmy is a 14-year-old Caucasian male who has been brought to a community mental health clinic by his mother. She is concerned about his change in attitude and behavior in the last 6 months or so. He recently refused to eat dinner with his family. She reports she is concerned and has "tried everything—even took his phone away and he doesn't care. He seems to be in a dark spot."

Jimmy is the middle child. He has one older brother who attends collage out of state and reports having a good relationship with him. His younger sister is 11 and frustrates Jimmy because "she gets whatever she wants whenever she wants it and my parents think she's perfect."

Jimmy is a ninth grader and a marginal student. School has never been "fun" but he tolerated it and received passing grades up until last year. Jimmy has a few friends, but most of his friends went to a different high school after last year. He spends most of his time in his room sleeping or in the basement of their home watching YouTube.

He recently has been smoking pot a few times a week. He does not consider it a big deal; he started smoking last year with some older guys after school. He got suspended once for smoking pot on the playground while "hanging out" after school. He reported to the school social worker that pot helps him to "chill out." She agreed to not share this with his parents this time, because he is generally such a good kid.

Clinical points to ponder:

1. Does grief have any impact on Jimmy's mood? If so, what are the factors to consider?
2. What is the impact of marijuana use on Jimmy's outlook?
3. Identify Jimmy's protective factors in his life.
4. Are there any ethical considerations in Jimmy's case?

ANXIETY

Prevalence

Anxiety disorders are among the most common mental disorders across the life span (lifetime prevalence estimates are usually in the 6–12% range) and typically have their onset much earlier in life than other commonly occurring behavior disorders (Kessler et al., 2009). Thus, it is not surprising that, among adolescents, anxiety disorders are highly prevalent, including often co-occurring among adolescents with an SUD (Blumenthal et al., 2011). The diverse range of problems represented by anxiety disorders complicates their relationships with substance use and SUD (Kushner et al., 2000). Several studies indicate that anxiety disorders are more frequent among female adolescents than in male adolescents (Kaminer et al., 2019).

There are several subtypes of anxiety disorders. Table 6.1 provides a summary of the prevalence rates of anxiety subtypes (Kaminer et al., 2019). Some of these disorders' onset is during pre-adolescence and their rate declines during adolescence. Another feature is that depression commonly accompanies anxiety disorders.

Table 6.1 PREVALENCE RATES OF ANXIETY DISORDERS AMONG ADOLESCENTS

Type of Anxiety Disorder	Approximate Prevalence Rate among Adolescents
Simple phobia	5.0%
Separation anxiety	4.0%
Social phobia	1.5%
Panic disorder	1.0%
Obsessive-compulsive disorder	1.0%
Generalized anxiety	1.0%
Agoraphobia	1.0%
Multiple anxiety disorders	25%

Characteristics

Similar to the problem of distinguishing common features of adolescence from clinical depression, it can be a challenge to determine when an adolescent is expressing normal stress and emotionality or showing signs of an anxiety disorder. When an adolescent is experiencing an anxiety disorder, the level of anxiety is severe and typically gets worse over time, and it interferes with daily activities at school and work and their relationships with peers and family members.

Anxiety *symptoms* take many forms: restlessness or feeling keyed up or on edge; being easily fatigued; difficulty concentrating or mind going blank; irritability; physical discomforts (e.g., muscle tensions; sweating); and difficulty falling or staying asleep. Within the category of anxiety disorders there are many symptoms that will overlap and anxiety conditions can sometimes be confused with one another. Also, these symptoms can be found in many mental health conditions listed in the DSM-5, such as within depressive disorders and eating disorders. But for all subtypes of anxiety disorders (described below), the symptoms have to be severe and persistent (lasting at least 1 month for some subtypes and 6 months for others), include anxious-related thinking, and negatively impact the person's daily functioning.

DSM-5 subtypes. The DSM-5 diagnostic system includes the following anxiety disorders: simple phobia, separation anxiety disorder, social anxiety, panic disorder, agoraphobia, and generalized anxiety disorder. Obsessive-compulsive disorder (OCD) and PTSD are assigned to separate categories as a major change from DSM-IV to DSM-5. These subtypes of anxiety disorders, as well as OCD and PTSD, are described below.

Features common to anxiety disorder subtypes in the DMS-5 are the following:

1. The disturbance is not better explained by another mental disorder (e.g., content of delusional beliefs in schizophrenia).

2. The disturbance is not attributable to the physiological effects of substance abuse or a medical condition.
3. Symptoms occur more days than not for at least 6 months.

Simple phobias. A specific phobia is an intense, persistent, and irrational fear of a well-defined object or situation. Some individuals suffer from several specific phobias simultaneously. People with a simple phobia know that their fear is irrational, is not based on fact, and does not make rational sense. Nevertheless, thoughts and feelings of anxiety persist and are chronic in nature. Phobias fall under four categories: natural (e.g., lightning), mutilation (e.g., needle injections), animal (e.g., snakes), and situational (e.g., heights). A phobia is distinguishable from a fear. Being phobic about a situation or object means that the person displays unreasonable and excessive fear that leads to immediate anxiety, and the afflicted person goes out of their way to avoid the object or situation or endures it with extreme distress.

Some common phobias:

- Acrophobia, fear of heights
- Aerophobia, fear of flying
- Arachnophobia, fear of spiders
- Astraphobia, fear of thunder and lightning
- Autophobia, fear of being alone
- Claustrophobia, fear of confined or crowded spaces
- Hemophobia, fear of blood
- Hydrophobia, fear of water
- Ophidiophobia, fear of snakes
- Zoophobia, fear of animals

Separation anxiety. Separation anxiety disorder is defined by excessive anxiety about separation from parents or other individuals to whom the adolescent is attached. Youth with separation anxiety disorder fear being lost from their family or fear something bad happening to a family member if they are separated from them. Symptoms of anxiety or fear about being separated from family members must last for a significant period. A separation anxiety disorder is different from stranger anxiety, which is normal and usually experienced by nearly every child at some point up to age 3.

Social anxiety. This is defined by the persistent fear of embarrassment and discomfort in situations involving social scrutiny. Whereas all of us have felt anxious on some social settings, those with a social anxiety disorder have a heightened fear of nearly all social interactions in all situations. The person is constantly worried about what others think of them (an excessive form of fear of being scrutinized) to the point that they avoid social interactions. This intense anxiety causes impairment in functioning and interferes significantly with the individual's life and relationships. At its extreme, the sufferer will not leave the house for fear of being judged by others. The negative impacts of a social anxiety disorder can be severe. The person may not be able to maintain friendships, find it hard to go to school or hold down a job, and may be a barrier to carrying out simple tasks that require leaving the house (e.g., collecting mail from the mailbox).

Common situations that trigger significant distress for people with social anxiety are the following:

- Speaking in public
- Being the center of attention
- Talking to strangers
- Going on dates
- Meeting new people
- Interviewing for a new job
- Going to work or school

Public Speaking

Comfortably and effectively communicating your ideas in a public forum is an essential component of success across many domains of life. Yet fear of public speaking is quite common; approximately 25% of people report experiencing it.

Your career and relationships can be advanced by being a good public speaker. It can help you promote ideas and motivate colleagues and others to engage to act. For many, this skill accelerates a person's professional and personal growth. Yet fear is a barrier for many to stand in front of a crowd and deliver an idea, a story, or one's body of work. Experts point to the value of practicing to overcome this fear.

Panic disorder. Panic disorder is defined by relatively short periods of intense fear that are not the result of exposure to a feared situation. This acute fear episode is a panic attack. Pain attacks are sudden waves of terror characterized by convulsing of the body, difficulty breathing, and thoughts that one is dying. They usually subside within 30 minutes, after which the person usually feels very fatigued. Those suffering from a panic disorder have panic attacks repeatedly.

Agoraphobia. Panic disorder is often accompanied by agoraphobia, a disorder in which the person has an extreme fear of being in situations where there is no easy way to escape or get help if the anxiety intensifies. The sufferer feels trapped, helpless, or embarrassed in such situations and a panic attack may occur. Those with this disorder fear situations such as being in a crowd, using public transportation, or being in open or enclosed spaces. The anxiety can be so severe that they may not leave home. To deal with these extreme fears, sufferers will often ask a friend or companion to accompany them when out in public places.

Generalized anxiety disorder. This type of anxiety involves excessive anxiety or worry over everyday events that for most people would not contribute to excessive worrying. For example, most of us worry that if a car raced through a red light, a serious car accident may happen. Such an event is possible but it is unlikely to happen to any individual person. Adolescents with generalized anxiety experience intense emotional stress that lasts for an extended period of time and display a range of anxiety-related symptoms (low self-esteem, frequent heart palpitations, trembling).

Other anxiety-related disorders. One type of disorder related to anxiety is *OCD*. Obsessions are persistent, *irrational*, or *distorted* thoughts that are experienced as intrusive, and compulsions are repetitive and intentional behaviors performed in response to obsessions. The obsessions and compulsions are so severe that they interfere with everyday living. An example of a "checking" OCD would be leaving your car worried that you left the door unlocked. Even after returning to your car several times, you are still not convinced that you locked the door. Other types of OCD rituals are contamination based (e.g., repeatedly washing one's hands over fear about germs and disease) and symmetry based (e.g., excessive need for orderliness or exactness).

The distinction between irrational and distorted thoughts is worth additional discussion. An *irrational thought* is based on a most extreme unlikely possibility and cannot be factually supported. It is irrational to believe that unless you immediately wash your hands, you will always get sick every time you touch a doorknob.

In contrast, a *distorted belief* is often based on a rational point of view but takes a very extreme or gross distortion of that point of view. Hoarders are an example. Whereas it is true that being thrifty and not being wasteful is of admirable value, it is a distortion to believe that *everything* has significant value and nothing should ever be discarded. These distinctions are important for treatment reasons. Trying to convince someone that an irrational thought is not sensible and harmful is easier than trying to refute a person's distorted thoughts. One type of treatment for OCD is exposure therapy, a technique in which the client is exposed to those things that they fear the most (triggers) (Foa, 2011).

A&E Television Networks has produced several seasons of *Hoarders*. Each episode focuses on a specific family dealing with a family member with a hoarding affliction. "*Hoarders* team of experts come together to help families understand the impact of this devastating mental disorder while racing against the clock to help clean the hoards and avert crisis."

Summary of season 2, episode 5: Julie is living a nightmare. A series of tragedies triggered massive hoarding, which in turn led to Julie's son moving in with her ex-husband. Now she must clean up or risk losing the two daughters who still live with her. Shannon, her husband Tim, and their four young children live in a house that is filled with garbage and infested with mice. Her dogs roam freely in the clutter, and there's a 2-foot hole in the bathroom floor. She was devastated when Animal Control removed 20 cats from the home 3 weeks ago. Now, as cameras are rolling, police arrive at the front door with Child Protective Services to remove her children.

SOURCE: https://www.aetv.com/shows/hoarders

Another type of anxiety-related disorder is *PTSD* (more on PTSD below). Many people who experience directly or indirectly a tragic event may experience a lasting effect that leads to a PTSD. PTSD among adolescents can be caused by a single traumatic event (acute trauma), such a witnessing or being a victim of a crime or the death of a parent, or by an ongoing traumatic event (chronic trauma), such as exposure to childhood abuse or gang violence. To qualify as a traumatic event for DSM-5, it can be experienced, or witnessed as it occurred to someone else, or the person learned about it where a close relative or friend experienced the actual event. Suffers may find it difficult to carry out normal daily activities because of periods of anger and depression, experience nightmares or flashbacks, and have reoccurring and upsetting memories of the trauma. The person frequently avoids reminders associated with the traumatic event, may block memories or important aspects of the event, and can be prone to blame themselves for the cause of it. Symptoms must be present for at least a month.

Not all individuals who are abused in childhood suffer serious impairments. Certain people seem behaviorally resilient despite a history of maltreatment. What then, is the difference, biologically, between those who are behaviorally susceptible and those who are resilient?

A recent study (Ohashi et al., 2019) compared these two groups and found that the resilient group had abnormalities in overall brain network architecture that were "at least as strong" as those seen in the susceptible group. But the resilient participants had additional abnormalities, which ironically appeared to have protected them. This, the researchers hypothesized, may partially isolate and limit the harmful impact of susceptible components in the network, resulting in no long-term impacts on behavior.

Treatment of Anxiety Disorders

At this time, recommendations for comorbid anxiety disorders and SUD in adolescents are based on little empirical study. But based on what extant research exists, effective treatments for adolescent anxiety disorders include several modalities: individual psychosocial interventions, family therapy, education of the adolescent and parents, and pharmacotherapy. As is the case with all treatments for coexisting disorders, there are potential complications when an SUD is present. The anxiety disorder may alter response to treatment for the SUD and vice versa. The major types of effective psychosocial treatments for anxiety disorders have utilized CBT approaches (Connolly & Bernstein, 2007). Banneyer and colleagues (2018) comprehensively reviewed this approach and concluded that CBT has been shown to be effective for a range of anxiety disorders in adolescents and is associated with long-term benefit. Key elements to effective individual or group CBT are cognitive restructuring, relaxation training, and exposure to the stimuli associated with the distress (Banneyer et al., 2018).

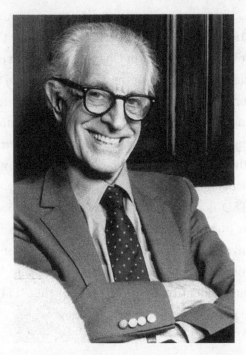

Albert Ellis is a famous American psychologist (1913–2007) acknowledged for developing a prominent behavior theory often used to treat anxiety disorders—rational emotive therapy (RET). This approach teaches the client to counter their anxieties with rational beliefs grounded in reality (e.g., "Flying is safer than traveling by car.").
© Albert Ellis Institute

Family interventions for anxiety disorders in adolescents typically focus on steering the parent–adolescent relationship to an appropriate balance between parental involvement and adolescent independence (AACAP, 2007). This counselling strategy to achieve a healthy "balance" needs to take into consideration the adolescent's self-regulation skills and the parents' capabilities for effective parenting.

Why are antidepressant medications effective for the treatment of anxiety disorders? Certain antidepressants affect levels of serotonin (selective) by preventing its absorption (reuptake) by nerve cells in the brain. By stabilizing levels of serotonin, these medications decrease feelings of anxiety.

The standard treatment for OCD is cognitive behavior therapy (CBT), a treatment strategy highlighted in Chapter 10. The aim of therapy is to increase the client's insights about the disabling effects of the obsessions and compulsions and practice specific strategies to counter them. These include systematic desensitization (e.g., pairing relaxation techniques while imagining the distressful obsession), cognitive restructuring (e.g., emphasizing that obsessive concerns can be ignored), and behavioral goals (e.g., practicing anti-compulsive alternatives).

Treating PTSD is complex. A contemporary approach is the dialectic behavior therapy (DBT), which we also discuss in Chapter 10. Briefly, DBT involves a CBT approach to help the person manage their painful emotions and decrease conflict in relationship. The treatment approach includes identifying the triggers of the PTSD arousal and improving the person's regulation of emotions.

Pharmacological approaches to adolescent anxiety disorders include traditional tricyclic antidepressants (e.g., Elavil, Tofrinal) and SSRIs (e.g., Celexa, Lexapro) (Leonte et al., 2018). The beneficial effects of medications on anxiety disorders in adolescents have also been shown to continue over an extended period (Leonte et al., 2018; Walkup et al., 2008). When tricyclic antidepressants and SSRIs have been compared, results have shown that it is advisable to try SSRIs first, given that the effectiveness of tricyclic antidepressant medications for anxiety disorders in children and adolescent is not impressive (Connolly & Bernstein, 2007). But in sum, psychosocial interventions are preferred over pharmacological interventions for initial treatment of youth with a coexisting anxiety disorder and SUD. The empirical literature is silent on the integration of psychosocial and pharmacotherapy, so it needs to be guided by clinical practice (Kaminer et al., 2019).

Case Illustration of Generalized Anxiety Disorder

Sloan; age: 14; ethnicity: Caucasian; gender: transgender female; sexual orientation: "I am not sure"; family situation: biological and biological parents distant; school: mainstream; clinical setting: school-based mental health clinic

The concern that Sloan would like to work on most is being able to fall asleep. She often goes to bed at about 10 PM and does not fall asleep until after 1:00 AM, only to get up at 6:30 AM, to get ready for school. She is often moody and irritable, a problem for which her family has little tolerance. She reports everything else is "fine."

Sloan is a 14-year-old who lives in an upper middle–class neighborhood with her parents and her 12-year-old brother. Sloan's mother describes Sloan as "always being pretty tightly wound up—but I guess we all are at times."

Sloan's parents recently had a meeting with school administrators to asked them not to distribute the most recent orchestra concert video. Sloan is a member of the junior high orchestra—she is the first chair violin. In the first 20 minutes of the performance Sloan got up and walked off stage—not to return. Sloan was horrified and does not want anyone else to recall the incident because it is so embarrassing. She missed the next week of orchestra and was moved to second chair.

Sloan has two to three close friends who she feels "good" with most of the time. She does not want to participate in sleep-overs even though she is invited to them on occasion.

Clinical points to ponder:

1. Is it helpful to Sloan to have her parents stop the distribution of the video?—Please discuss your reasoning.
2. How does sleep impact Sloan?
3. Is Sloan potentially a candidate for anti-anxiety medication? Explain the reasons on both sides of the debate.
4. Could her gender be a factor in social situations? Please discuss your reasoning.

OTHER DISORDERS

Post-Traumatic Stress Disorder

Subsequent to being impacted by a tragic event, a person may experience lasting effects. In some instances, this trauma can elicit a PTSD. Tragic events for adolescents can include accidents, natural disasters, fires, crimes, the loss of a parent or other family member, and being victimized by physical, sexual, or emotional abuse (often referred to adverse childhood experiences). Both "acute" trauma and "chronic" trauma can lead to PTSD. An *acute trauma* is a single tragic event, such as seeing a violent crime. *Chronic trauma* is being exposed to ongoing trauma; examples include exposure to childhood abuse, domestic violence, or gang violence. The DSM-5 (American Psychiatric Association, 2013) diagnosis of PTSD includes the following criteria:

- Direct, witnessed or indirect exposure to a traumatic event
- The traumatic event is persistently re-experienced via unwanted and upsetting memories and/or nightmares
- Negative thoughts or feelings that began or worsened after the trauma
- Symptoms lasting more than a month that interfere with normal functioning

As many as two in three adolescents report having been exposed to traumatic stressors at some point in their lives, including directly experiencing or witnessing violence, abuse, injury, or loss, war and terrorism, and life-threatening disasters (see Masten & Narayan, 2012, for a review). Trauma-exposed adolescents are at risk for not only PTSD but also major depressive disorder and related behavioral and psychosocial problems (e.g., Ford et al., 2010). Also, how an adolescent responds to stress may be related to the biologically based stress response (Kuhlman et al., 2018).

SUD is a common comorbidity of PTSD among adolescents, which suggests that a major subgroup of adolescents have coexisting SUD and PTSD. In the National Survey of Adolescents, approximately one-quarter of girls and boys who had PTSD also met criteria for an SUD, and among youth with an SUD, 25% of girls and 14% of boys had coexisting PTSD (Kilpatrick et al., 2000). The research on effective treatment for coexisting SUD and PTSD with adolescents is limited (Kaminer et al., 2019). The adult SUD–PTSD treatment literature suggests that concurrently treating both domains will produce better outcomes than a sequential treatment strategy (McCauley et al., 2012).

Seeking Safety is a psychosocial intervention initially tested in girls with coexisting SUD and PTSD. It uses a range of behavioral strategies (cognitive behavioral therapy and motivational enhancement therapy), as discussed in Chapters 10 and 11. A small pilot study showed promise in reducing sexual concerns and distress and problems with anorexia, somatization, and depression (Najavits et al., 2006).

Case Illustration of PTSD

Terry; age: 17; ethnicity: African American; gender: male; sexual orientation: heterosexual; family situation: biological mother distant; foster family involved; 10-year-old brother; school: Individual Education Plan.

Terry is a 17-year-old junior, starting football player, and who has average school grades. His family has had county child protective services involved with their family off and on for as long as he can remember. Two years ago, Terry entered the foster care system. At this point, one of his teachers took him in and obtained a temporary foster care license to do so. Terry has a county child protection social worker and an individual therapist who sees him on a semi-regular basis. He missed sessions for sports and has a hard time getting back on track.

Terry is the oldest of three children in his family. He has a history of sexual abuse and witnessing open drug use and violence in the home by his mother and mother's friends. Terry has only spoken to his father once, when he was 7, and wishes to never do that again because he was "just set up." Before he was placed outside the home he would "protect [his] little brother and sister from all the craziness." His siblings have been returned to the care of his mother and he does not have the opportunity to see them. The last time he saw his 10-year-old brother, his brother spit on him and told him to get away from him. Terry went on to say, "I don't really blame him, it's kind of my fault that they had to go to foster care when my mom went to prison."

Terry's mom will text him frequently during the week and ask if he is "happy breaking up the family?", if he is a "good man by putting him mom in jail," and announcing to him, "you're a horrible role model to your brother and sister." She will also call him disparaging names and on occasion tells him she never wants to see him again—he is dead to her. Terry's mother's parental rights have not been terminated and it is uncertain if he will even go back to live with her.

Recently, Terry has been moodier, "having a harder time bouncing back" when things are a challenge. He has started to cut when he gets overwhelmed—because he reports "I just feel numb—I know it's crazy but I feel nothing." His therapist recently learned that there are pending charges against Terry for perpetrating sexual acts on a girl in his apartment building when he was 12. When the therapist inquired about things that where bothering him, he told his therapist that his lawyer told him he couldn't talk about any of that.

In Terry's last therapy session, he discloses about the cutting and reports some thoughts of passive suicidal thoughts. He states that when he can't sleep at night, it's due to not wanting to have nightmares. When he lies awake, he wishes that he just would get hit by the bus or get his neck broken in football. He thinks it would all just be a relief to not have to think about it all anymore.

Clinical points to ponder:

1. Who should the therapist be communicating with about Terry and why?

   County social worker?

   Foster parent?

   Biological mother?

   Lawyer?

2. Based on the interventions covered in the text, what is a promising therapeutic approach for Terry and his therapist?

3. What are Terry's strengths?

Bipolar Disorder

Bipolar disorder is defined by periods or episodes of extreme disturbances of a person's mood, thoughts, and behavior. There are two main types of bipolar disorder: bipolar I and bipolar II. As described in the DSM-5 (American Psychiatric Association, 2013), bipolar I disorder involves episodes of severe mania and often depression. Bipolar II disorder involves a less severe form of mania called *hypomania*. During a manic phase, the person over the course of several days may engage in risky or reckless behavior (e.g., make impulsive decisions), have feelings of euphoria, have less need for sleep, and have a marked increase in energy. All of these symptoms can be part of normal adolescence. What distinguishes these manic episodes is that they occur at a very high level of intensity for several days on end and are not transitory.

The link between bipolar disorder and creativity has received attention by researchers. Based on the study of the personal historical accounts of several famous people, the following notable individuals appear to have suffered from bipolar disorder (Jamison, 1993).

- Richard Dryfuss
- Ernest Hemingway
- Vincent Van Gogh
- Mark Vonnegut

Autism

Autism is not a single construct but a spectrum of interrelated disorders that have a common set of symptoms. These core symptoms include persistent deficits in social communication and social interaction across numerous and different situations (e.g., poor or absence of verbal response during conversation; lack of response to social), stereotyped or repetitive motor movements (e.g., repeating simple hand motor movements), and insistence on sameness (e.g., rigid thinking patterns). In years past, there were several separate autism-related disorders (e.g., Asperger's syndrome, pervasive developmental disorder, Rett's disorder). DSM-5 (American Psychiatric Association, 2013) now defines this construct with one disorder—the autism spectrum disorder. Whereas every individual with this disorder has problems to some degree with social interaction, empathy, communication, and flexible behavior, those afflicted vary considerably in terms of the level of severity and disability of their symptoms.

It is estimated that about 10% of people with the autism spectrum disorder have special "savant" skills. Common savant skills involve remarkable mathematical calculations, musical abilities, and incredible displays of memory. Examples of autistic savants receiving attention in the media include the ability to multiply large numbers in their head, playing a piano concerto after hearing it once, or quickly memorizing pages of the telephone book.

Based on two real-life savants, Barry Levinson's 1988 *Rain Man* portrayed a savant (portrayed by Dustin Hoffman) whose remarkable memory skills are used to help his younger brother (played by Tom Cruise) win big at blackjack by counting cards.

MINI-REVIEW

- Internalizing disorders represent mental or behavioral conditions that are dominated by emotionality. Emotions are an adaptive tool to deal with life's challenges. Adolescence is a development period when emotions can be extreme when elicited by both positive and negative experiences. The major internalizing disorders are depressive disorders and anxiety disorders; related ones in this domain include PTSD, bipolar disorder, and autism.

- Treatment effectiveness for teenagers with SUD and a coexisting internalizing disorder is optimized when both domains are addressed. Behavioral-based treatment approaches and, in some circumstances, concurrent psychotropic medication are part of the treatment plan.

- One of the most common mental and behavioral disorders among adolescents in the United States is depression. For those suffering from a major depressive disorder, symptoms include a period of at least 2 weeks of a very persistent low mood accompanied with low self-esteem, loss of interest in normally enjoyable activities, and problems with sleep, energy, and concentration.

- Anxiety disorders are also a common mental disorder among adolescents. The several subtypes of anxiety disorders include simple phobias, separation anxiety, social anxiety, generalized anxiety, and obsessive-compulsive disorder. Symptoms of an anxiety disorder include restlessness, being easily fatigued, irritability, and difficulty concentrating.

- PTSD (exposure to trauma that contributes to such distress that functioning is impaired), bipolar disorder (episodes of extreme disturbances of mood elevation and bizarre behavior), and autism (a spectrum of behaviors that impair social functioning) are other disorders within the internalizing disorder class.

DISCUSSION POINTS

1. What do you think are reasons contributing to the rising rate of adolescent depression in recent years? How might the negative impact of COVID-19 pandemic also contribute to an increase in the prevalence of depression?
2. What can parents do to help a teenager suffering from depression? Here are two recommendations from experts.
   i. Focus on listening.
   ii. Push for social interactions.
   What would you add to the list?
3. As noted in the chapter, a common fear is public speaking. How can a person conquer this fear? What approaches work well in terms of building skills and boosting confidence?
4. Experts recommend that the treatment of SUD accompanied by social anxiety should be conducted individually and not in a group setting until significant improvement of this anxiety disorder has been reached. Discuss the reasons for this recommendation.
5. Modern times pose stressors and sources of trauma. What are modern-day examples of trauma that likely would not be a contributor to PTSD in prior generations?

FURTHER CURIOSITY AND DIGGING

General

National Association of Mental Illness (NAMI). (2022). Kids, teens and young adults.
https://www.nami.org/Find-Support/Teens-and-Young-Adults
NAMI provides advocacy, education, support, and public awareness for individuals and
families affected by mental illness.

Depression

American Psychological Association. (2022). *Depression assessment measures and
instruments*. https://www.apa.org/depression-guideline/assessment/
How Gary Gulman Emerged From a 'Spiral' of Depression With 'The Great Depresh': https://
www.bing.com/videos/search?q=How+comedian+Gary+Gulman+overcame+dep
ression&docid=608050443200251393&mid=C748FDE768250928187BC748FDE76
8250928187B&view=detail&FORM=VIRE
Video on Adolescent Depression by National Institute of Health: https://www.bing.com/
videos/search?q=adolescent+depression+video+from+NIMH&docid=60802041708
7865710&mid=8844F7070D07ED3E5CCF8844F7070D07ED3E5CCF&view=det
ail&FORM=VIRE

Anxiety

Berman, E. D. (2018). *Anxiety: Recent advances in anxiety—Children/adolescents*. [Video].
YouTube. https://www.youtube.com/watch?v=yc9TS89qxlQ

PTSD

Uniformed Services University of the Health Sciences, Center for Developmental
Psychology. (n.d.). *Post-traumatic Stress Disorder (PTSD)*. https://deploymentpsych.
org/disorders/ptsd-main
A diverse amount of PTSD-related resources for practitioners, clients, family members,
and policymakers: https://www:nctsn.org

Bipolar Disorder

Jamison, K. R. (2015). *An unquiet mind*. Vintage Books.

Autism

A wide range of information and resources are provided by The Autism Society: https://
www.autism-society.org/

Gender Spectrum

Gender Spectrum offers resources to empower your relationships, work, and interactions
with youth and children: https://www.genderspectrum.org/resources/

REFERENCES

American Psychiatric Association. (2013). *Diagnostic and statistical manual of mental disorders* (5th ed.). American Psychiatric Association Press.

Banneyer, K. N., Bonin, L., Price, K., Goodman, W. K., & Storch, E. A. (2018). Cognitive behavioral therapy for childhood anxiety disorders: A review of recent advances. *Current Psychiatry Reports, 20*, 65. doi:10.1007/s11920-018-0924-9

Blue Cross Blue Shield Association. (2018). *Major depression: The impact on overall health.* https://www.bcbs.com/the-health-of-america/reports/major-depression-the-impact-overall-health

Blumenthal, H., Leen-Feldner, E. W., Badour, C. L., & Babson, K. A. (2011). Anxiety psychopathology and alcohol use among adolescents: A critical review of the empirical literature and recommendations for future research. *Journal of Experimental Psychopathology, 2*, 318–353.

Buckner, J. D., Schmidt, N. B., Lang, A. R., Small, J. W., Schlauch, R. C., & Lewinsohn, P. M. (2008). Specificity of social anxiety disorder as a risk factor for alcohol and cannabis dependence. *Journal of Psychiatric Research, 42*, 230–239.

Carrellas, N. W., Biederman, J., & Uchida, M. (2017). How prevalent and morbid are subthreshold manifestations of major depression in adolescents? A literature review. *Journal of Affective Disorders, 210*, 166–173.

Connolly, S. D., & Bernstein, G. A. (2007). Practice parameter for the assessment and treatment of children and adolescents with anxiety disorders. *Journal of the American Academy of Child & Adolescent Psychiatry, 46*, 267–283.

Curry, J., Silva, S., Rohde, P., Ginsburg, G., Kennard, B., Kratochvil, C., . . . Feeny, N. (2012). Onset of alcohol or substance use disorders following treatment for adolescent depression. *Journal of Consulting and Clinical Psychology, 80*, 299–312.

Curtin, S. C., & Heron, M. P. (2019). *Death rates due to suicide and homicide among persons aged 10–24: United States, 2000–2017* (no. 352, October, 2019). National Center for Health Statistics.

Foa, E. B. (2011). Prolonged exposure therapy: Past, present, and future. *Depression and Anxiety, 28*, 1043–1047.

Ford, J. D., Elhai, J. D., Connor, D. F., & Frueh, C. (2010). Poly-victimization and risk of posttraumatic, depressive, and substance use disorders and involvement in delinquency in a national sample of adolescents. *Journal of Adolescent Health, 46*, 545–552.

Goodwin, R. D., Fergusson, D. M., & Horwood, L. J. (2004). Early anxious/withdrawn behaviours predict later internalising disorders. *Journal of Child Psychology and Psychiatry, 45*, 874–883.

Groenman, A. P., Janssen, T. W., & Oosterlaan, J. (2017). Childhood psychiatric disorders as risk factor for subsequent substance abuse: A meta-analysis. *Journal of the American Academy of Child & Adolescent Psychiatry, 56*, 556–569.

Hawke, J. M., Kaminer, Y., Burke, R., & Burleson, J. A. (2008). Stability of comorbid psychiatric diagnosis among youths in treatment and aftercare for alcohol use disorders. *Substance Abuse, 29*, 33–41.

Hersh, J., Curry, J. F., & Kaminer, Y. (2014). What is the impact of comorbid depression on adolescent substance abuse treatment? *Substance Abuse, 35,* 364–375.

Hill, R. M., Pettit, J. W., Lewinsohn, P. M., Seeley, J. R., & Klein, D. N. (2014). Escalation to major depressive disorder among adolescents with subthreshold depressive symptoms: Evidence of distinct subgroups at risk. *Journal of Affective Disorders, 158,* 133–138.

Hollenstein, T., Colasante, T., & Lougheed, J. P. (2021). Adolescent and maternal anxiety symptoms decreased but depressive symptoms increased before to during COVID-19 lockdown. *Journal of Research on Adolescence, 31,* 517–530.

Jamison, K. R. (1993). *Touched with fire: Manic-depressive illness and the artistic temperament.* The Free Press.

Kaminer, Y., Connor, D. F., & Curry, J. F. (2008). Treatment of comorbid adolescent cannabis use and major depressive disorder. *Psychiatry (Edgmont), 5,* 34–39.

Kaminer, Y., & Winters, K. C. (Eds.). (2019). *Clinical manual of adolescent addictive disorders* (2nd ed.). American Psychiatric Association.

Kaminer, Y., Zajac, K., & Winters, K. C. (2019). Assessment and treatment of internalizing disorders (depression, anxiety disorders and PTSD). In Y. Kaminer & K. C. Winters (Eds.), *Clinical manual of adolescent addictive disorders* (2nd ed., pp. 375–412). American Psychiatric Association.

Kessler, R. C., Ruscio, A. M., Shear, K., & Wittchen, H. U. (2009). Epidemiology of anxiety disorders. In M. B. Stein & T. Steckler (Eds.), *Behavioral neurobiology of anxiety and its treatment* (pp. 21–35). Springer.

Kilpatrick, D. G., Acierno, R., Saunders, B., Resnick, H. S., Best, C. L., & Schnurr, P. P. (2000). Risk factors for adolescent substance abuse and dependence: Data from a national sample. *Journal of Consulting and Clinical Psychology, 68,* 19–30.

Kuhlman, K. R., Geiss, E. G., Vargas, I., & Lopez-Duran, N. (2018). HPA-axis activation as a key moderator of childhood trauma exposure and adolescent mental health. *Journal of Abnormal Child Psychology, 46,* 149–157.

Kushner, M. G., Abrams, K., & Borchardt, C. (2000). The relationship between anxiety disorders and alcohol use disorders: A review of major perspectives and findings. *Clinical Psychology Review, 20,* 149–171.

Leonte, K. G., Puliafico, A., Na, P., & Rynn, M. A. (2018). Pharmacotherapy for anxiety disorders in children and adolescents. *UpToDate.* https://www.uptodate.com/contents/pharmacotherapy-for-anxiety-disorders-in-children-and-adolescents

Low, N. C., Dugas, E., O'Loughlin, E., Rodriguez, D., Contreras, G., Chaiton, M., & O'Loughlin, J. (2012). Common stressful life events and difficulties are associated with mental health symptoms and substance use in young adolescents. *BMC Psychiatry, 12,* 116.

Masten, A. S., & Narayen, A. J. (2012). Child development in the context of disaster, war, and terrorism: Pathways of risk and resilience. *Annual Review of Psychology, 63,* 227–257.

McCance-Katz, E. F. (2019). *The National Survey on Drug Use and Health: 2017.* Substance Abuse and Mental Health Services Administration. https://www.samhsa.gov/data/sites/default/files/nsduh-ppt-09-2018.pdf

McCauley, J. L., Killeen, T., Gros, D. F., Brady, K. T., & Back, S. E. (2012). Posttraumatic stress disorder and co-occurring substance use disorders: Advances in assessment and treatment. *Clinical Psychology: Science and Practice, 19*, 283–304.

Miller, A. B., & Prinstein, M. J. (2019). Adolescent suicide as a failure of acute stress-response systems. *Annual Review of Clinical Psychology, 15*, 425–450.

Miu, A. C., Homberg, J. R., & Lesch, K. P. (Eds.). (2019). *Genes, brain, and emotions: Interdisciplinary and translational perspectives.* Oxford University Press.

Najavits, L. M., Gallop, R. J., & Weiss, R. D. (2006). Seeking safety therapy for adolescent girls with PTSD and substance use disorder: A randomized controlled trial. *Journal of Behavioral Health Services Research, 33*, 453–463.

Ohashi, K., Anderson, C. M., Bolger, E. A., Khan, A., McGreenery, C. E., & Teicher, M. H. (2019). Susceptibility or resilience to maltreatment can be explained by specific differences in brain network architecture. *Biological Psychiatry, 85*, 690–702.

Riggs, P. D., Mikulich-Gilbertson, S. K., Davies, R. D., Lohman, M., Klein, C., & Stover, S. K. (2007). A randomized controlled trial of fluoxetine and cognitive behavioral therapy in adolescents with major depression, behavior problems, and substance use disorders. *Archives of Pediatrics & Adolescent Medicine, 161*, 1026–1034.

Rohde, P., Brière, F. N., & Stice, E. (2018). Major depression prevention effects for a cognitive-behavioral adolescent indicated prevention group intervention across four trials. *Behaviour Research and Therapy, 100*, 1–6.

Walkup, J. T., Albano, A. M., Piacentini, J., Birmaher, B., Compton, S. N., Sherrill, J. T., . . . Iyengar, S. (2008). Cognitive behavioral therapy, sertraline, or a combination in childhood anxiety. *New England Journal of Medicine, 359*(26), 2753–2766.

Externalizing and Related Disorders

CHAPTER OUTLINE

INTRODUCTION

This chapter addresses the other large domain of disorders that coexist with adolescent substance use disorder (SUD)—the externalizing disorders. This set consists of attention-deficit/hyperactivity disorder (ADHD), oppositional defiant disorder (ODD), and conduct disorder (CD). We will also discuss two externalizing-related disorders—schizophrenia and personality disorders. Many factors may lead to a child developing any of these disorders—genetic vulnerability, exposure to child abuse or neglect, traumatic life experiences, and disruptive family environment. The epidemiology, clinical characteristics, and treatment for each will be discussed, and case examples will also be provided.

INTERSECTION OF EXTERNALIZING DISORDERS AND SUBSTANCE USE DISORDER

This core group of externalizing disorders (ADHD, CD, and ODD) is the most common co-occurring group of behavioral/mental disorders in young people with SUDs (American Academy of Pediatrics, 2011). For example, meta-analyses have shown an overall prevalence rate of 28% of ADHD among youth with an SUD (Brewer et al., 2017). As is the case with internalizing disorders, discussed in the previous chapter, there are increased rates of substance use and related problems, as well as significant negative impact in terms of personal, societal, and economic costs, for youth with an externalizing disorder compared to youth without any of these disorders (Groenman et al., 2017). More specifically, youth with an externalizing disorder display an earlier onset of drug use, their level of use is heavier, they have a higher risk of developing an SUD, and they show a poorer response to treatment than youth without an externalizing disorder (Ignaszewski & Waslick, 2018).

ADHD

Prevalence

In developed countries, the estimated prevalence rate of ADHD among adolescents is 5–12% (Zulauf et al., 2014), although more conservative estimates place the high-end prevalence rate at 7% (American Psychiatric Association, 2013). ADHD occurs more often in boys than in girls, and behaviors can be different based on gender. For example, boys may show more of the hyperactive symptoms (e.g., be on the go, in constant motion), and girls may tend to reveal the inattentive symptoms (e.g., fail to pay close attention to details). Although originally thought to be a disorder of childhood, between 46 and 66% of individuals diagnosed with ADHD will continue to experience significant impairment into adolescence and early adulthood (Barkley et al., 2006), and an estimated 50–60% will continue to experience symptoms into adulthood (Faraone et al., 2006). ADHD youth with a coexisting SUD are about 3.5 times more likely to suffer from additional coexisting disorders, including depression and anxiety disorders, antisocial personality disorder, conduct disorder, and oppositional defiant disorder (Biederman et al., 2012; Van Emmerik-van Oortmerssen et al., 2014).

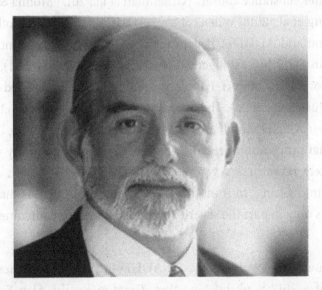

Russell Barkley, Ph.D., is probably best known for his theoretical and empirical work on the etiology of ADHD.
Photo courtesy of Russell Barkley.

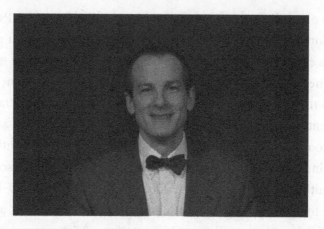

Timothy Wilens, M.D., has focused much of his research on the interrelationship of ADHD and substance use disorder.
Photo courtesy of Timothy Wilens.

Controversy about the ADHD–SUD connection. Experts have debated as to whether ADHD alone or its coexistence with CD poses a significant risk for later substance abusers (Groenman et al., 2017; Molina & Pelham, 2014; Wang et al., 2018; Wilens et al., 2011). In some reports, both ADHD in isolation and ADHD–CD appear to be related to significantly higher rates of an SUD (e.g., Rodgers et al., 2015; Wilens et al., 2011), whereas other reports show that ADHD alone is not linked to an elevated SUD risk (e.g., August et al., 2006). The interesting aspect of the August et al. study is that their ADHD sample was recruited from the community, instead of the normal procedure of recruiting from a clinic. Community-recruited youth likely reveal less severe ADHD symptoms than youth recruited from a clinic setting. In sum, this range of findings suggests that ADHD influences only in part the severity of substance-related outcomes.

The issue of the overdiagnosis of ADHD in the United States is the focus of a 2017 book by *New York Times* journalist Alan Schwarz, *ADHD Nation: Children, Doctors, Big Pharma, and the Making of an*

American Epidemic. A major thesis of his book is that the pharmaceutical industry is a driving force behind the increase in diagnosing and treating ADHD.

Is ADHD overdiagnosed and overtreated? Professionals from numerous disciplines in the child mental health arena have raised concerns that ADHD is overdiagnosed and overtreated (Giuliano & Geyer, 2017). The main thrust of this view is that whereas some children andadolescents are appropriately diagnosed with ADHD and will benefit from medication (e.g., psychostimulants, such as Ritalin or Concerta), many children are overdiagnosed. In recent years there has been a troubling trend to liberally apply the ADHD diagnostic criteria to many youth who are being mislabeled as having ADHD and, consequently, being erroneously prescribed psychostimulant medication (Cohen et al., 2017).

Characteristics

There are three main behavioral dimensions of ADHD, all of which have onset during childhood and may persist into adulthood. *Inattention* means the youth commonly wanders off task, lacks persistence, has difficulty sustaining focus, and is disorganized. These features are not due to defiance or lack of comprehension. *Hyperactivity* is characterized by the person moving about constantly and excessively fidgeting, tapping, or talking. These symptoms occur in situations in which it is not appropriate (e.g., the classroom). The final feature is *impulsivity*. This refers to making hasty decisions or taking actions in the absence of first thinking about the consequences or harm of the actions, a desire for immediate rewards, and an inability to delay gratification. These three features are the key behaviors of ADHD. Some youth with ADHD only have problems with one of these behavioral domains, while others exhibit all behaviors. During adolescence, hyperactivity seems to lessen and may show more often as feelings of restlessness or fidgeting, but inattention and impulsivity may remain.

DSM-5 diagnostic criteria for ADHD. For a child or adolescent to receive a diagnosis of ADHD, the symptoms of inattention and/or hyperactivity-impulsivity must be long-lasting (chronic), impair the person's functioning, and cause the person to fall behind normal development for their age. The symptoms need to be distinguished from another medical or behavioral condition. Symptoms of ADHD can be mistaken for emotional or disciplinary problems or missed entirely in quiet, well-behaved children, leading to a delay in diagnosis. Also, a diagnosis of ADHD requires that the symptoms have been present prior to age 12, and the symptoms can appear as early as between the ages of 3 and 6 and can continue through adolescence and adulthood. Thus, it is not surprising that most youth who get a diagnosis of ADHD usually get their first diagnosis during the elementary school years. Provided below are more detailed features of the diagnostic criteria of ADHD's main behaviors.

DSM-5 ADHD criteria of inattention: Core features of the inattention component of ADHD are noted below.

- Overlooks or misses details, makes careless mistakes in schoolwork, at work, or during other activities
- Has problems sustaining attention in tasks or play, including conversations, lectures, or lengthy reading
- Does not seem to listen when spoken to directly
- Does not follow through on instructions and fails to finish schoolwork, chores, or duties in the workplace, or starts tasks but quickly loses focus and gets easily sidetracked
- Has problems organizing tasks and activities, such as what to do in sequence, keeping materials and belongings in order, having messy work and poor time management, and failing to meet deadlines
- Avoids or dislikes tasks that require sustained mental effort, such as schoolwork or homework, or for teens and older adults, preparing reports, completing forms or reviewing lengthy papers

- Loses things necessary for tasks or activities, such as school supplies, pencils, books, tools, wallets, keys, paperwork, eyeglasses, and cell phones
- Is easily distracted by unrelated thoughts or stimuli
- Is forgetful in daily activities, such as chores, errands, returning calls, and keeping appointments

DSM-5 ADHD criteria of hyperactivity-impulsivity. Core features of the hyperactivity-impulsivity subtype of ADHD are described below.

- Fidgets and squirms in their seat
- Leaves their seat in situations when staying seated is expected, such as in the classroom or in the office
- Runs or dashes around or climbs in situations where it is inappropriate or, in teens and adults, often feels restless
- Is unable to play or engage in hobbies quietly
- Is constantly in motion or "on the go," or acts as if "driven by a motor"
- Talks nonstop
- Blurts out an answer before a question has been completed, finishes other people's sentences, or speaks without waiting for a turn in conversation
- Has trouble waiting their turn
- Interrupts or intrudes on others, for example, in conversations, games, or activities

Can ADHD symptoms be reduced by avoiding certain foods? Some studies indicate that avoiding certain food colorings and preservatives may decrease temporarily some ADHD behaviors in some children. The U.S. Food and Drug Administration (FDA) Food Advisory Committee and the national advocacy organization, Children and Adults with Attention-Deficit/Hyperactivity Disorder, have cautioned that consistent empirical evidence is lacking to support a link between avoiding certain food coloring and a reliable reduction in hyperactivity.

Some children appear to have an allergy to certain food artificial colors and preservatives.

More rigorous research is needed to find out if limiting or avoiding certain food additives will contribute to a reduction in ADHD symptoms.

SOURCE: https://www.mayoclinic.org/diseases-conditions/adhd/expert-answers/adhd/faq-20058203

Treatment

The treatment of ADHD has a long history. There is a range of available treatments that can ameliorate symptoms. The main treatment approaches for ADHD are summarized below.

An important brain chemical believed to be a factor in ADHD is norepinephrine. This is an important neurotransmitter—a chemical released by brain nerve cells that facilitates neurochemical communication among nerve cells. Norepinephrine influences brain function related to attention and decision making. ADHD is a disorder believed to result from a deficiency in this neurotransmitter, and ADHD medications raise the level of norepinephrine within the brain.

SOURCE: https://www.additudemag.com/adhd-neuroscience-101/

Medication. Psychostimulants (e.g., Ritalin, Concerta) are the most common group of medication used for treating ADHD. It may seem counterintuitive to treat ADHD with a medication that is considered a stimulant. Yet these medications work because they are administered in doses that do not normally pose an addictive threat, and they improve brain chemical activity that plays an important role in attention and decision making. A youth taking psychostimulant medications needs to be monitored closely and carefully by their prescribing physician. While considered safe when taken as prescribed, there are risks and side effects (e.g., increase in blood pressure), especially when misused or taken in excess of the prescribed dose.

Are there nonstimulant medications for ADHD? Yes; examples are Strattera and Wellbutrin. However, their effectiveness is typically weaker than that of stimulant medication; one problem is that these medications take longer to start working than psychostimulants. When a child or adolescent has troubling side effects from psychostimulants, a nonstimulant is often prescribed.

Psychotherapy. There is growing consensus in the research and clinical practice arenas that the optimal treatment for ADHD involves a combination of behavioral therapy with medication (Pelham et al., 2016). The aim of behavioral therapy is to help the adolescent with ADHD to change the various maladaptive behaviors that are characteristic of the disorder. Such changes include building skills and providing strategies for monitoring one's behavior, organizing tasks, completing schoolwork, resisting impulses to act or talk abruptly, controlling anger and risk taking, and dealing with emotionally difficult situations. Adding a family therapy component helps to support the adolescent's goals. Family members are taught effective ways to handle disruptive behaviors, improve communication with the adolescent, establish clear expectations, and provide structured routines.

Education and training. A supplement to family members participating in psychotherapy is to provide the parents with education about how ADHD affects the family, skills for parenting, and strategies for stress management. ADHD education involves a primer on the disorder, its expected course, and the importance of treatment. A good example is Russell Barkley's *Taking Charge of ADHD: The Complete, Authoritative Guide for Parents* (Barkley, 2013). Barkley presents a science-based, eight-step behavior management plan for the home that is specifically designed for 6- to 18-year-olds with ADHD. Education of parents of a child with ADHD focuses on teaching parents the skills that will likely encourage positive behaviors and reduce the likelihood of negative behaviors in their adolescent. Parents are taught the basic principle of cognitive behavioral therapy (discussed in detail in Chapter 10)—that is, to give immediate and positive feedback for behaviors they want to encourage, and to ignore or redirect behaviors that they want to discourage. Stress management techniques benefit parents by increasing their ability to cope with frustration so that they will respond calmly to their adolescent's disruptive behavior. Strategies include relaxation techniques, meditation, and cognitive restructuring.

Case Illustration of ADHD

Jovita; age: 16; ethnicity: African American; gender: female; sexual orientation: heterosexual; family situation: biological mother; step-father; 10-year-old brother; 8-year-old brother; school: Individual Education Plan

Jovita was brought into the emergency room after joyriding in a stolen car that was in a car accident. When she and her friends where pulled over by the police, her blood alcohol level was 0.28%. The nurses were surprised to be talking to Jovita at the time of admission. When her mom arrived to pick her up, it was determined that her physical health was fine, but the medical team did have concerns about her alcohol levels. The discharge recommendations were for a diagnostic assessment and to follow the directions.

Jovita's mom insisted that they do what the hospital recommended, and they received a diagnostic assessment. At the end of the diagnostic assessment, Jovita was referred for further ADHD testing and a substance use evaluation because of drug use history. Jovita reported that she drank a few times a week; she didn't "care what or how much." She also reported, "I smoke weed when I want to and tried some pills every so often."

At the diagnostic assessment it was revealed that Jovita often is seen as the class clown and "fun one" in her peer group. She is in 10th grade and struggles academically. Her mom reports "she gets barely passing grades, but she is smart as whip!—she just don't care—just like this car thing—she just don't care!"

Jovita competed the evaluations but with resistance and irritation. After four visits to the community mental health clinic, she completed the following:

- Diagnostic interview with her mom
- Conners Rating Scale (completed by Jovita, her mom, and two teachers)
- Substance Abuse Subtle Screening Inventory (SASSI)–Adolescent Version
- Millon Clinical Multiaxial Inventory Personality Inventory (MACI)–Adolescent version
- Wechsler Adult Intelligence Scale–IV (WAIS-IV)
- Test of Variables of Attention (TOVA)
- Brief test of attention

The result was a diagnostic picture of an above-average intelligent teen with attention deficit disorder and an alcohol dependence.

Clinical points to ponder:

1. How might have adverse childhood experiences been a factor with the onset and continuation of attention problems reported by Jovita?
2. Was *all* the testing needed? Couldn't the results be just as easily found through free online screening tools?
3. In what ways does parenting play a role in helping a teen deal with ADHD?
4. Is s person born with ADHD or is it acquired?

CONDUCT DISORDER

Prevalence

Conduct disorder (CD) is more common among boys than girls; in the general population, the rate among boys ranges from 6 to 16%, whereas the rate among girls ranges from 2 to 9% (Boat et al., 2015). These figures are based on a data-analytic procedure called a *meta-analysis*, in which investigators synthesized prevalence of behavioral and mental disorders in youth from more than 50 international community surveys published between 2004 and 2013. Among both boys and girls, CD is one of the disorders most frequently diagnosed in mental health settings. And this disorder continues to be the most common externalizing disorder in adolescents with SUD; it is present among almost three-quarters of youth with an SUD (Brewer et al., 2017), even though the prevalence of behaviors associated with CD has decreased for males in the last 25 years (Johnston et al., 20198).

There are indications that some conduct disorder–related problems are on the decline. A downturn in the rates of adolescent risk behaviors, including violence, crime, and drug use, has been observed in the United States in recent years. Specifics include the following (Grucza et al., 2018):

- Arrest rates for both assault and theft dropped by 75% between 1992 and 2010.
- Self-reported survey data show declines in
  - Bullying and fighting;
  - Binge drinking, cigarette smoking, and use of most classes of illicit drugs (as discussed in Chapter 4); and
  - Early sexual involvement

Characteristics

CD is a repetitive and persistent pattern of behavior in youth that by most standards constitutes violations of the rights of others or basic social rules and laws. Adolescents with CD frequently do not follow rules, fail to show empathy, and behave inappropriately in social situations. These delinquent behaviors cause significant disruptions in the youth's social and academic functioning and usually occur across a variety of settings (e.g., at home and school). When CD starts during childhood and includes an aggressive component (e.g., frequent fighting), the risk is greater for persistent delinquent behavior and more severe functioning problems (e.g., academic difficulties; future criminality) (Lahey et al., 2005; Loeber et al., 1995). But research indicates that when adolescents with CD show desistance of their problem behaviors during adolescence or young adulthood, they can function well as law-abiding adults (Loeber et al., 1991).

One of the authors (KCW) is personally familiar with such a case of "delinquency desistance." Jon (not real name), as a teenager, joined his delinquent friends in serial thefts. They would break into vacant homes, steal property, and then fence it for cash. Jon had the role of the look-out person. The group was eventually caught and each received some jail time. Jon matured out of his delinquent ways. He persuaded the local university to admit him by agreeing to the condition that if he did not keep his grades above a B average, the school could dismiss him. He went on to get a professional degree in the behavioral sciences. His area of research expertise—adolescent delinquency.

Diagnostic criteria. To receive a diagnosis CD, the adolescent must show a repetitive and persistent pattern of behavior as manifested by the presence of at least 3 of any of the following 15 criteria across four categories. These behaviors, listed below, must have occurred within the past 12 months and had their onset before age 10 years (Substance Abuse and Mental Health Services Administration, 2016).

DSM-5 criteria for conduct disorder:

Aggression to People and Animals

1. Bullies, threatens or intimidates others
2. Starts physical fights
3. Has used a weapon that could cause serious physical harm to others (e.g., a bat, brick, broken bottle, knife, or gun)
4. Has been physically cruel to people
5. Has been physically cruel to animals
6. Steals from a victim while hurting them
7. Forces someone into sexual activity

Destruction of Property

8. Deliberately engages in fire setting with the intention to cause damage
9. Deliberately destroys others' property

Deceitfulness, Lying, or Stealing

10. Has broken into someone else's building, house, or car
11. Lies to obtain goods or favors or to avoid obligations
12. Steals items without confronting a victim (e.g., shoplifting, but without breaking and entering)

Serious Violations of Rules

13. Often stays out at night despite parental objections
14. Has run away from home overnight at least twice
15. Frequently is truant from school

Treatment

Without treatment, adolescents with a CD are likely to have continuing social and work-related adjustment problems into adulthood. Early research pointed to mixed effectiveness when treating adolescents with CD.

Consider the significant challenges: the adolescent my harbor an unco-operative attitude and express distrust of adults; the intensive parenting requirements toward implementing treatment goals may be perceived by the parents as too burdensome; and treatment progress may be frustrat-ingly slow.

An important clinical question regarding CD is to what extent a youth with this diagnosis continues to display problem behaviors into adult-hood and meet criteria for an antisocial personality disorder (APD). A group of researchers at the University of Pittsburgh studied this issue with boys (Lahey et al., 2005). The best predictor of adult APD among boys with a CD diagnosis was the predominance of *covert* CD symptoms as opposed to a majority of *overt* CD symptoms. Covert symptoms of CD include aggression, violence, and destruction of pro-perty. Overt symptoms are lying, being deceitful, and committing se-rious violations of rules.

Fortunately, several recent reviews of the literature have identified promising approaches (American Academy of Child and Adolescent Psychiatry, 1997). The most successful approaches involve intervening as early as possible (before the young person reaches adolescence), are in-tensive and structured, and address the problem behaviors in the wide variety of situations and settings in which they occur (e.g., home, school, neighborhood). We review in subsequent chapters the most effective treatment approaches, such as functional family therapy, multisystemic therapy, and cognitive behavioral approaches. All of these approaches focus on building skills in the adolescent, such as anger management and resisting peer influences, and strengthening parent skills in monitoring, disciplining, and support. There are no pharmacological interventions that directly address the delinquent behaviors underlying CD, but some youth with CD are medicated for secondary problems, such as inattention or depression.

Case Illustration of Conduct Disorder

Billy; age: 16; ethnicity: Caucasian; gender: male; sexual orientation: heterosexual; family situation: biological mother; father not connected to the family; no siblings; school: mainstream high school

Billy is a 16-year-old Caucasian male referred to the school health clinic because of persistent disruptive behavior in the classroom. There have been several complaints about his behavior from numerous teachers. The problematic behavior includes yelling at other students, being defiant of classroom rules, and physical altercations with students. He has been disciplined before by teachers (e.g., being sent to the vice-principal's office). Given that Billy's behavior has not changed over the semester, school officials recommended that the school's behavioral health counselor evaluate the situation.

Bill is an only child who is being raised by his single mother. His biological father, who divorced Billy's mother right after he was born, has not been involved at all in Billy's upbringing. As a 10th grader, Billy gets average grades but puts in minimal effort. He shows many signs of being bright but thinks school is a "waste of time."

Billy is part of a "tough" group of students, all of whom have been in trouble with school officials. Billy's extroverted personality puts him at being a leader of the group.

In addition to disruptive school behavior, Billy admits to the school counselor that he and his friends have committed several unlawful acts (e.g., damaging property, shoplifting). He likes to play video games and often uses alcohol and cannabis on weekends, which he does not see as a problem.

Clinical points to ponder:

1. Does substance use contribute to Billy's delinquent behavior? If so, how?
2. Does Billy's delinquent behavior contribute to his substance use? If so, how?

3. What strategies would you use to address Billy's delinquent behavior?

4. If Billy and his mother agreed to seeing a family counselor, what major goals might be important to work on?

OPPOSITIONAL DEFIANT DISORDER

Prevalence

The rate of oppositional defiant disorder (ODD) among adolescents is estimated to be 2.8% (National Research Council and Institute of Medicine, 2009). As is the case with its related disorder—CD—ODD is common among youth with other coexisting disorders. It is present in about half of children with ADHD, and among a very high percentage of those with an SUD (Groenman et al., 2017). Although more commonly diagnosed in boys, girls can develop ODD.

An interesting issue with the ODD–SUD relationship is that it may be bidirectional. Youth with early-onset ODD may be more likely to use substances because of their willingness to act in oppositional ways. Or there is the possibility that substance use contributes to engaging in disruptive behavior, because of the effects of intoxication.

As noted in the text, some youth with ODD transition to CD. This pattern occurs more commonly in boys than in girls (Rowe et al., 2010). Another key difference is the outcomes seen in young adulthood. Findings regarding adolescents with pure ODD versus those with combined ODD followed by CD (ODD/CD) were this: pure ODD youth showed more emotional disorders in young adulthood, whereas ODD/CD youth showed more behavioral problems (e.g., aggression, continued law-breaking, and destruction of property) (Rowe et al., 2010).

Characteristics

It can be expected that many adolescents will be defiant at times, particularly when stressed or unhappy (American Academy of Child & Adolescent Psychiatry, 2019). As discussed in Chapter 3, behaviors such as talking back, disobeying rules, and openly displaying outbursts of anger are a normal part of development. Normal defiance is a "phase" of adolescence that does not persist past adolescence for most teenagers. Also, some teenagers may become defiant in an attempt to deal with an anxiety disorder or having experienced trauma. What distinguishes ODD from normal behavior is that the adolescent with ODD displays oppositional behaviors that are so frequent and severe that they disrupt the person's social and academic functioning and become a problem to those around the adolescent. ODD's symptoms typically begin before adolescence and they persist well into adulthood. Some adolescents with ODD escalate their delinquency and subsequently meet criteria for CD.

Diagnostic criteria. Adolescents who meet DSM-5 diagnostic criteria for ODD show an ongoing pattern of uncooperative, defiant, and hostile behavior toward authority figures that seriously interferes with the child's day-to-day functioning and occurs multiple settings. The official criteria require a pattern of at least four of the symptoms listed below, and that such behaviors are present for a period of at least 6 months, their severity must be greater than "normal" adolescent angst or defiance, and they were displayed in the presence of at least one person who is not a sibling. *DSM-5 diagnostic criteria for ODD:*

1. Often loses temper
2. Is often touchy or easily annoyed
3. Is often angry and resentful
4. Often argues with authority figures or, for children and adolescents, with adults
5. Often actively defies or refuses to comply with requests from authority figures or with rules

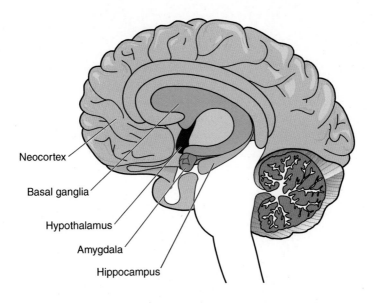

Neocortex

Basal ganglia

Hypothalamus

Amygdala

Hippocampus

Unfortunately, bullying is fairly common during adolescence. Experts estimate that about 25–50% of teenagers in the United States report have been a victim of bullying or have bullied others. Neuroscientists are learning that adolescents who bully other teens tend to display a different pattern of brain activity in response to certain facial expressions. Swartz and colleagues (Swartz et al., 2019) examined the brain activity among a group of adolescents in the brain region known as the amygdala, which plays a key role in emotional processing and responding to threats. The adolescents had their brain activity measured with functional magnetic resonance imaging technique while they completed an emotional face-matching task. The adolescents who reported engaging in more either physical bullying behavior or relational bullying (purposefully excluding a peer or spreading rumors) tended to display higher amygdala activity in response to angry faces and lower amygdala activity in response to fearful faces. The authors interpreted the finding as follows: higher amygdala activity to angry faces could suggest that these teens are more sensitive to signals of anger from other people (which may be a trigger to act as a bully), whereas lower amygdala activity to fearful faces could suggest that the brains of these teens are less responsive to signals of distress and thus are not sensitive to the concerns of the teen being victimized by the bullying.

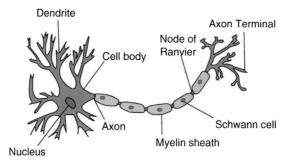

Figure 3.1 Myelin sheath surrounding the nerve cell connections (axons).

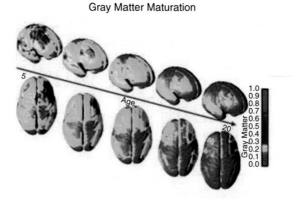

Figure 3.3 Maturation of the brain's gray matter from age 5 to 20 years.

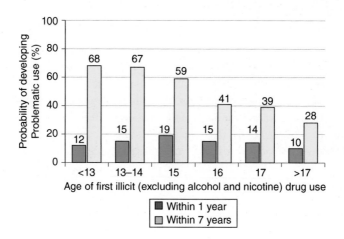

Figure 3.8 Earlier onset of illicit drug use is associated with a greater likelihood of future problematic use.

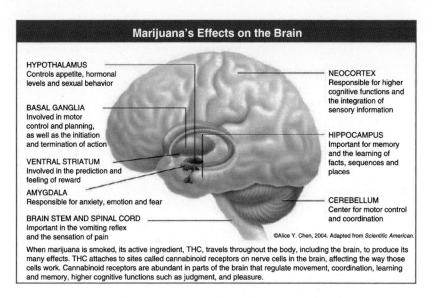

Figure 3.9 Cannabis binds to cannabinoid receptors located throughout the brain.

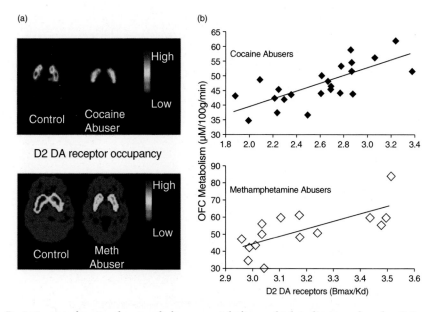

Brain images showing decreased glucose metabolism, which indicates reduced activity, in the orbitofrontal cortex (OFC) in a control subject (a) and a cocaine- addicted subject (b).

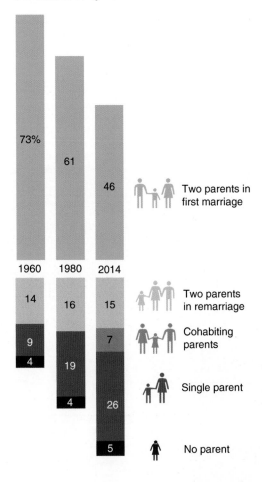

For children, growing diversity in family living arrangements

% of children living with...

73%
61
46 — Two parents in first marriage

1960 1980 2014

14
16
15 — Two parents in remarriage

9
7 — Cohabiting parents

4
19

4
26 — Single parent

5 — No parent

Note: Based on children under 18. Data regarding cohabitation are not available for 1960 and 1980; in those years, children with cohabiting parents are included in "one parent." For 2014, the total share of children living with two married parents is 62% after rounding. Figures do not add up to 100% due to rounding.

Figure 12.1 Percent of children living in various family arrangements.

6. Often deliberately annoys others
7. Often blames others for their mistakes or misbehavior
8. Has been spiteful or vindictive at least twice within the past
   6 months

Treatment

Left untreated, an adolescent with ODD is at risk of developing a CD and additional coexisting disorders. As is the case for CD, effective treatment protocols for ODD center on individual and counseling approaches. Individual-focused counseling may include anger management, social skills training, and problem-solving techniques to address stress and frustrations and to deal with peer influences that contribute to negative behaviors. When medications are used, they are prescribed for the adolescent's secondary problems (e.g., anxiety, depression).

Parent counseling often is the primary focus of treatment for adolescent ODD. Strategies include praising and reinforcing positive behaviors; setting reasonable age-appropriate limits with consequences that can be enforced; monitoring how the adolescent spends their free time; prioritizing responses when the adolescent overly misbehaves (e.g., not all acts of defiance need to trigger a disciplining response); and modeling good behavior by taking personal time-outs or breaks and by not overreacting to stressful situations.

PERSONALITY DISORDERS

The DSM-5 (American Psychiatric Association, 2013) recognizes 10 diagnosable personality disorders (PDs). Each is characterized by a personality style that is so extreme that it creates problems for the sufferer to have healthy and normal relations with others. A PD is not simply a minor quirk in a person's personality. A PD's features are so troubling that they cause conflict with other people, cause relationships to fail or prevent them from developing in the first place, and interfere in the person's ability to reach life goals. Those who meet criteria for one PD often meet criteria for at least one additional one. The relevance of PDs and adolescence is significant: PDs tend to emerge during adolescence or early adulthood and continue for many years. Table 7.1 provides a brief description of the 10 PDs, organized by the three clusters or subgroups as described in the DSM-5.

Table 7.1 DSM-5 PERSONALITY DISORDERS

Type of Personality Disorder (PD)	Features
Cluster A	*These personality disorders are characterized by odd or eccentric behavior.*
• Paranoid PD	Pervasive distrust and suspicion of other people; feel exploited by others
• Schizoid PD	Social isolation and indifference toward other people
• Schizotypal PD	Odd speech, behavior, and appearance; strange beliefs
Cluster B	*Dramatic, erratic, and impulsive behaviors are the essential elements of these personality disorders.*
• Antisocial PD	Disregard for rules and social norms; lack of empathy for other people
• Borderline PD	Emotional instability, intense interpersonal relationships, and impulsive behaviors
• Histrionic PD	Over-dramatization of feelings and situations; need to be the center of attention
• Narcissistic PD	Grandiosity about oneself and one's achievements; lack of empathy for others.
Cluster C	*These personality disorders are associated with pervasive anxiety and fearfulness.*
• Avoidant PD	Disregard for rules; lack of empathy and remorse
• Dependent PD	Fear of being alone; often seek help from others
• Obsessive-Compulsive PD	Preoccupation with orderliness, perfection, and control of relationships

Treatment

PDs are very difficult to treat. This is not surprising, considering that these disorders, by definition, are long-standing personality traits. The National Alliance on Mental Illness (NAMI; https://www.nami.org/Home) and the National Institute on Mental Health (NIMH; https://www.nimh.nih.gov) list two forms of psychotherapy that may be useful for treating personality disorders (both of these treatments are described in more detail in Chapter 10).

Cognitive behavioral therapy (CBT). The goal of CBT is to learn effective coping strategies by changing negative thoughts and behaviors to positive thoughts and rational problem-solving behaviors. Thus, the premise of CBT is that a person's thoughts and behaviors influence negative emotions, such as anxiety and depression, and health can be obtained if the person reframes their thinking pattern. Here is an example. A counselor who is faced with a client who is thinking, "I cannot get anything right and I am a disappointment to my family," will try to steer the person's thinking to be more constructive, such as, "Let's focus on your strengths and come up with a realistic plan of what goals you can achieve. You have already accomplished a lot in life and let's build on that."

Dialectical behavior therapy (DBT). The term *dialectical* is the Buddhist concept of opposing forces. As applied to a counseling technique, it refers to how making changes and wanting to make changes sometimes are at odds with a person and can create opposite inclinations. DBT involves components of CBT, along with added features that focus on building skills to regulate emotions, improve interpersonal relationships, and cope with extreme distress. DBT sessions typically involve the clinician helping the client understand that emotions, while genuine, should not dictate how to cope with and solve problems.

SCHIZOPHRENIA

Schizophrenia, which occurs in approximately 1% of the population (National Institute of Mental Health, 2020), involves a range of problems with thinking, behavior, or emotions that severely impair the individual's ability to function. Its symptoms, which can begin during adolescence or young adulthood, reflect trouble processing personal emotions and can lead the person to become completely detached from reality. Common early signs of adolescent-onset schizophrenia are withdrawal from friends and family, a drop in performance at school, sudden loss in interest in hobbies, strange behavior, and substance use. A differential diagnosis to establish the presence of schizophrenia requires determining if these symptoms become worse as time goes on and the adolescent's functioning significantly deteriorates. (In a subsection below we discuss in more detail early-onset schizophrenia and the importance of differentiating it from normal features of adolescence.)

There is considerable debate in the research literature as to the extent that use of cannabis contributes to the onset of schizophrenia. We concur with the conclusion by many experts: Heavy and frequent use of cannabis does not directly cause schizophrenia in a person with no biological risk for this disorder. But for high-risk individuals, prolonged cannabis use likely contributes to an earlier onset and a more severe course of schizophrenia (Miller, 2018). Another related issue is the association of cannabis use and conduct disorders. A prevailing thought is that early-onset conduct problems are a risk factor to use cannabis, and then continued use of cannabis further accentuates conduct-related symptoms (Hawes et al., 2020).

At its severe end, a person with schizophrenia experiences hallucinations (seeing or hearing things that do not exist), expresses delusions (false beliefs), displays disorganized speech (e.g., answers to questions may be partially or completely unrelated), and exhibits what are referred to as "negative symptoms" (e.g., neglects personal hygiene, appears to lack emotion, speaks in a monotone).

Treatment

Schizophrenia, as a chronic condition, requires lifelong treatment. Because people with schizophrenia have a difficult time understanding information and processing lessons, the goal of schizophrenia treatment is to help the person understand the disease and work hard to keep it under control. Treatment typically requires hospitalization, intensive counseling, and medication. Antipsychotic medications include chlorpromazine, haloperidol, fluphenazine, risperidone, and olanzapine.

An emerging form of treatment for schizophrenia is cognitive remediation (CR). CR addresses an intervention method used to address the client's cognitive dysfunction. CR is unlike other treatment methods in that it targets neurocognition directly by training the schizophrenic to improve cognitive domains impaired by the disorder: perception, working memory, attention, executive functions, long-term memory, and social cognition (Barlati et al., 2013).

Early-Onset Schizophrenia

Some individuals show subtle signs of schizophrenia during adolescence, some of whom go on to develop full-blown schizophrenia with discernable symptoms of delusions and hallucinations. These early signs can be so subtle that they are hardly noticeable. It is important for the individual to have a thorough medical and psychological assessment to rule out any physical illness that may be the cause of symptoms that mimic psychosis.

Common early signs of schizophrenia, which vary among individuals in this phase, are the following:

- Reduced concentration
- Decreased motivation
- Withdrawal from friends and family

- Sleep problems
- Deterioration in functioning
- Unusual beliefs/magical thinking.

Risk factors associated with early-onset psychosis span biological and environmental factors, but these factors linked to psychosis are far from definitive. Experts place an emphasis on a number of brain chemicals, including the neurotransmitters dopamine and serotonin, which may play a role in how psychosis develops. Also, a stressful event may trigger psychotic symptoms in a person who is vulnerable. It is estimated that a first-episode psychosis will occur within 12 months among 15–30% of individuals with high-risk symptoms, and after 3 years, over 36%. These "transition rates" are several-hundred-fold above that of the general population (National Institute of Mental Health, 2015).

Caregivers of schizophrenics are often taught about the importance of expressed emotion (EE) when communicating with their schizophrenic relative or friend. Negative (or undesired) EE refers to being hostile, critical, and overinvolved; positive (or desired) EE refers to expressing warmth and positive regard.

The relapse rate of schizophrenics in families with "high" EE (more negative features than positive) is about 50%, which is in stark contrast to a relapse rate of about 20% in families with low EE (Butzlaff & Hooley, 1998).

Why is high EE deleterious to a patient's course? High EE

- overstimulates the patient;
- impairs their ability to cope;
- contributes to social withdrawal; and
- leads to the perception of poor family support.

Identifying and initiating treatment for adolescents with early-onset schizophrenia may significantly improve the youth's long-term outcome.

As noted above for CBT, DBT and cognitive remediation are applicable therapy strategies for these youth.

MINI-REVIEW

- The traditional disorders that comprise the cluster of externalizing disorders are attention-deficit/hyperactivity disorder (ADHD), oppositional defiant disorder (ODD), and conduct disorder (CD). We consider schizophrenia and personality disorders as affiliated externalizing disorders.
- Generally, the risk of developing an SUD among youth with an externalizing disorder is greater than the risk of developing an SUD if the youth has an internalizing disorder.
- There are three main behavioral dimensions of ADHD, all of which have onset during the person's childhood and may persist into adulthood. *Inattention* refers to difficulty sustaining focus and to being disorganized. *Hyperactivity* is manifested by the youth moving about constantly and excessively fidgeting. *Impulsivity* means being hasty with decisions and having difficulty delaying gratification.
- CD and ODD are related, with ODD being a milder version of CD. Common features of CD are exhibiting repetitive and persistent patterns of behavior that by most standards are violations of the rights of others or of basic social rules and laws. Behaviors include repeatedly being involved in physical fights and damaging property of others. Symptoms of ODD include often being angry and argumentative, being noncompliant when asked to honor a request, and being defiant of adults.
- There are 10 personality disorders described in DSM-5. Each disorder shares this common feature: the personality impairments are so disruptive that the sufferer's relationships with others are negatively affected in significant ways.

- Schizophrenia is a chronic, debilitating disorder that often starts during late adolescence or young adulthood. It is characterized by delusions (holding beliefs that are most certainly false, such as persistent thoughts that someone is out to harm the individual) and hallucinations (experiencing false sensory perceptions, such as hearing voices).

DISCUSSION POINTS

1. Symptoms of ADHD can be difficult to distinguish from normal adolescent behaviors. What of the following questions are valid questions when attempting to distinguish bona-fide ADHD symptoms from normal adolescent behavior?
   - Does the behavior meaningfully disrupt social and role functioning?
   - Are the behaviors persistent?
   - Does the teenager's best friend say it's normal behavior?
   - Do the behaviors cause distress to the individual and others?
   - To what extent does context (e.g., type of situation or setting) elicit the behaviors?
2. Research indicates that children who have been diagnosed with ADHD based on rigorous procedures and who are properly treated with stimulant-based medication (e.g., Ritalin) are at *lower* risk of developing an SUD as a teenager than are children with ADHD who do not receive medication-based treatment. Why might this be the case?
3. Imagine you are counseling a teenager with oppositional defiant disorder (ODD). What skills would be good to work on during the counseling sessions with the aim of reducing or eliminating the ODD-related problem behaviors?
4. Choose one of the personality disorders listed in Table 7.1. Discuss how symptoms of that disorder can negatively impact an interpersonal relationship with a parent, and one with a friend.

FURTHER CURIOSITY AND DIGGING

ADHD

Web-based resource for parents of and those afflicted with ADHD: https://chadd.org/

Online magazine and resource for youth and adults with ADHD: https://www.additude mag.com/

National Institute of Mental Health. (2016). *Mental health medications.* https://www. nimh.nih.gov/health/topics/mental-health-medications/index.shtml

Learn the basics about psychostimulants to treat ADHD on this website.

Is ADHD Over-diagnosed and Over-treated?: https://www.medicalnewstoday.com/ articles/is-adhd-overdiagnosed-and-overtreated

Conduct Disorder

The progression of conduct disorder to antisocial personality disorder:

Lahey, B. B., Loeber, R., Burke, J. D., & Applegate, B. (2005). Predicting future antisocial personality disorder in males from a clinical assessment in childhood. *Journal of Consulting and Clinical Psychology, 73,* 389–399.

Schizophrenia

An online site for adolescents and parents that offers information about schizophrenia:

Mental Health Literacy: Schizophrenia https://mentalhealthliteracy.org/mental-disord ers/schizophrenia/

A study from Europe linking use cannabis and risk for psychosis:

Di Forti, M., Morgan, C., Dazzan, P., Pariante, C., Mondelli, V., Marques, T. R., . . . Butt, A. (2009). High-potency cannabis and the risk of psychosis. *The British Journal of Psychiatry, 195,* 488–491.

REFERENCES

American Academy of Child & Adolescent Psychiatry. (1997). Practice parameters for the assessment and treatment of children and adolescents with conduct disorder. *Journal of the American Academy of Child and Adolescent Psychiatry, 36* (Suppl.); 122S–139S.

American Academy of Child & Adolescent Psychiatry. (2019). *Oppositional defiant disorder.* https://www.aacap.org/AACAP/Families_and_youth/Facts_for_Families/ FFF-Guide/Children-With-Oppositional-Defiant-Disorder-072.aspx

American Academy of Pediatrics (AAP). (2011). Subcommittee on Attention-Deficit/ Hyperactivity Disorder, Steering Committee on Quality Improvement and Management. ADHD: Clinical practice guideline for the diagnosis, evaluation, and treatment of Attention-Deficit/Hyperactivity Disorder in children and adolescents. *Pediatrics, 128,* 1007–1022.

American Psychiatric Association. (2013). *Diagnostic and statistical manual of mental disorders* (5th ed.). American Psychiatric Association Press.

August, G. J., Winters, K. C., Realmuto, G., Fahnhorst, T., Botzet, A., & Lee, S. (2006). Prospective study of adolescent drug abuse among community samples of ADHD and non-ADHD participants. *Journal of the American Academy of Child and Adolescent Psychiatry, 45,* 824–832.

Barkley, R. A. (2013). *Taking charge of ADHD: The complete, authoritative guide for parents.* Guilford Press.

Barkley, R. A., Fischer, M., Smallish, L., & Fletcher, K. (2006). Young adult outcome of hyperactive children: Adaptive functioning in major life activities. *Journal of the American Academy of Child & Adolescent Psychiatry, 45,* 192–202.

Barlati, S., Deste, G., De Peri, L., Ariu, C., & Vita, A. (2013). Cognitive remediation in schizophrenia: Current status and future perspectives. *Schizophrenia Research and Treatment, 2013,* 1–12.

Biederman, J., Petty, C. R., Woodworth, K. Y., Lomedico, A., Hyder, L. L., & Faraone, S. V. (2012). Adult outcome of attention-deficit/hyperactivity disorder: A controlled 16-year follow-up study. *Journal of Clinical Psychiatry, 73,* 941–950.

Boat, T. F., Wu, J. T., Sciences, S., & National Academies of Sciences, Engineering, and Medicine. (2015). Prevalence of oppositional defiant disorder and conduct disorder. In *Mental disorders and disabilities among low-income children.* National Academies Press.

Brewer, S., Godley, M. D., & Hulvershorn, L. A. (2017). Treating mental health and substance use disorders in adolescents: What is on the menu? *Current Psychiatry Reports, 19,* 5. https://doi.org/10.1007/s11920-017-0755-0

Butzlaff, R. L., & Hooley, J. M. (1998). Expressed emotion and psychiatric relapse: A meta-analysis. *Archives of General Psychiatry, 55,* 547–552.

Faraone, S. V., Biederman, J., Spencer, T., Mick, E., Murray, K., Petty, C., . . . Monuteaux, M. C. (2006). Diagnosing adult attention deficit hyperactivity disorder: are late onset and subthreshold diagnoses valid?. *American Journal of Psychiatry, 163,* 1720–1729.

Groenman, A. P., Janssen, T. W., & Oosterlaan, J. (2017). Childhood psychiatric disorders as risk factor for subsequent substance abuse: A meta-analysis. *Journal of the American Academy of Child & Adolescent Psychiatry, 56,* 556–569.

Grucza, R. A., Krueger, R. F., Agrawal, A., Plunk, A. D., Krauss, M. J., Bongu, J., . . . Bierut, L. J. (2018). Declines in prevalence of adolescent substance use disorders and delinquent behaviors in the USA: A unitary trend? *Psychological Medicine, 48,* 1494–1503.

Giuliano, K., & Geyer, E. (2017). ADHD: Overdiagnosed and overtreated, or misdiagnosed and mistreated. *Cleveland Clinic Journal of Medicine, 84,* 873–880.

Hawes, S. W., Pacheco-Colon, I., Ross, J. M., & Gonzalez, R. (2020). Adolescent cannabis use and conduct problems: The mediating influence of callous-unemotional traits. *International Journal of Mental Health and Addiction, 18,* 613–627.

Ignaszewski, M. J., & Waslick, B. (2018). Update on randomized placebo-controlled trials in the past decade for treatment of major depressive disorder in child and adolescent patients: A systematic review. *Journal of Child and Adolescent Psychopharmacology, 28,* 668–675.

Johnston, L. D., Miech, R. A., O'Malley, P. M., Bachman, J. G., Schulenberg, J. E., & Patrick, M. E. (2019). *Monitoring the Future national survey results on drug use,*

1975–2018: Overview, key findings on adolescent drug use. University of Michigan, Institute for Social Research.

Lahey, B. B., Loeber, R., Burke, J. D., & Applegate, B. (2005). Predicting future antisocial personality disorder in males from a clinical assessment in childhood. *Journal of Consulting and Clinical Psychology, 73*, 389–399.

Loeber, R., Green, S. M., Keenan, K., & Lahey, B. B. (1995). Which boys will fare worse? Early predictors of the onset of conduct disorder in a six-year longitudinal study. *Journal of the American Academy of Child & Adolescent Psychiatry, 34*, 499–509.

Loeber, R., Stouthamer-Loeber, M., Van Kammen, W., & Farrington, D. P. (1991). Initiation, escalation and desistance in juvenile offending and their correlates. *Journal of Criminal Law & Criminology, 82*, 36–82

Miller, C. L. (2018). Cannabis and mental health. In K. A. Sabet & K. C. Winters (Eds.), *Contemporary health issues on marijuana* (pp. 122–164). Oxford University Press.

Molina, B. S., & Pelham Jr, W. E. (2014). Attention-deficit/hyperactivity disorder and risk of substance use disorder: Developmental considerations, potential pathways, and opportunities for research. *Annual Review of Clinical Psychology, 10*, 607–639.

National Institute of Mental Health. (2015). *Fact sheet: First episode psychosis.* https://www.nimh.nih.gov/health/topics/schizophrenia/raise/fact-sheet-first-episode-psychosis.shtml

National Institute of Mental Health. (2020). *Schizophrenia.* https://www.nimh.nih.gov/health/topics/schizophrenia/index.shtml

National Research Council and Institute of Medicine. (2009). *Preventing mental, emotional, and behavioral disorders among young people: Progress and possibilities.* The National Academies Press.

Pelham Jr, W. E., Fabiano, G. A., Waxmonsky, J. G., Greiner, A. R., Gnagy, E. M., Pelham III, W. E., . . . Karch, K. (2016). Treatment sequencing for childhood ADHD: A multiple-randomization study of adaptive medication and behavioral interventions. *Journal of Clinical Child & Adolescent Psychology, 45*, 396–415.

Rodgers, S., Müller, M., Rössler, W., Castelao, E., Preisig, M., & Ajdacic-Gross, V. (2015). Externalizing disorders and substance use: empirically derived subtypes in a population-based sample of adults. *Social Psychiatry and Psychiatric Epidemiology, 50*, 7–17.

Rowe, R., Costello, E. J., Angold, A., Copeland, W. E., & Maughan, B. (2010). Developmental pathways in oppositional defiant disorder and conduct disorder. *Journal of Abnormal Psychology, 119*, 726–738.

Substance Abuse and Mental Health Services Administration. (2016). *DSM-5 changes: Implications for child serious emotional disturbances.* Author.

van Emmerik-van Oortmerssen, K., van de Glind, G., Koeter, M. W., Allsop, S., Auriacombe, M., Barta, C., . . . Schoevers, R. A. (2014). Psychiatric comorbidity in treatment-seeking substance use disorder patients with and without attention deficit hyperactivity disorder: Results of the IASP study. *Addiction, 109*, 262–272.

Wang, C. H., Mazursky-Horowitz, H., & Chronis-Tuscano, A. (2014). Delivering evidence-based treatments for child attention-deficit/hyperactivity disorder (ADHD) in the context of parental ADHD. *Current psychiatry reports, 16*, 1–8.

Wilens, T. E., Martelon, M., Joshi, G., Bateman, C., Fried, R., Petty, C., & Biederman, J. (2011). Does ADHD predict substance-use disorders? A 10-year follow-up study of young adults with ADHD. *Journal of the American Academy of Child & Adolescent Psychiatry, 50*, 543–553.

Zulauf, C. A., Sprich, S. E., Safren, S. A., & Wilens, T. E. (2014). The complicated relationship between attention deficit/hyperactivity disorder and substance use disorders. *Current Psychiatry Reports, 16*, 1–11.

Behavioral Addictions

CHAPTER OUTLINE

INTRODUCTION

The concept of addictive behaviors can be extended to include a group of disorders that does not involve any intoxicant but is characterized by compulsive-like behaviors in the face of negative consequences. Commonly referred to *behavioral* or *process addictions*, this group of addictions occurs when a person repeatedly engages in an activity or behavior despite efforts to stop and suffers from resulting negative effects on the their ability to function normally in daily life and on their overall health (https://ameri canaddictioncenters.org/behavioral-addictions). The personal impact includes feeling remorse after engaging in the compulsive behavior. As is the case with substance use disorder (SUD), many individuals with a behavioral addiction and indulgences need professional help to address their problem. Examples of behavioral addictions discussed in this chapter are the following: gambling, internet/video gaming, social media, eating, sex, and shopping. Some of these are not common among adolescents (e.g., sex addiction, compulsive shopping), but there is educational value in learning about these types of addictions given that pre-disorder behavior patterns often occur during adolescence.

THE DSM AND BEHAVIORAL ADDICTIONS

Not all behavioral addictions have made their way to the most recent official diagnostic manual, authored by a team from the American Psychiatric Association (APA), the *Diagnostic and Statistical Manual of Mental Disorders* (5th ed.) (DSM-5; American Psychiatric Association, 2013). For inclusion in the DSM, an extensive research literature needs to exist documenting the disorder's validity. Relatively rare mental and behavioral disorders may not attract much attention from the scientific field, and thus it can be a long process for enough research to accumulate. The behavioral addiction literature is characterized by case reports and studies with very small samples and, thus, many of them are not in the manual.

The one behavioral addiction with the longest DSM history is gambling disorder (GD), as labeled in DSM-5 (prior versions of the DSM termed this disorder *compulsive gambling* and *pathological gambling*). GD is included in the DSM-5 disorder class of Substance-Related and Addictive Disorders, owing to the vast research that GD is a behavioral addiction with many similarities to the symptoms of SUD (see Box 8.1 for the DSM-5 criteria for GD).

The DSM issues pertaining to the other behavioral addictions are summarized below.

BOX 8.1

A DESCRIPTION OF THE NINE DSM-5 CRITERIA FOR GAMBLING
DISORDER (AMERICAN PSYCHIATRIC ASSOCIATION, 2013)

Persistent involvement in gambling activities that leads to significant negative consequences indicated by four or more of the following during a
12-month period:

1. Needs to gamble with increasing amounts of money in order to experience the desired excitement
2. Becomes restless or irritable when attempting to reduce or stop
   gambling
3. Numerous efforts to control, cut back, or stop gambling are unsuccessful.
4. Frequently preoccupied with gambling; examples include often reliving
   past gambling experiences, planning the next gambling occasion or betting opportunity, or planning ways to get money with which to gamble.
5. Often gambles when feeling negative emotions, such as helplessness,
   guilt, anxiety, or depression
6. Frequently "chases losses," that is, keeps gambling or returns another
   day to win back earlier losses
7. Lies to conceal the extent of time spent gambling or the extent of financial problems due to gambling
8. Excessive gambling has resulted in significant negative personal
   consequences (e.g., jeopardized a relationship; led to loss of a job or
   educational or career opportunity).
9. Gambling-related financial problems are so severe that others are asked
   to provide money or other types of financial relief.

- Sex addiction is not a formal DSM category, which has surprised
  some experts given that earlier DSM versions included "sexual
  disorders not otherwise specified" and "hypersexual disorder" is
  expected to be included in the 12th edition of a diagnostic system
  similar to the DSM, the International Classification of Diseases
  (ICD) (Krueger, 2016).

- Food addiction is not formally featured in DSM-5, but many of its characteristics are part of the definition of the DSM-5's feeding and eating disorders.
- Internet gaming addiction was discussed by the DSM-5 authors and it was decided that more clinical research is needed before consideration as a formal disorder. In the end, the DSM-5 authors placed internet gaming disorder in the Appendix among those conditions viewed as a potential diagnosis requiring further research. But the upcoming edition of the ICD will include gaming disorder as a new disorder. In some countries, including South Korea and China, video gaming has been recognized as a disorder and treatment programs have been established.

For future editions of the DSM to include a new behavioral addiction, the following will be required: 1) defining features of the addiction have been identified; 2) reliability and validity of specific behavioral addiction criteria have been obtained; 3) prevalence rates of the addiction are determined in representative national epidemiological samples; and 4) research has evaluated the etiology and associated biological features of the addiction.

ADOLESCENTS AND ADDICTIVE DISORDERS

All of the addictive disorders we review below can occur at varying levels of severity during adolescence. Some youth may show subclinical indulgence in a particular addictive-like behavior pattern that falls short of meeting a clinical definition of the respective disorder. Whether a person's symptoms escalate to the point of a full-blown disorder will depend on many individual and environmental risk and protective factors.

There is a substantive research literature on adolescent psychosocial risk and protective factors that are significantly associated with excessive gambling during adolescence. For the most part, the following variables have consistently been identified as characteristic of youth who gamble frequently: being a male; history of ADHD; parent or parents with a gambling problem; and pattern of substance abuse (Winters & Stinchfield, 2012).

Adolescence is a developmental period characterized by overinvolvement in certain social and reward-seeking activities, as we discussed in Chapter 2. But in most instances, the adolescent matures and learns to moderate prior indulgences. The typical trajectory of substance use among modern-day youth in the United States is an example of this—on average, adolescence is a period of escalating substance use, and by around age 25 this pattern shows a declining trend (Brown et al., 2008). Yet a favorable path is not always the case. Some youth develop a serious behavioral addiction during the teen years and also find themselves with a continuing problem into adulthood.

General Features

The main features of behavioral addictions consist of the core components of all addictions—excessive and compulsive-like involvement in the behavior, continuation of the behavior in the face of negative social and personal consequences, and the need to escalate the behavior in order to achieve the same rewarding result as earlier experienced. One way to demonstrate this is the comparability of the symptoms of an SUD and behavioral addictions. Signs and symptoms of behavioral addictions match many characteristics of an SUD, including the two "physical-based" SUD symptoms—tolerance and withdrawal. In Table 8.1 we show this comparison between SUD and GD diagnostic criteria.

Is it a behavioral addiction or overindulgence? The behavioral addictions are a controversial concept among researchers and those who work in the addiction field. Some experts adhere to the position that unless the behavior involves the use of a psychoactive substance, then the behavior cannot be a legitimate addiction. Then there is also the issue that some behavioral addictions represent normal and necessary behaviors (e.g., eating disorders

Table 8.1 COMPARISON OF DSM-5 CRITERIA FOR SUBSTANCE USE DISORDER AND
GAMBLING DISORDER

DSM-5 Criteria of a Substance Use Disorder	Comparable DSM-5 Criteria of a Gambling Disorder
Taking the substance in larger amounts or for longer than a person is meant to	Gambling is frequently on the person's mind—both reliving past gambling experiences and planning future gambling events
Wanting to cut down or stop using the substance but not managing to	Keeps trying to reduce or stop gambling without success
Spending a lot of time getting, using, or recovering from use of the substance	Gambling is frequently on the person's mind—both reliving past gambling experiences and planning future gambling events
Cravings and urges to use the substance	Gambling is frequently on the person's mind—both reliving past gambling experiences and planning future gambling events
Not managing to do what one should at work, home, or school because of substance use	Loses not only money but also relationships, their job, or a significant career opportunity as a result of gambling
Continuing to use, even when it causes problems in relationships	Lies to cover up how much they are gambling
	Becomes dependent on other people to give them money to deal with financial problems that have been caused by gambling
Giving up important social, occupational, or recreational activities because of substance use	Loses not only money but also relationships, their job, or a significant career opportunity as a result of gambling
Using substances again and again, even when it puts the person in danger (hazardous use)	Loses not only money but also relationships, their job, or a significant career opportunity as a result of gambling

Table 8.1 CONTINUED

DSM-5 Criteria of a Substance Use Disorder	Comparable DSM-5 Criteria of a Gambling Disorder
Continuing to use, even when the person knows they have a physical or psychological problem that could have been caused or made worse by the substance	Gambles when feeling depressed, guilty, or anxious
Needing more of the substance to get the effect the person wants (tolerance)	Needing to gamble with more money to get the same excitement from gambling as before
Development of withdrawal symptoms, which can be relieved by taking more of the substance	Feels restless or irritable when trying to reduce or stop gambling
	DSM-5 Criteria of a Gambling Disorder Not Comparable to SUD Criteria
	Tries to win back gambling losses

and sex addiction). Some are vital to our survival (e.g., eating and sex), and others are enjoyed as recreational outlets (e.g., shopping and exercise). The normality and abnormality of the behaviors that underlie behavioral addictions lie on a continuum from appropriate to inappropriate behavior, and this continuum may be distinctly different across a range of cultures.

We agree that the line between what is healthy involvement and unhealthy indulgence is not always clear. For example, there are many individuals who gamble frequently and do so for entertainment. Some may be high-frequency gamblers (e.g., playing fantasy sports daily or weekly) and their involvement is kept in check, does not involve large amounts of money, and does not result in interpersonal conflicts. Such individuals do not let their gambling interfere with work or other responsibilities. One can argue that the person is not using their money wisely, but if the person limits their losses to a minimum and shows other signs of self-control (e.g., plays only one fantasy sport), this behavior pattern would not fit a definition of addiction. This example of fantasy sports players fits what might be considered a "healthy indulgence": the person engages in the behavior for psychological enjoyment but the involvement falls short of causing harm, and the person demonstrates control over the behavior (e.g., stops or cuts down the behavior when circumstances dictate).

But there are now theoretical and empirical reasons why behavioral addictions can be viewed as valid addictions. When the involvement is excessive, has ritualistic features (e.g., repeats a behavior pattern prior to engaging in the addiction), leads the person to later feel remorse, and the behavior causes harm to oneself or others, the indulgence may be an indication of a behavioral addiction. Other signs of behavioral addictions are the following:

- Strong cravings to engage in the behavior, even when it's not appropriate to do so.
- The person is unable to stop engaging in the behavior despite several negative consequences resulting from or aggravated by the addictive behavior.
- Negative consequences resulting from a behavioral addition include problems with mental health, physical illness, disruptions in relationships with significant others and co-workers, financial or legal problems, and other negative effects as a direct result of continuing the problem behavior.

GAMBLING DISORDER

Gambling disorder (GD), as it is referred to in the DSM-5, has also been referred to as problem gambling, compulsive gambling, pathological gambling, and gambling addiction. It refers to playing games of chance for some payout or reward (typically money) at a compulsive-like level that causes the gambler significant personal, legal, and financial consequences. As we detailed in Box 8.1, the symptoms of GD include the following: placing bets more and more frequently; betting more than originally intended; "chasing" losses by continually betting beyond the ability to pay; feeling irritable or aggressive when unable to gamble or when losing; and being preoccupied with gambling.

Research surveys indicate that most adolescents report some gambling. The most popular games played by teenagers are cards, sports betting, and informal betting (e.g., betting which friend will be the first to get a driver's license) (Calado et al., 2017; Welte et al., 2002, 2008). Gambling by adults is as popular as it is with adolescents; games most commonly played by adults are casino games, lotteries and sports betting.) Recently, researchers have noted the increased popularity of social casino gaming by teenagers (Derevensky & Gainsbury, 2016). These games are generally free to play (although some offer opportunities to play for money), are easy to play, and offer social and competitive features.

There is a debate among experts as to the prevalence of *problem gambling* among adolescents. Some reports indicate that the adolescent rate of problem gambling is higher than among adults, and the other side of the argument is that survey data are prone to false positives (Derevensky et al., 2003). We turn to recent U.S. surveys of gambling behavior by Welte and colleagues (Welte et al., 2002, 2008). Drawing from both of their publications, the prevalence of problem gambling across seven age groups are reported in Table 8.2. The prevalence of recent (past year) problem gambling was highest among those in the 31- to 40-year-old group (5.2%) and lowest in the young and old age groups (14–18 age, 1.3%; 61+ age, 1.2%) (Welte et al., 2002, 2008).

Table 8.2 Past-Year Problem Gambling Prevalence Rate by Age Group, U.S. National Sample (Welte et al., 2002, 2008)

Age Group (years)	Percent Problem Gamblers
14–18	1.3
19–25	2.1
26–30	4.3
31–40	5.2
41–50	3.3
51–60	3.3
61+	1.2

A relevant topic regarding adolescent gambling is that most adults who develop a gambling problem started their gambling habit during adolescence, and the onset of clinical symptoms did not emerge until adulthood (Winters & Stinchfield, 2012). This point of view includes the notion that adolescent gambling involvement may lead to some "soft signs" of a problem with gambling, but bona fide, clinical-level gambling problems typically do not emerge until adulthood. This perspective is supported by data from a U.S. survey of mental health among a national sample of adults; the survey included gambling and problem gambling questions (Kessler et al., 2008). Figure 8.1 shows two sets of bars. The *orange bars* show the mean age of gambling onset across groups defined by the number of gambling symptoms already experienced by respondents. There is a clear and statistically significant relationship: more gambling problems are associated with a younger the age of gambling onset. The *seaweed green* bars speak to the issue of the relationship of number of problem gambling symptoms as a function of the age the first symptom was experienced. The green bars indicate that regardless of how many DSM-level symptoms have been experienced, the onset of the first symptom generally occurs in the mid-20s (the mean age of onset across severity groups hovers around age 24). These data confirm what other researchers have reported: The origins of an adult gambling problem involve adolescent onset of gambling involvement, and a serious gambling problem, if it occurs, starts to reveal itself in the mid-20s.

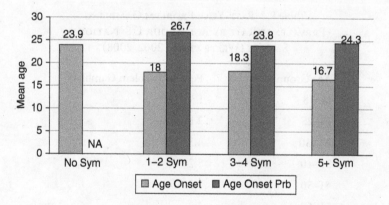

Figure 8.1 Onset of Gambling Variables and Number of Lifetime Symptoms (Kessler et al., 2008)

INTERNET AND VIDEO GAMING ADDICTION

The internet is a major part of most of our daily lives, and this is also the case for adolescents. They use the internet to communicate with their friends, keep up-to-date with current events, and to find information (and perhaps too often, misinformation). The most popular online platforms among adolescents are YouTube, Instagram, and Snapchat. The popularity of once "go-to sites," Twitter and Facebook, has dropped in recent years as these more recent online platforms have shifted the popularity trends (see Figure 8.2 for a comparison of internet platforms among adolescents).

YouTube, Instagram and Snapchat are the most popular online platforms among teens

% of U.S. teens who...

	Say they use ...	Say they use __ most often
YouTube	85%	32%
Instagram	72	15
Snapchat	69	35
Facebook	51	10
Twitter	32	3
Tumblr	9	<1
Reddit	7	1
None of the above	3	3

Note: Figures in first column add to more than 100% because multiple responses were allowed. Question about most-used site was asked only of respondents who use multiple sites; results have been recalculated to include those who use only one site. Respondents who did not give an answer are not shown.
Source: Survey conducted March 7-April 10, 2018.
"Teens, Social Media & Technology 2018'

PEW RESEARCH CENTER

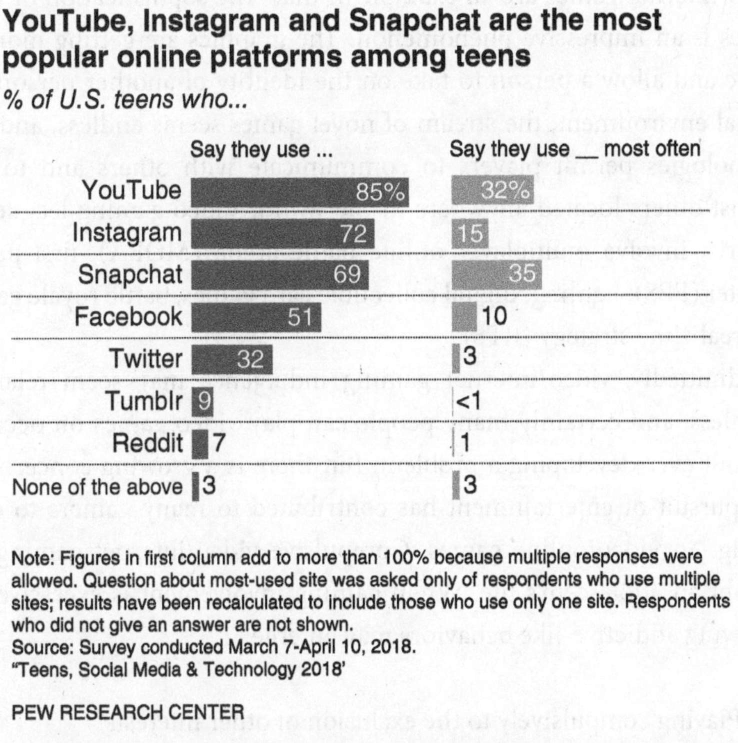

Figure 8.2 Most Popular Internet Platforms Among Teenagers
SOURCE: "TEENS, SOCIAL MEDIA & TECHNOLOGY 2018" Pew Research Center, Washington, D.C. (MAY 29, 2018) https://www.pewresearch.org/internet/2018/05/31/teens-social-media-technology-2018/pi_2018-05-31_teenstech_0-01/

There are several colleges that now support varsity eSports programs. As of 2018, 63 universities and colleges had a program;
this is up from 7 in 2016. Often started as the college's popular stu-
dent-run eSports club, many varsity programs offer elite gamers
scholarships. Supporters of this trend cite these advantages: it's another
avenue in which colleges can attract students; the sport celebrates the
diversity of interests on campus; and investments in training facilities
and other costs are much less than investments in most collegiate
sports. The NCAA is already considering their role in the sport.

Another purpose of the internet is as a source of entertainment, and
video/internet games are an example of that. The sophistication of video
games is an impressive phenomenon. The graphics are getting more realistic and allow a person to take on the identity of another person in a
virtual environment, the stream of novel games seems endless, and new
technologies permit players to communicate with others and to play
against others located anywhere in the world. Video gaming leagues, or
eSports, involve multiplayer online battle arena (MOBA), first-person
shooter (FPS), fighting, digital collectible card games, battle royale games,
and real-time strategy (RTS).

Admittedly, video/internet gaming indulgence may seem relatively
harmless, and certainly many people can play video games on occasion
without ever developing a problem. But there is a growing concern that
this pursuit of entertainment has contributed to many gamers to over-
indulge in video/online games. Compulsive video/internet gaming can
disrupt an adolescent's life. When gaming involvement is excessive, the
following addictive-like behaviors may emerge:

- Playing compulsively to the exclusion of other interests
- Persistent gaming results in clinically significant impairment
- Amount of time spent playing contributes to impairment in one's
  academic or job functioning

- Withdrawal symptoms occur when kept from gaming
- Inability to cut down or stop
- The need to spend more time gaming to satisfy the urge

The Entertainment Software Association and others in the industry called on the World Health Organization to reverse its decision, saying "gaming disorder" is not based on sufficiently robust evidence to justify inclusion." This reaction by an industry that provides the agent or source of a product that has been linked to addiction is not new. Decades ago, the tobacco industry advanced the claim that their product was safe (of course, they no longer support these types of claims). Some observers also include the casino industry as another example. However, the American Gaming Association (AGA), the main lobbyist group for the gaming industry, promotes a public health view of gambling (e.g., AGA supports the view that when gambling, "know your limits and bet safely").

Video/internet games can be highly engrossing, but can adolescents and others get addicted to them? Simply spending a lot of time playing video/internet games is not sufficient to consider it a disorder; the gaming needs to interfere with the adolescent's daily life. There is no consensus among experts for assigning "gaming addiction" as a formal diagnostic category. Yet evidence for its inclusion was viewed as strong enough by the World Health Organization (WHO); "gaming disorder" is now a mental health condition in the WHO's ICD-11 (11th edition of the International Classification of Diseases). In some support of the ICD, the U.S.-based DSM-5 system, which is authored by the APA, lists internet gaming disorder as a provisional disorder that requires more research (see Box 8.2).

The research that does exist on video addiction is mainly based on studies conducted in Asian countries and Australia. A common finding is that among gamers, young males are by far the most prevalent

---

BOX 8.2

DSM-5 PROVISIONAL CRITERIA FOR INTERNET GAMING DISORDER*

1. Preoccupation with gaming
2. Withdrawal symptoms when gaming is taken away or not possible (sadness, anxiety, irritability)
3. Tolerance, the need to spend more time gaming to satisfy the urge
4. Inability to reduce playing, unsuccessful attempts to quit gaming
5. Giving up other activities, loss of interest in previously enjoyed activities due to gaming
6. Continuing to game despite problems
7. Deceiving family members or others about the amount of time spent on gaming
8. The use of gaming to relieve negative moods, such as guilt or hopelessness
9. Risk having jeopardized or lost a job or relationship due to gaming

*Five or more symptoms experienced within any given year are required. The condition can include gaming on the internet or on any electronic device.

---

demographic group (Griffiths & Pontes, 2020; Van Rooij et al., 2014). But there are no reliable statistics as to what percent of youth who play these games develop an addiction.

SOCIAL MEDIA INDULGENCE

Social media involves websites and applications that allow users to create and share content or to participate in social discussions. Numerous online sites are the source of social media. A representative survey of adolescents conducted in 2018 showed that 97% of respondents said they used at least one popular *online social media sites*, the most popular being YouTube, Instagram, and Snapchat (as we show above in Figure 8.2).

In 2004, the successful social networking site, Facebook, was established as a closed virtual community for Harvard students. The site expanded very quickly and Facebook currently has more than 500 million users, of whom 50% log on to it every day. But Facebook was not the first social networking site. What was the first?

Answer: SixDegrees, launched in 1997, based on the idea that everybody is linked with everybody else via six degrees of separation, and initially referred to as the "small world problem."

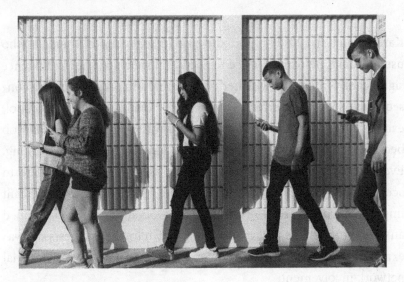

SOURCE: Rawpixel.com/Shutterstock.

"Social media addiction" is not recognized in any of the formal diagnostic classification systems (DSM and ICD) and its prevalence as a bona-fide addiction is a topic for debate. There are case reports and qualitative studies suggesting that excess involvement in social media leads to the classic addictive behaviors we described above. Experts have noted that chronic social media users report mental preoccupation with social networking, check their mobile phone nearly all the time, and report discomfort and agitation if they are unable to connect (Kuss &

Griffiths, 2011). But problems can arise when a young person compulsively posts mundane details of one's daily life, is spending hours on the various sources of social media, and is using this form of communication to bully others. The lure of social media can be significant for a teenager; it offers a buffer for those who lack secure social relationships, numerous opportunities to communicate and establish relationships through social networks, and the ability to manage one's self-presentation in ways not possible with person-to-person contact. Social media can provide a social retreat for teens who experience or perceive deficits in their social relationships.

Karaiskos et al. (2010) report the case of a 24-year-old female who used a social network service to such an extent that her indulgence significantly interfered with her professional and private life. As a consequence, she was referred to a psychiatric clinic. She used Facebook excessively for at least 5 hours a day and was dismissed from her job because she continuously checked her account instead of working. Even during the clinical interview, she used her mobile phone to access Facebook. In addition to excessive use that led to significant impairment in a variety of areas in the woman's life, she developed anxiety symptoms as well as insomnia, which further suggests she was experiencing a clinical-level problem associated with excessive social network involvement.

In terms of prevalence studies, we found only two studies that *directly* measured criteria for social media addiction among youth. Both are studies of college students in China and are limited by use of only self-report measures to measure addiction. In each study, respondents were administered the Internet Addiction Test (Young, 1996) to rate their involvement with a popular Chinese social networking site. Rates of social media addiction (based on elevated test score) were 24% (Zhou & Leung, 2012) and 34% (Wan, 2009).

Research indicates that teens are getting less sleep than in prior years. Experts contend that one reason is the excessive use of smartphone and other electronic devices before bedtime. The blue light emitted by smartphones and tablets simulates daylight, inhibiting the brain's production of melatonin, a hormone important for regulating normal sleep.

A related research issue is the extent of *smartphone use* and if excessive use of one's phone can be considered an addiction (Biang & Leung, 2014; Billieux et al., 2015). A recent survey suggests that the prevalence of "problematic smartphone use" (i.e., excessive use) is relatively high. The 2018 survey of adolescents by Pew Research indicated that 54% of adolescents say they worry they spend too much time on their smartphone (Schaeffer, 2019). And other surveys point to the association between excessive smartphone use and sleep disturbance (Lemola et al., 2015; Semenza et al., 2020) and interpersonal problems (O'Reilly, 2020; Smetaniuk, 2014; Thomée et al., 2011).

Screen Time

Whether or not an adolescent is addicted to social media, there is the health issue of being connected and online for extended periods of time (e.g., Babic et al., 2017). Longitudinal studies suggest that increases in recreational screen time precede lower psychological well-being among adolescents. For example, a large U.S. ($n = 40,337$) national random sample in 2016 of 2- to 17-year-old youth included comprehensive measures of screen time (including cell phones, computers, electronic devices, electronic games, and TV) and an array of psychological well-being measures (Twenge & Campbell, 2018). Among 11- to 13-year-olds, the average time spent on electronic devices (primarily smartphones) was 2 hours per day; for 14- to 17-year-olds, average time spent on electronic devices was 2.7 hours per day. Table 8.3 shows the survey results for two types of screen

Table 8.3 MEAN HOURS OF DAY OF SCREEN USE BY AGE GROUP, U.S., 2016
(TWENGE & CAMPBELL, 2018; $N = 40,337$)

	2 to 5 years	6 to 10 years	11 to 13 years	14 to 17 years
TV and video games	1.46	1.53	1.80	1.89
Electronic device	0.82	1.25	2.00	2.70
Total screen time	2.28	2.78	3.80	4.59

sources (TV/video games and electronic devices) for various child and early teenage age groups.

An average of more than 1 hour/day of smartphone use, compared to nonusers or low users, reported these health issues (Twenge & Campbell, 2018):

- Less psychological well-being;
- Less self-control, emotional stability;
- More difficulty to finish tasks; and
- More difficulty making friends

Can abstaining or reducing screen time improve a person's well-being? Tromholt (2016) recruited over 1,000 adults in Denmark to agree to abstain from Facebook for a week. By comparing the treatment group (participants who took a break from Facebook) with the control group (participants who kept using Facebook), it was demonstrated that taking a break from Facebook had positive effects on two dimensions of well-being: life satisfaction increases and emotions become more positive. Furthermore, it was demonstrated that these effects were significantly greater for Facebook users who reported that they tend to envy others on Facebook.

Those with an average of more than 7 hours/day of smartphone use were twice as likely to ever have been diagnosed with depression or anxiety or treated by mental health professional. Also, nonusers and low users were generally equal on well-being measures, suggesting that some use of smartphone use is not linked to poor health.

Hutton and colleagues (Hutton et al., 2019) examined with a cross-sectional design the associations between screen-based media use and brain structures known to support language and literacy skills in preschool-aged children. Based on parent estimate of their child's screen time, lower integrity of brain white matter tracts supporting language and emergent literacy skills in prekindergarten children was linked to increased children's time spent on screen-based media devices. "Lower integrity" in the brain's white matter suggests a decrement in brain development. The findings suggest that excessive screen time at very early stages of brain development can be harmful to neurodevelopment.

The same research group analyzed data from two representative surveys of U.S. adolescents (ages 13 to 18; $N = 506,820$) in order to compare national statistics on depressive symptoms, suicide rates, and time spent on "new media" (including social media and electronic devices such as smartphones) (Twenge et al., 2018). The researchers found that adolescents who had more screen time were more likely to report mental health issues, and adolescents who spent more time on non-screen activities (in-person social interaction, sports/exercise, homework, print media, and attending religious services) were less likely to report such issues. Cyclical economic factors such as unemployment and other economic signs were not associated with suicide rates when matched by year.

DISORDERED EATING

Of course, all of us need to eat, yet for some, overeating is a problem. Referred to as disordered eating or a food addiction, chronic overeating can be a struggle for some individuals and lead to serious health problems. Those who cannot control their compulsive eating behaviors tend to crave unhealthy foods, such as those high in fats, sugar, and salt. Sufferers often describe feeling an intoxicating "high" during binge eating, develop a tolerance for food (as seen in drug addiction), experience low self-esteem and even shame, and may gain weight to the point of becoming obese (although many with a food addiction have normal body mass indexes [BMIs]). This problem is not simply a deficit with the physiological basis of feeling full; the excessive eating occurs when the person no longer feels hungry.

How is obesity defined? Informally, it refers to being well above one's normal weight. Most experts consider "well above" if a person is more than 20% over their ideal weight. Obesity has been more precisely defined by the National Institutes of Health Body Mass Index (BMI) of 30 and above. A BMI of 30 is about 30 pounds overweight.

SOURCE: https://www.medicinenet.com/script/main/art.asp?articlekey=11760

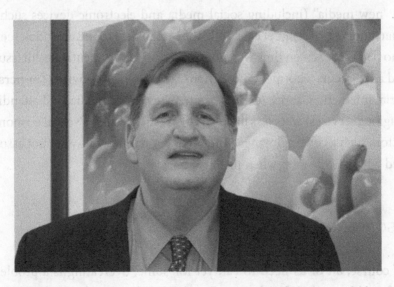

SOURCE: Kelly Brownell, Ph.D., an internationally renowned scholar known for his work on obesity and food policy. Photo courtesy of Kelly Brownell.

Appearance-related teasing was the focus of survey of 1,344 students ages 11 to 14 from five public middle schools near Hartford, Connecticut (Klinck et al., 2020). The students were asked if friends, peers, or family members had teased them about their weight, body shape, or eating during the prior 6 months. More than half (55%) of the students reported teasing of this type, including three out of four overweight girls (76%), 71% of overweight boys, 52% of girls who weren't overweight, and 43% of boys who weren't overweight. The survey also found that frequent weight-based teasing was associated with higher levels of total alcohol use, binge drinking, and marijuana use. This research suggests that weight-based teasing and bullying are common and have many negative effects for adolescents.

The notion that a person can get addicted to food is supported by several lines of evidence. The characteristics of excessive food eating are consistent with other behavioral addictions (e.g., compulsive-like behavior in the face of negative consequences, preoccupied with the behavior, difficulty stopping or reducing the behavior, accelerating the behavior due to developing tolerance). Also, brain imaging studies provide some insight. The effects of any eating will activate the pleasure or reward regions in the brain. These regions of the brain involve dopamine-rich neural networks in the amygdala (emotion region), nucleus accumbens (motivation region), and hippocampus (memory region) (for more on this issue, see Chapter 3). Yet when a person eats highly "palatable" foods, the dopamine system is activated with higher intensity (Blumenthal & Gold, 2010; Brownell & Walsh, 2017). Palatable foods are very attractive to our taste buds, and as you might expect, examples are the junk foods (salty snakes, chocolate, non-diet soda, most fast foods). Once people experience this intense pleasure from eating highly palatable foods, the likelihood is increased that they will feel the need to eat these unhealthy foods again. And when palatable foods are the mainstay of a person's diet, the result may be a food addiction. But because nonpalatable foods are also rewarding and can potentially be binged, researchers have also looked at the way foods are overconsumed (e.g., alternating access and restriction) as a contributing source to this problem

(Pelchat, 2009). Also, food addiction does not always play a role in obesity. Normal-weight individuals may exhibit food addiction but avoid gaining weight by increasing physical exercise or because of genetic factors that allow them to accommodate a high-caloric diet.

Types of Eating Disorders

The DSM-5 (American Psychiatric Association, 2013) describes three eating-related disorders. *Anorexia* is characterized by excessive restriction of energy intake relative to requirements, a significantly low body weight, and intense fear of gaining weight. *Bulimia* involves recurrent and distinct episodes of uncontrollable binge eating and recurrent inappropriate compensatory behavior in order to prevent weight gain (e.g., self-induced vomiting). The main characteristic of a *binge eating disorder* is binge eating without the compensatory behavior. Whereas some characteristics of food addiction overlap with bulimia and binge eating disorder (Rosa et al., 2015), many features of a food addiction can be present without a person meeting diagnostic criteria for any of the DSM-5 eating-related disorders.

How big a problem is disordered eating among adolescents? Based on a DSM-defined disorder, the lifetime prevalence of any eating disorder (i.e., anorexia, bulimia, and binge eating) among adolescents in the United States is estimated to be approximately 6% (Swanson et al., 2011). The majority of positive cases are girls and some only had a diagnosable problem during childhood. If the definition of eating disorder is broadened to include *adolescent obesity*, the prevalence rate is much higher than 6%.

SEX ADDICTION

The characteristics of the proposed hypersexual disorder discussed by the DSM committee are the following:

- Repetitive and intense preoccupation with sexual fantasies, urges, and behaviors

- Adverse consequences or impairments in social, occupational, or other important areas resulting from the preoccupation
- Repeated unsuccessful attempts to control or diminish the amount of time spent in sexual thoughts
- The excessive sexual behavior is in response to negative mood states or stressful life events.

Also referred to as compulsive sexual behavior or hypersexuality, the signs of this addiction include the following: persistent sexual impulses or urges; these urges are so strong that the person engages in repetitive sexual behaviors; the repetitive sexual behavior is so frequent that the person neglects health and responsibilities and it contributes to social and personal adverse consequences (e.g., school disruption, other areas of functioning); and repeated and unsuccessful efforts to control or reduce the sexual behaviors (Kraus et al., 2016). Other characteristics are sex with multiple and sometimes anonymous partners; sex acts that are designed to maximize stimulation; a tendency to not use protection and thus elevating one's risk for contracting sexually transmitted infections (STIs), including deadly viruses like HIV; and compulsive use of internet pornography.

Is love addiction real? Feeling emotionally attached to a partner, even a strong emotional attachment, most certainly does not meet the definition of an addiction associated with maladaptive behaviors. But consider a serial monogamist who spends time ensuring that the partner will be a positive partner and craves the love and attention of the prospective partner. Yet before long it is clear that the person is not interested in a long-lasting genuine connection and then moves on to seeking another partner.

As noted above, sex addiction is not a formal DSM-5 category, although it was seriously considered by the APA committee (as "hypersexuality disorder"). Some experts make a case that sexuality is so complicated and controversial that the APA committee wanted to steer clear of the topic. Included in this argument is the concern that a sex addiction disorder will be too often used as an excuse for a person's excessive and perceived immoral behavior. This notion is referred to as "functional attribution of misbehavior." In this light, the person's problem behavior is claimed to be due to a behavioral or mental disorder. The other side of the argument is that the concept of sex addiction has some research backing (as evidenced by the fact that it's being considered for the next edition of ICD), and characteristics of excessive sexual behavior dovetail with other behavioral addictions—that is, compulsive behavior that continues in the face of negative consequences, intense preoccupation (in this case with sexual fantasies and urges and behaviors), and the inability to control the behavior).

SHOPPING ADDICTION

Like many other behavioral addictions, shopping addiction (or referred to as compulsive buying behaviors) is not currently listed in DSM-5 as an addictive disorder, nor as a stand-alone impulse control disorder (Granero et al., 2016). Shopping addiction is characterized by the excessive, impulsive, and uncontrollable purchasing of products and goods despite the presence of numerous and severe psychological, social, occupational, and financial consequences (Müller et al., 2015). Common statements or thoughts from a compulsive shopper are as follows: "It was a great deal I couldn't pass up." "I can use this later on." "My friends will think this is so cool." "You can never have too many of these."

Another feature pertains to the underlying functional value of shopping. When noncompulsive consumers shop, the value and usefulness of the purchase are the primary consideration. However, for a compulsive shopper, the activity addresses motivations related to improving mood, coping with stress, and managing self-image (McQueen et al., 2014). Yet, as is the case with most behavioral addictions, the person feels regret and remorse after the binge activity (Thege et al., 2015).

Is there a neurological component to compulsive shopping? As is the case with substance use disorders, brain imaging studies in people who are compulsive shoppers reveal activation of the reward processing region of the brain, or referred to as the limbic system, as seen with other addictions (e.g., Hartston, 2012). This finding provides further support that behavioral addictions are mediated by important neurological structures and processes. (See Chapter 4 for a discussion of the brain's reward processing region and addiction.)

The prevalence of shopping addiction is a point of debate. There is some indication that it has increased worldwide during recent times, perhaps owing to the ease at which online shopping can facilitate urges to binge shop. A recent meta-analysis estimated a pooled prevalence rate of 4.9% for compulsive shopping among adults (with higher rates among women), and higher rates among university students (Maraz et al., 2015) and older adults (Mueller et al., 2010). However, other prevalence studies place estimates as low as 1% and as high as 30% (Basu et al., 2011). These wide ranges are likely due to the variability in how surveys have defined compulsive shopping, as well as the variability of particular contextual factors affected by current economic conditions, availability of goods, disposable income, and materialistic values (Unger et al., 2014).

A self-admitted "shopping addict" is Elton John. At the end of the 2019 movie *Rocket Man*, his extended recovery from drug addiction is celebrated. But what follows is a photo of him smiling, surrounded by numerous boxes and bags of merchandise, with this subtitle: "I'm still a shopping addict."

Does shopping addiction typically show early signs during adolescence? Many experts believe so (Maraz et al., 2015), but there are no studies that have rigorously documented this connection. But it is noteworthy that most adults addicted to shopping report that the habit began during adolescence or young adulthood.

TREATMENT ISSUES

Treatment options in the United States specifically for behavioral addictions is, at best, available to some degree in large urban areas and virtually nonexistent elsewhere. A handful of problem gambling treatment facilities exist; the National Center on Problem Gambling lists eight outpatient or residential programs (see https://www.ncpgambling.org/help-treatment/treatment-facilities/). None of these indicate that they have a specific adolescent component. The authors know of a small handful of treatment facilities in the United States that specialize in sexual addictions, yet we are not aware of any that specifically focus on social messaging, shopping, and exercise addictions.

Treatment for Disordered Eating

On the other hand, there exists a vast system of treatment programs for adolescents with disordered eating and there is a substantial research literature on this topic (Mayo Clinic, 2017). Binge eating disorder and anorexia are both addressed by most programs. For medically unstable adolescents whose disordered eating has resulted in serious medical problems (e.g., a very low admission weight), a course of inpatient treatment is indicated until medical stability is achieved. For medically stable adolescents with a binge eating disorder, two strategies are commonly integrated in the clinical practice arena. One is the use of cognitive behavioral therapy (CBT) strategies for developing a weight reduction plan (typical plans include detailed meal and food instructions), developing eating control strategies, increasing the adolescent's physical activity, and restoring normal adolescent development interests and tasks. The other strategy is family-based treatment, with the focus on ways parents can support the adolescent's goals, including the use of rewards and consequences based on the adolescent's compliance with the treatment plan.

Self-Help for Behavioral Addictions

When early signs of a behavioral addiction emerge, a starting point for getting help can be initiated when a significant other or friend has a conversation with the person. Expressing concern and suggesting that person seek professional help can be a powerful motivator for behavior change. A list of common early signs for any of the behavioral addictions we discussed in this chapter are noted below.

- The behavior becomes an obsession.
- The behavior becomes frequent—daily and/or multiple times per day.
- The person chooses to engage in the behavior rather than do school work, go to school, spend time with family or friends, or engage in other activities that were once enjoyed.
- Relationships are harmed by the person's chronic engagement in the behavior.
- Other serious consequences result from an inability to stop the behavior (e.g., problems at work or school, health problems, legal issues, money problems).

There are a growing number of self-help programs for behavioral addictions, most of which are based on the 12-step model that has its origins in treating alcoholism and drug addiction (see Chapter 13 for details of the 12-step model). Examples include Gamblers Anonymous, SMART Recovery's Gambling Addiction, Food Addicts Anonymous, Food Addicts in Recovery, Sex Addicts Anonymous, and Shopaholics Anonymous. Some SMART Recovery programs, an alternative to the 12-step model, welcome those with behavioral addictions at their meetings.

MINI-REVIEW

- Behavioral (or process) addictions are defined as addictions when an individual repeatedly engages in a behavior that leads to negative effects on their ability to function normally in daily life and has a deleterious effect on their overall health.
- Core features of behavioral addictions are similar to symptoms of a substance use disorder: compulsive-like behavior; continuing of the behavior in the face of negative consequences; and difficulty in cutting back or halting the addictive-like behavior.
- Behavioral addictions and indulgences discussed in this chapter are gambling, internet/video gaming, social media, eating, sex, and shopping. The DSM-5 (American Psychiatric Association, 2013) recognizes gambling disorder and eating disorders as an official diagnostic category; internet gaming disorder is a provisional category at this time.
- Some behavioral addictions are very rare among adolescents (e.g., sex addiction, compulsive shopping) but there is educational value in learning about all of them given that pre-disorder behavior patterns often occur during adolescence (e.g., excessive involvement in playing video games).
- Eating disorders are the one behavioral addiction that is most relevant among youth. This domain includes bulimia, anorexia, and binge eating disorder.
- Many individuals with a behavioral addiction need professional help to address their problem.

DISCUSSION POINTS

1. In what ways do behavioral addictions differ from an obsessive-compulsive disorder, which is discussed in Chapter 7?

2. Can virtually any behavior be an "addiction"? This question is an ongoing debate among experts. Discuss these two questions:
   - What are the key issues of defining if a behavior pattern is an addiction?
   - Is the term *addiction* overused (e.g., addicted to TV watching; work addiction)?

3. Many drug addiction treatment programs are abstinence based. But with some behavioral addictions, total abstinence is not a consideration (e.g., sex addiction and shopping addiction). Discuss non-abstinence treatment goals for a client with a shopping addiction.

4. What techniques are used by social media platforms to keep users drawn to them? Are these techniques similar to marketing techniques used in other areas of the economy?

FURTHER CURIOSITY AND DIGGING

Addictions

Web-based research resource from Harvard on addictions: Brief Addiction Science Information Source: https://www.basisonline.org/about_the_basis.htmlReferences

Behavioral Addictions

Scholarly book on the behavioral addictions:
Rosenberg, K. R., & Feder, L. C. (Eds.). (2014). *Behavioral addictions: Criteria, evidence, and treatment.* Academic Press.

Problem Gambling

Web-based resource on problem gambling research: International Center on Responsible Gaming: https://www.icrg.org

Eating Disorder

Web-based resource for eating disorders: National Eating Disorders Association: https://www.nationaleatingdisorders.org/

Indulgence with Social Media

Netflix: *The Social Dilemma* (2020).

REFERENCES

American Psychiatric Association. (2013). *Diagnostic and statistical manual of mental disorders* (5th ed.). American Psychiatric Association Press.

Babic, M. J., Smith, J. J., Morgan, P. J., Eather, N., Plotnikoff, R. C., & Lubans, D. R. (2017). Longitudinal associations between changes in screen-time and mental health outcomes in adolescents. *Mental Health and Physical Activity, 12*, 124–131.

Basu, B., Basu, S., & Basu, J. (2011). Compulsive buying: An overlooked entity. *Journal of the Indian Medical Association, 109*, 582–585.

Biang, M., & Leung, L. (2014). Smartphone addiction: Linking loneliness, shyness, symptoms and patterns of use to social capital. *Media Asia, 41*, 159–176.

Billieux, J., Maurage, P., Lopez-Fernandez, O., Kuss, D. J., & Griffiths, M. D. (2015). Can disordered mobile phone use be considered a behavioral addiction? An update on current evidence and a comprehensive model for future research. *Current Addiction Reports, 2*, 156–162.

Blumenthal, D. M., & Gold, M. S. (2010). Neurobiology of food addiction. *Current Opinion in Clinical Nutrition & Metabolic Care, 13*, 359–365.

Brown, S. A., McGue, M., Maggs, J., Schulenberg, J., Hingson, R., Swartzwelder, S., Martin, C., Chung, T., Tapert, S. F., Sher, K., Winters, K. C., Lowman, C., & Murphy, S. (2008). A developmental perspective on alcohol and youth ages 16–20. *Pediatrics, 121*, S290–S310.

Brownell, K. D., & Walsh, B. T. (Eds.). (2017). *Eating disorders and obesity: A comprehensive handbook*. Guilford Publications.

Calado, F., Alexandre, J., & Griffiths, M. D. (2017). Prevalence of adolescent problem gambling: A systematic review of recent research. *Journal of Gambling Studies, 33*, 397–424.

Derevensky, J. L., & Gainsbury, S. M. (2016). Social casino gaming and adolescents: Should we be concerned and is regulation in sight? *International Journal of Law and Psychiatry, 44*, 1–6.

Derevensky, J., Gupta, R., & Winters, K. C. (2003). Prevalence rates of youth gambling: Are the current rates inflated? *Journal of Gambling Studies, 19*, 405–426.

Granero, R., Fernández-Aranda, F., Mestre-Bach, G., Steward, T., Baño, M., del Pino-Gutiérrez, A., . . . Tárrega, S. (2016). Compulsive buying behavior: clinical comparison with other behavioral addictions. *Frontiers in Psychology, 7*, 914. https://doi.org/10.3389/fpsyg.2016.00914

Griffiths, M. D., & Pontes, H. M. (2020). The future of gaming disorder research and player protection: What role should the video gaming industry and researchers play? *International Journal of Mental Health and Addiction, 18*, 784–790.

Hartston, H. (2012). The case for compulsive shopping as an addiction. *Journal of Psychoactive Drugs, 44*, 64–67.

Hutton, J. S., Dudley, J., Horowitz-Kraus, T., DeWitt, T., & Holland, S. K. (2019). Associations between screen-based media use and brain white matter integrity in preschool-aged children. *JAMA Pediatrics*, e193869–e193869.

Karaiskos, D., Tzavellas, E., Balta, G., & Paparrigopoulos, T. (2010). P02-232-Social net-work addiction: A new clinical disorder? *European Psychiatry, 25*, 855. https://doi. org/10.1016/S0924-9338(10)70846-4

Kessler, R., Hwang, I., LaBrie, R., Petukhova, M., Sampson, N., Winters, K. C., & Shaffer, H. (2008). The prevalence and correlates of DSM-IV pathological gambling in the National Comorbidity Survey Replication Study. *Psychological Medicine, 38*, 1351–1360.

Klinck, M., Vannucci, A., Fagle, T., & Ohannessian, C.M. (2020). Appearance-related teasing and substance use during early adolescence. *Psychology of Addictive Behaviors, 34*(4), 541–548. DOI:10.1037/adb0000563

Kraus, S. W., Voon, V., & Potenza, M. N. (2016). Should compulsive sexual behavior be considered an addiction? *Addiction, 111*, 2097–2106.

Krueger, R. B. (2016). Diagnosis of hypersexual or compulsive sexual behavior can be made using ICD-10 and DSM-5 despite rejection of this diagnosis by the American Psychiatric Association. *Addiction, 111*, 2110–2111.

Kuss, D. J., & Griffiths, M. D. (2011). Online social networking and addiction—A review of the psychological literature. *International Journal of Environmental Research and Public Health, 8*, 3528–3552.

Lemola, S., Perkinson-Gloor, N., Brand, S., Dewald-Kaufmann, J. F., & Grob, A. (2015). Adolescents' electronic media use at night, sleep disturbance, and depressive symptoms in the smartphone age. *Journal of Youth and Adolescence, 44*, 405–418.

Maraz A., Griffiths M. D., & Demetrovics Z. (2015). The prevalence of compulsive buying: A meta-analysis. *Addiction, 111*, 408–419.

Mayo Clinic. (2017). *Eating disorder treatment: Know your options.* https://www.mayocli nic.org/diseases-conditions/eating-disorders/in-depth/eating-disorder-treatment/art-20046234

McQueen, P., Moulding, R., & Kyrios, M. (2014). Experimental evidence for the in-fluence of cognitions on compulsive buying. *Journal of Behavior Therapy and Experimental Psychiatry, 45*, 496–501.

Mueller, A., Mitchell, J. E., Crosby, R. D., Gefeller, O., Faber, R. J., Martin, A., . . . de Zwaan, M. (2010). Estimated prevalence of compulsive buying in Germany and its association with sociodemographic characteristics and depressive symptoms. *Psychiatry Research, 180*, 137–142.

Müller A., Mitchell J. E., & de Zwaan, M. (2015). Compulsive buying. *American Journal of Addictions, 24*, 132–137.

O'Reilly, M. (2020). Social media and adolescent mental health: the good, the bad and the ugly. *Journal of Mental Health, 29*, 200–206.

Pelchat, M. L. (2009). Food addiction in humans. *Journal of Nutrition, 139*, 620–622.

Rosa, M. A. C., Collombat, J., Denis, C. M., Alexandre, J. M., Serre, F., Auriacombe, M., & Fatseas, M. (2015). Overlap between food addiction and DSM-5 eating disorders in a treatment seeking sample. *Drug and Alcohol Dependence, 100*, e19.

Schaeffer, K. (2019, August 23). Most U.S. teens who use cellphones do it to pass time, connect with others, learn new things. Pew Research Center. https://www.pewresea

rch.org/fact-tank/2019/08/23/most-u-s-teens-who-use-cellphones-do-it-to-pass-time-connect-with-others-learn-new-things/

Semenza, D. C., Jackson, D. B., Testa, A., & Meldrum, R. C. (2020). Adolescent sleep problems and susceptibility to peer influence. *Youth & Society*, *54*(2), 179–200. https://doi.org/10.1177%2F0044118X20969024

Smetaniuk, P. (2014). A preliminary investigation into the prevalence and prediction of problematic cell phone use. *Journal of Behavioral Addictions*, *3*, 41–53.

Swanson, S. A., Crow, S. J., Le Grange, D., Swendsen, J., & Merikangas, K. R. (2011). Prevalence and correlates of eating disorders in adolescents: Results from the national comorbidity survey replication adolescent supplement. *Archives of General Psychiatry*, *68*, 714–723.

Thege, B. K., Woodin, E. M., Hodgins, D. C., & Williams, R. J. (2015). Natural course of behavioral addictions: A 5-year longitudinal study. *BMC Psychiatry*, *15*, 4. https://doi.org/10.1186/s12888-015-0383-3

Thomée, S., Härenstam, A., & Hagberg, M. (2011). Mobile phone use and stress, sleep disturbances, and symptoms of depression among young adults—A prospective cohort study. *BMC Public Health*, *11*, 66. https://doi.org/10.1186/1471-2458-11-66

Tromholt, M. (2016). The Facebook experiment: Quitting Facebook leads to higher levels of well-being. *Cyberpsychology, Behavior, and Social Networking*, *19*, 661–666.

Twenge, J. M., & Campbell, W. K. (2018). Associations between screen time and lower psychological well-being among children and adolescents: Evidence from a population-based study. *Preventive Medicine Reports*, *12*, 271–283.

Twenge, J. M., Joiner, T. E., Rogers, M. L., & Martin, G. N. (2018). Increases in depressive symptoms, suicide-related outcomes, and suicide rates among US adolescents after 2010 and links to increased new media screen time. *Clinical Psychological Science*, *6*, 3–17.

Unger A., Papastamatelou J., Yolbulan Okan E., & Aytas S. (2014). How the economic situation moderates the influence of available money on compulsive buying of students—A comparative study between Turkey and Greece. *Journal of Behavioral Addiction*, *3*, 173–181.

Van Rooij, A. J., Kuss, D. J., Griffiths, M. D., Shorter, G. W., Schoenmakers, T. M., & Van De Mheen, D. (2014). The (co-) occurrence of problematic video gaming, substance use, and psychosocial problems in adolescents. *Journal of Behavioral Addictions*, *3*, 157–165.

Wan C. (2009). *Gratifications & loneliness as predictors of campus-SNS websites addiction & usage pattern among Chinese college students*. MS Thesis, Chinese University of Hong Kong.

Welte, J. W., Barnes, G. M., Tidwell, M. C. O., & Hoffman, J. H. (2008). The prevalence of problem gambling among US adolescents and young adults: Results from a national survey. *Journal of Gambling Studies*, *24*, 119–133.

Welte, J. W., Barnes, G. M., Wieczorek, W. F., Tidwell, M. C., & Parker, J. (2002). Gambling participation in the US—Results from a national survey. *Journal of Gambling Studies*, *18*, 313–337.

Winters, K.C. & Stinchfield, R. D. (2012). Youth gambling: Prevalence, risk and protective factors and clinical issues. In C. Reilly (Ed.), *Increasing the odds (Vol. 7): What clinicians need to know about gambling disorders* (pp. 14-25). National Center on Responsible Gaming.

Young K. (1996). Internet addiction: The emergence of a new clinical disorder. *Cyber Psychological Behavior, 3,* 237–244.

Zhou, S. X., & Leung, L. (2012). Gratification, loneliness, leisure boredom, and self-esteem as predictors of SNS-game addiction and usage pattern among Chinese college students. *International Journal of Cyber Behavior, Psychology and Learning, 2,* 34–48.

INTERVENTIONS AND
TREATMENTS

Continuum of Care and Treatment Planning

INTRODUCTION

As discussed in Chapter 2, adolescence is a development period during which many youth start to use alcohol and other drugs. Such early onset of use increases the likelihood of negative effects on cognitive, physical, and psychosocial development (Brown et al., 2008). And as discussed in Chapter 4, early onset of substance use increases the likelihood of developing a substance use disorder (SUD) (Winters & Lee, 2008). Recent trends in the United States to legalize marijuana for recreational or medical purposes (https://learnaboutsam.org) may contribute to both a rise in the rate of use of marijuana at a young age and the onset of a marijuana use disorder during adolescence (Volkow et al., 2014).

Treatment Need

For youth who are using substances, some form and intensity of intervention or treatment may be appropriate. In 2016, approximately half a million youth ages 12 to 25 received treatment for substance use issues at a specialty facility in the United States (Substance Abuse and Mental Health Services Administration, 2017). Yet this represents only about 10% of those estimated to need treatment. There are several reasons for this large gap between treatment utilization by youth and those with an SUD: inadequate local treatment options; poor health insurance coverage; parents disinterested or unsupportive in a treatment option; stigma about drug treatment; and low motivation of youth to seek help.

Treatment studies that investigate post-treatment youth outcomes indicate that many positive treatment benefits exist, including positive changes in substance use and improvement in psychosocial functioning outcomes. But many benefits for some youth quickly diminish post-treatment (Winters et al., 2018). For example, relapse is relatively common. Studies show that 65–70% of youth return to some level of drug use during the initial 3 months after treatment, and 1 year out, the relapse rate rises to approximately 80%; up to two-thirds of these youth move in and out of treatment during this 1-year-out period (Waldron & Turner, 2008; Winters et al., 2018).

Many people have a SUD relapse after a period of abstinence, especially if they return to places where they previously used the drug. This phenomenon is known as *context-driven relapse*. New research has brought insight regarding the significance of a biological mechanism known as *neurogenesis* to the basis of context-driven relapse. Neurogenesis is the development of new neurons in the brain and is an essential process for learning. For example, newly formed circuits may link rewards, such as food or a drug, to reward-associated memories, such as the physical location or other setting characteristics where the reward was received. Based on a recent study with rats (Galinato et al., 2018a, 2018b), the investigators found that when neurogenesis occurs in the hippocampus (the brain's memory region), memories tied to the prior drug-seeking behavior may strengthen. They also found that neurogenesis during *abstinence* strengthened drug-associated memories that promote context-driven reinstatement of drug use. The implication of this research is that patients seeking a drug-free recovery need to develop strategies to prevent the influence of context-driven triggers.

We agree with the progressive view held by many SUD treatment service providers that relapse is normative and best approached as an opportunity to engage in further, and perhaps alternative, services and to troubleshoot where potential sources of support for the teenager (e.g., parents, siblings, non–drug-using peers) can be enhanced. And whereas most treatment programs have abstinence as the goal, there is room for treatment goals that consider a range of non-abstinence outcomes.

Treatment Planning

Treatment planning for adolescents with SUDs starts with a screening or comprehensive assessment and follows with a determination of a treatment response. A treatment plan needs to consist of what is the most suitable treatment setting, treatment intensity (e.g., number of sessions or length of stay), form of treatment, behavior change goals, and personalization that is needed (e.g., adjusting treatment if there are client special needs). Thus, treatment placement is dictated by the results of the assessment and takes into account that one size does not fit all (Fishman, 2019).

DEVELOPMENTAL ISSUES

A core theme of contemporary treatment approaches for adolescents is that developmental issues must be taken into consideration. Adolescent drug use patterns, reasons for substance use, willingness to self-examine, and motivation for behavior change differ significantly from those of adults (National Institute on Drug Abuse, 2014). Consider the last issue. It can be difficult enough to get an adult into treatment, despite the likelihood that the adult has faced numerous and serious negative consequences as a result of substance use, has the benefit of many life experiences, and presumably has a relatively realistic view of the world. Most adolescents do not view their drug use as a problem and lack the insight that they are not making healthy decisions. Moreover, many adolescents are coerced or mandated into seeking treatment. Thus, it is not unexpected that a significant challenge of any counselor working with a teenager is to address the less-than-optimal motivation to change the mindset of the adolescent.

Does participating in group therapy contribute to secondary (contagion) negative effects? Potential harms thought to be elicited by affiliation with delinquent peers in group counseling has been a controversy among adolescent treatment providers and researchers of adolescent SUD. A recent scholarly review of this topic concluded that the "lion's share of two decades of comparative studies indicates that group treatment is a safe and effective modality for adolescent substance use treatment—particularly when incorporating cognitive behavior therapy—that poses no greater risk of harmful outcome than any other form of treatment" (Hogue et al., 2019, p. 9). As the authors suggest, there are several clinical strategies to employ to reduce the likelihood of contagion effects, including actively discouraging deviant talk, minimizing informal socialization, and addressing negative stigma related to participating in treatment.

Another age-specific treatment issue is that advice alone from an adult counselor may not be very effective, which suggests that peer interactions are important to changing an adolescent client's behavior (Riggs et al., 2007). Thus counseling with a teenager is likely strengthened when adults are not the sole change agent and when group therapy is included.

KEYS TO EFFECTIVE TREATMENT

The majority of adolescent drug treatment programs employ a range of behavior change strategies that typically address these treatment goals: promote personal strengths; teach strategies to identify and resist triggers of substance use, and address underlying coexisting problems.

What makes a good therapist? It is likely that qualifications, experience, and training are important. A study that equated these characteristics among counselors still found that they varied widely in effectiveness (Gaume et al., 2009). The more effective counselors seemed to arise from more use of an accepting, nonjudgmental spirit and approach, which embodies motivational interviewing strategy (we discuss this interviewing strategy in Chapter 11).

What does research say about the most effective form of treatment? There is no single approach that can be cited as superior when treating adolescent substance abuse. Yet there are several approaches indicated by research to be most suitable for adolescents. We agree with the conclusions from Hogue and colleagues' review of literature (Hogue et al., 2018) that the handful of well-established and effective approaches are the following: cognitive behavioral therapy, motivational enhancement therapy, family-based treatment, and a 12-step approach. In subsequent chapters (Chapters 10, 11, 12 and 13), we review each of these approaches.

Are there common elements to these effective treatment approaches? Experts convened by the National Institute of Drug Abuse addressed this question. In their report (National Institute on Drug Abuse, 2014), 13 key principles were identified as being important to optimizing treatment effectiveness. These "essentials" are summarized in Table 9.1. Briefly, the principles emphasize the importance of developmentally trained staff, the use of evidence-based and adolescent-appropriate assessment tools and treatment strategies, tailoring treatment to the unique needs of the youth, and the importance of addressing the disorders that coexist with SUD.

Table 9.1 PRINCIPLES OF EFFECTIVE ADOLESCENT DRUG TREATMENT (NATIONAL INSTITUTE ON DRUG ABUSE, 2014)

Principle	Description
1. Identify and address substance use as soon as possible.	Identifying and addressing adolescent substance use as soon as possible is important because of the negative effects early use can have on the brain. Additionally, adults with substance use disorders often report using drugs as adolescents or young adults.
2. Adolescents do not have to be addicted to benefit from a substance use intervention.	Interventions can successfully treat a range of substance use disorders, from problematic use to severe addiction. Youth in particular can benefit from intervention at early stages. Even use that does not seem problematic can lead to heavier use and other risky behaviors.
3. Medical visits are an opportunity to ask about drug use.	Medical doctors (e.g., pediatricians, emergency room doctors, dentists) can use standardized screenings to determine if an adolescent is using substances and if an intervention is warranted. In some instances, it is possible to provide a brief intervention in the physician's office, and in other cases referral to treatment is more appropriate.

Table 9.1 CONTINUED

Principle	Description
4. Legal or family pressure may be an important influence on an adolescent's involvement in treatment.	Most adolescents with a substance use disorder do not think they need treatment and rarely look for treatment. Treatment can be successful even if the adolescent is legally mandated to treatment or goes because of family pressures.
5. Treatment should be tailored to the adolescent's needs	Many factors need to be considered when developing a treatment plan for an adolescent, including sex, family, peer relationships, and community environment. Therefore, it is necessary to begin with a comprehensive assessment.
6. Treatment should not focus on just substance use.	Treatment is most successful when it focuses on the whole person. Treatment should address housing, medical, social, and legal needs.
7. Behavioral therapies can effectively treat substance use disorders.	Behavioral therapies have been shown to be an effective treatment. These therapies help build motivation to change by providing incentives for abstinence, teaching skills to deal with cravings, and finding positive and rewarding activities.
8. Family and community support are important features of treatment.	There are several evidence-based interventions for adolescent substance use that involve family members and individuals in the community. These interventions try to improve family communication and provide the adolescent with support.
9. Mental health conditions need to be addressed in order to effectively treat substance use.	Adolescents with a substance use disorder often have co-occurring mental health conditions. It is important that adolescents are screened and treated for these other conditions in order for substance abuse treatment to be successful.

(continued)

Table 9.1 CONTINUED

Principle	Description
10. Sensitive issues should be addressed and confidentiality maintained when possible.	It is common for adolescents with substance use disorders to have a history of abuse or other trauma. Whereas maintaining confidentiality with respect to sensitive issues is important in the therapeutic setting, appropriate authorities need to be informed if abuse is suspected.
11. Drug use should be monitored during treatment.	It is important to monitor an adolescent's drug use while in treatment and identify a relapse early on. The relapse could indicate that treatment should be intensified or needs to be altered to better meet the adolescent's needs.
12. Completing treatment and having a continuing care plan are important.	The length of treatment will vary based on the severity of the adolescent's substance use disorder; however, studies have shown outcomes are best when an individual is in treatment 3 months or longer. The adolescent can also benefit from continuing care.
13. Adolescents should be tested for sexually transmitted diseases.	Drug-using adolescents are at an increased risk for sexually transmitted and blood-borne diseases (e.g., human immunodeficiency virus, hepatitis B and C) because of the increase in high-risk behaviors that result from drug use. Addressing this in treatment can help decrease high-risk behaviors, thereby reducing the likelihood of infection.

From the National Institute on Drug Abuse. (2014). *Principles of adolescent substance use disorder treatment: A research-based guide.* https://www.drugabuse.gov/publicati ons/principles-adolescent-substance-use-disorder-treatment-research-based-guide/pri nciples-adolescent-substance-use-disorder-treatment10

ADDRESSING ADOLESCENT SUBSTANCE ABUSE ALONG THE CONTINUUM OF CARE

The nature of a response to an adolescent's drug involvement depends on many individual characteristics: the severity of drug involvement; mental health condition; current and past medical condition; environment support for recovery; and readiness to change. We support the principle that parents and a primary care physician can provide front-line intervention when adolescent substance use is in its early stages. Yet when drug involvement reaches a serious level (e.g., the adolescent meets DSM-5 criteria for SUD), it is advisable to initially place an adolescent into a level of treatment that matches the severity of the adolescent's drug involvement. A well-known system used to identify a continuum of levels of care is provided by the American Society of Addiction Medicine (ASAM; Mee-Lee et al., 2014). The ASAM Criteria provide a consensus roadmap of the various levels of care and the service elements within each level of care. The expectation is to match an adolescent's level or depth of problem severity with the appropriate level of care. In addition to the ASAM system, we have identified additional levels of care not directly addressed by ASAM. But before we describe each of the levels of care, some context is needed.

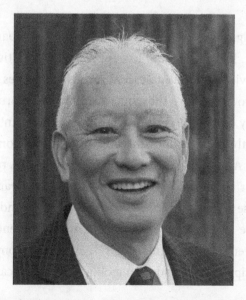

David Mee-Lee, M.D., has been the Chief Editor of all editions of ASAM's criteria. Photo courtesy of David Mee-Lee.

Current interventions for adolescent SUDs typically demonstrate relatively low rates of long-term abstinence. Thus, non-abstinence-oriented goals, even interventions that focus on non-abstinence, are worthy of discussion. However, a harm reduction treatment philosophy may lead to conflicts and resistance among providers and may be particularly problematic for youth involved in the juvenile justice system and those with coexisting mental or behavioral disorders (Bagot & Kaminer, 2018).

Non-abstinent, harm reduction goals for an adolescent can include the following:

- Reducing quantity of use
- Reducing frequency of use
- Reducing or eliminating poly-drug use
- Not using before or during school
- Not using when negative consequences are likely (e.g., not using when driving a vehicle)

General Principles of Treatment Planning and Referral

The task of assigning or referring an adolescent to a particular level of care is complex. It is misleading to expect that a definitive outcome will be achieved by virtue of the adolescent receiving services in a single level of care. Many youth require subsequent referrals to more intensive services before they achieve long-term health. Multiple interventions and treatments (both multicomponent and multidimensional approaches) may be needed. As national expert Marc Fishman, M.D., put it, the course of treatment for an adolescent consists of "a waxing-waning, remitting-relapsing course over a prolonged period of time and across several episodes of care at different levels of care, with different kinds of services and interventions" (Fishman, 2019). And it is common for some youth to participate in extended, ongoing continuing care or to receive maintenance treatment. As we discuss in Chapter 13 (12-step treatment), there are numerous self-help resources for adolescents that can provide indefinite support.

An important distinction should be made between multicomponent treatments and multidomain treatments. *Multicomponent treatments* refer to intervention models or packages that contain multiple intervention components, such as combining individual counseling with family therapy. *Multidomain treatments* contain at least one component that specifically targets a co-occurring disorder or behavioral problem other than SUD. An example would be pharmacotherapy for an adolescent with a coexisting depressive disorder.

Also, treatment planning needs to be realistic, based on availability, the family's resources, and proximity to treatment, and it needs to suitable given the level or severity of the adolescent's problems. Regarding the latter issue, the initial assignment to a level of care needs to match the severity and impairment of the clinical picture. Increased level of care will follow from increased intensity of the adolescent's problem. We favor the general principle of a stepped-care approach: Begin with a relatively convenient and acceptable level of intervention, and only "step-up" to a more intense service if there is no or little improvement.

Does the notion of the continuum of care apply to all youth, regardless of socioeconomic status? We contend so. The ASAM criteria and our additional levels of care apply to all youth suspected of a substance use problem. It is not the case that only privately funded programs provide the upper echelon of intensive services. Publicly funded programs span the range of services in the United States. But we recognize that the more intensive services are the most expensive and may be difficult for by rural families, low-income families, and homeless youth to access.

Addressing coexisting disorders. Services for adolescents with coexisting disorders require more complexity than the therapy plan for a single disorder. Not only are a variety of services needed for the adolescent with coexisting disorders—spanning psychiatric, behavioral, and medical domains—but these services need to be coordinated. As noted above, a multidomain approach is optimal. A recommended form of the multidomain approach is the case management model (National Institute on Drug Abuse, 2014). This model seeks to address a client's comprehensive health needs via a collaboration among a range of service providers that provide a road map for options and services of available resources in the client's community.

The American Society of Addiction Medicine (ASAM) and Additional Treatment Placement Criteria

As noted above, the ASAM has developed a system, called the ASAM Criteria (Mee-Lee et al., 2014), for assessment of level and type of treatment placement decisions. This system consists of decision rules for adolescent treatment placement. These rules are distinct from those for adults, which is important given the unique developmental issues of adolescence. There is a debate as to whether the adolescent or adult criteria are preferred for young adults (e.g., age 19–24). In such instances, perhaps the functional maturity of the individual is more important than chronological age. The variability of behavioral and emotional maturity of youth in this "emerging adult" age group is considerable. For such cases, clinical judgment is needed to evaluate which treatment criteria are best suited for the young person.

Eight Stages of Treatment Along the Continuum of Care

Below we describe eight stages in our broad view of the continuum of care for adolescents (some of which are part of the ASAM Criteria for treatment placement), beginning with parent involvement and ending in aftercare.

A recently developed program is aimed at training parents to facilitate their treatment-resistant adolescent's treatment entry and to manage their adolescent after entry into community-based treatment. The Community Reinforcement and Family Training program (CRAFT; Kirby et al., 2015) is adapted from an adult version. The adolescent program is tailored for parents of adolescents; content is based on the behavioral parent training literature and motivational interview principles.

Childhood maltreatment, defined as being victimized by physical, sexual, or psychological abuse, is associated with future adolescent health. Individuals having experienced childhood maltreatment report drinking more frequently and using illicit substances more frequently as an adolescent compared to those who do not report childhood maltreatment (Clark & Winters, 2002).

A related factor is caregiver attachment style. Adolescents who report that they experienced insecure and unstable attachment from their parents during childhood are more likely to report substance use (Hayre et al., 2019).

1. *Parents*. Parents can exert significant influence on adolescent substance use. They play an important role in enforcing family expectations, and the strength of the parent–adolescent relationship can reduce the likelihood of their son or daughter using substances, or, if use has started, can influence desistance of use (Andreas et al., 2016; Rusby et al., 2018). The authors appreciate the reality that it is unlikely that most parents will engage in any formal type of home-based intervention when they learn that their teenager is using drugs. Yet consider these advantages when parents are a "behavior change agent" in home: (1) the socializing influence of parents during the adolescent years can be significant; (2) the parent has ongoing access to the child (over 70% of adolescents live at home with at least one of their biological parents) and thus has multiple teachable moments to

influence their teenager's attitudes and behaviors; and (3) routine parenting practices (e.g., setting clear expectations, supporting appropriate behaviors) are also relevant to addressing adolescent drug involvement. Also, if an adolescent needs professional treatment, the parent will necessarily play a vital role in facilitating a referral.

2. Primary care and school health clinics. Preventive interventions are vital approaches to address early-stage drug use. Given that more than 80% of adolescents see a primary care provider yearly, and with the growing popularity of school health clinics (SHCs), these are opportunistic settings for adolescents to have a confidential discussions with professionals about the dangers of substance use (National Center for Health Statistics, 2016). Adolescents view health officials and experts as a legitimate source of information about substance use and thus may be open to discussing this topic (Harris et al., 2009; Winters et al., 2007).

The overall aims of the SBIRT model are the following:

- Increase early identification of adolescents at risk for substance use problems.
- Build awareness and educate adolescents on the risks associated with substance use.
- Motivate those at risk to reduce unhealthy, risky use, and adopt health-promoting behavior.
- Motivate individuals to seek help and increase access to care for those with (or at risk for) a substance use disorder.
- Link those high-risk individuals to more intensive treatment services.
- Foster a continuum of care by integrating prevention, intervention, and treatment services.

An emerging approach gaining popularity in primary health clinics and is called Screening, Brief Intervention, and Referral and Treatment (SBIRT) (Ozechowski et al., 2016). The SBIRT approach has many clinic-friendly features: (1) quick screening (e.g., CRAFFT; see Chapter 4), (2) a motivational interviewing approach to promote behavior change in a relatively short period of time (e.g., within a single 60-minute session), and (3) determination of need for possible follow-up services (Winters, 2016). SBIRT is recommended by the American Academy of Pediatrics (AAP) and the National Institute on Alcohol Abuse and Alcoholism (NIAAA), and some protocols and manualized versions exist (see http://www.norc.org/Research/Projects/Pages/national-addiction-technology-transfer-center-screening-brief-intervention-and-referral-to-treatment-focus.aspx).

Two brief intervention approaches have been developed by professional organizations:

1. American Academy of Pediatrics Committee on Substance Abuse: *Substance Use Screening, Brief Interventions and Referral to Treatment* (https://publications.aap.org/pediatrics/article/138/1/e20161210/52573/Substance-Use-Screening-Brief-Intervention-and?searchresult=1)
2. National Institute on Alcohol Abuse and Alcoholism: *Alcohol Screening and Brief Intervention for Youth* (https://www.niaaa.nih.gov/sites/default/files/publications/YouthGuide.pdf)

Both of these national organizations provide brief interventions that include providing praise and encouragement for individuals who have not yet used any substances, promoting the adolescent's strengths, providing clear advice and education about risks for adolescents with previous use, and offering possible referral to treatment for those with high-risk use.

The model's effectiveness? Literature reviews for the brief intervention component provide support for its effectiveness (e.g., Sterling et al., 2015;

Tanner-Smith & Lipsey, 2015), but there is less research on the use of the full SBIRT model with adolescents (Levy & Shrier, 2015).

In the 1990s, juvenile drug courts were introduced. Their aim is to divert youth from incarceration by providing services, such as mental health and substance use treatment, and regular monitoring. The Office of Juvenile Justice and Delinquency Prevention published in 2018 the Juvenile Drug Treatment Court Guidelines (https://www. ojjdp.gov/Juvenile-Drug-Treatment-Court-Guidelines.html). Several key guidelines are listed below.

1. Focus the court's philosophy on reducing substance abuse and recidivism, rather than on punishment.
2. Ensure equitable treatment for all youth.
3. Base the case management plan around a comprehensive assessment.
4. Employ evidence-based strategies, such as contingency management and community supervision.

3. *Juvenile justice diversion programs.* The United States continues to process a very large number of youth in the juvenile justice system (JJS). It is estimated that approximately 31 million youth are involved in the JJS each year, and about 1 million of them are involved for the first time (Hockenberry & Puzzanchera, 2018). A specialized JJS diversion program, juvenile drug courts, served an estimated 30,000 adolescents in 2015 among 409 such programs. Among adjudicated youth, approximately two-thirds report a history of substance use (Belenko & Logan, 2003), and the rates of other behavioral and mental disorders are also high (Zajac et al., 2019).

Whereas the JJS provides an excellent opportunity as a setting for early intervention and treatment (Teplin et al., 2002), only 25% of youth on probation receive treatment for drug abuse or mental health services, and the likelihood of receiving evidence-based care when it occurred was for only 7% of youth (White, 2017). Admittedly, the main priority of JJS is public safety, and rehabilitation of juvenile offenders may take a back seat in the minds of officials. Many practical and organizational barriers prevent many adolescents in JJS from receiving counseling for underlying behavioral problems (e.g., lack of expertise among JJS staff; funding priorities are placed elsewhere; few, if any, suitable service providers are in the local community; White, 2017). Nonetheless, providing evidence-based services to JJS-involved youth can improve recidivism rates and thus have a positive impact on public safety (Hoeve et al., 2014).

A comprehensive resource on best practices for juvenile diversion programs was developed by the National Council of Juvenile and Family Court Judges (http://www.ncjfcj.org/our-work/juvenile-drug-courts). Some features available on this site are the following:

- Juvenile Drug Treatment Court Guidelines
- Guidelines for Screening, Brief Intervention, Referral to Treatment
- Online Learning Center
- Learning Collaborative

Examples of programs described in the literature include Scared Straight, or prison visitation programs; Guided Group Interaction; Positive Peer Culture; military-style boot camps; and wilderness challenges (Dodge et al., 2006). But comprehensive reviews of these and other substance use treatments have found mixed results for JJS-involved youth (Hogue et al., 2019).

4. *Outpatient treatment (ASAM Criteria).* Adolescents suitable for outpatient treatment are not at risk of harm, show mild or minimal impairment and difficulties, and are not at significant risk of deterioration. They are likely to maintain abstinence or reduce use, and the family and environment can support recovery with minimal outside assistance.

5. *Intensive outpatient (ASAM Criteria).* This level of care is needed for adolescents experiencing mild or minimal withdrawal symptoms or who are at risk of withdrawal, are at low risk of harm, display mild or moderate

impairment and difficulties but can sustain responsibilities, but are likely to need near daily monitoring or counseling. These adolescents show variable interest in treatment, are at significant risk for relapse, and do not receive much, if any, support from the family and environment.

6. *Inpatient/residential (ASAM Criteria).* Adolescents aligned with this level of care are experiencing mild withdrawal or at risk of withdrawal and would reveal the following features: low risk of harm; moderate interference and impairment with daily activities due to substance abuse but able to carry out major responsibilities; and history of treatment suggesting the need for near daily monitoring and counseling. A structured program that emphasizes improving motivation to change, awareness of the harms if substance use continues, and relapse prevention is needed. Substantial daily monitoring will be needed if the adolescent's environment is dangerous.

7. *Medically managed hospital-based treatment (ASAM Criteria).* This most intensive level of care is considered when the adolescent is experiencing severe withdrawal (or is at risk of withdrawal) and requires 24-hour intensive active medical management by nursing staff at a licensed hospital. Additional features are that the adolescent is at severe risk of harm, their functioning is so impaired that treatment participation in a less intensive level would be unlikely, and the adolescent's history with prior services predicts destabilization without medical management.

Recovery-oriented services of care (ROSC), which is a relatively new concept in the substance use disorder field, provides an aftercare framework to create an infrastructure or "system of care" with the resources to effectively address the full range of substance use problems within communities. Basic principles of ROSC include the following:

• Embraces the possibility of recovery and well-being created by the inherent strengths and capacities of all people who experience an SUD and related mental health issues

- Maximizes self-determination and self-management of well-being and involves person-first, person-centered, strengths-based, and evidence-informed treatment, rehabilitation, and support
- Acknowledges the diversity of people's values and is responsive to people's gender, age, and developmental stage, culture, and families, as well as people's unique strengths, circumstances, needs, preferences, and beliefs
- Helps families or support people to understand their family member's experiences and recovery processes and how they can assist in their recovery
- Understands that people who have lived experience of unresolved trauma struggle to feel safe, considers the possibility of unresolved trauma in all service settings, and incorporates the core principles of trauma-informed care into service provision

SOURCE: https://www.samhsa.gov/sites/default/files/rosc_resource_guide_book.pdf

8. Aftercare. Continuing support services by the treatment program and community-based services are important after an adolescent is discharged from a program. The purpose of aftercare is to prevent relapse by providing services and, in some instances, supervision to help the adolescent make a successful transition back into the community and to promote health and well-being. Aftercare services can include participation in the treatment program's aftercare program, intensive supervision by a case manager, and participation in self-help or peer-recovery programs. Aftercare goals typically focus on promoting school involvement, learning to recreate without the use of drugs, dealing with negative peer influences, strengthening connections to the family, and promoting personal assets.

ASSESSING THE CONTINUUM OF CARE

Several well-established assessment tools exist that can be used along with clinical judgment in determining an adolescent's level of care. In Chapter 5, we listed several *comprehensive interviews,* all of which can be useful for this task. One clinical interview that is particularly helpful with evaluating level of care for adolescents is the Comprehensive Adolescent Structured Interview (CASI; Meyers et al., 1995). The CASI is a comprehensive, semi-structured, clinical assessment and outcomes interview. It consists of 10 independent modules, each incorporating objective, focused, and concrete questions. Modules include health, family, stressful life events, legal status, sexual behavior, substance use, mental health functioning, peer relationships, education, and use of leisure time. Questions are formatted to identify whether certain behaviors have ever occurred regularly, how old the adolescent was when they first occurred regularly, whether they occurred regularly during the past 12 months, and the extent to which the issue is viewed by the teenager as causing problems or discomfort. The interview also includes questions designed to assess strengths and assets of the adolescent. The CASI, which requires about 45 to 90 minutes to administer, has both paper-and-pencil and computer-administration formats.

EMERGING TREATMENTS

Neuroscience-Based Treatment

Developments in neuroscience have been translated into promising treatment approaches. How these treatments will be incorporated into the continuum of care is still to be determined. At this early stage point, they typically augment other forms of treatment or are used in cases where medication has not been effective.

Brain stimulation (or *neuromodulation*) techniques include various noninvasive ways of simulating the brain with the aim of treating various neurological and psychiatric disorders. Examples include repetitive transcranial magnetic stimulation (TMS), transcranial direct current stimulation, and deep brain stimulation (DBS). Emerging research is investigating neuromodulation as a treatment for SUDs (Coles et al., 2018). The research shows that these techniques are beginning to show promise in reducing *drug* craving, which is a key factor for promoting recovery (Coles et al., 2018).

Deep brain stimulation (DBS) is also approved to treat several movement-related conditions (epilepsy, essential tremor, Parkinson's disease, and dystonia) and is being investigated as treatment for chronic pain, cluster headache, dementia, Huntington's disease, multiple sclerosis, Tourette syndrome, and traumatic brain injury.

TMS is a noninvasive form of brain stimulation that involves the use of magnetic fields to stimulate nerve cells to improve mood, particularly symptoms of depression. TMS is typically used when other depression treatments for are ineffective. A more invasive example is DBS. DBS consists of implanting electrodes within certain areas of the brain, which produces electrical impulses that regulate abnormal impulses. A pacemaker-like device placed under the skin in the person's upper chest, with a wire that connects this device to electrodes in the brain, controls the intensity of the stimulation. DBS is already approved for obsessive-compulsive disorder and is being studied as a potential treatment for an SUD, as well as for those whose depression does not respond to TMS (Scangos et al., 2021).

Medications

There are various medications to address various aspects of addiction, including craving reduction, aversive therapy, substitution therapy, and treatment of underlying psychiatric disorders. Specifically, medications can be used to treat addiction to opioids, alcohol, or nicotine in adults, but there are no medications approved by the U.S. Food and Drug

Administration (FDA) to treat cannabis, cocaine, or methamphetamine abuse. Research is quite limited on this treatment strategy for adolescents, and there are no "addiction" medications currently approved by the FDA to treat adolescents.

Medications are currently available to treat several SUDs, and scientists are developing others. We summarize below those currently available.

Opioid use disorder: Methadone (Dolophine®, Methadose®), buprenorphine (Suboxone®, Subutex®, Probuphine®, Sublocade™), and naltrexone (Vivitrol®) are used to treat opioid addiction. Acting on the same targets in the brain as heroin and morphine, methadone and buprenorphine suppress withdrawal symptoms and relieve cravings. Naltrexone blocks the effects of opioids at their receptor sites in the brain and should be used only in patients who have already been detoxified.

Nicotine addiction: Nicotine replacement therapies include the patch, spray, gum, and lozenges. These products are available over the counter. The U.S. Food and Drug Administration (FDA) has approved two prescription medications for nicotine addiction: bupropion (Zyban®) and varenicline (Chantix®). The medications are more effective when combined with behavioral treatments.

Alcohol use disorder: These three medications have been FDA approved for treating alcohol addiction:

1. Naltrexone blocks opioid receptors in the brain that are involved in the rewarding effects of drinking and in the craving for alcohol. It reduces relapse to heavy drinking and is highly effective in some patients.
2. Acamprosate (Campral®) is probably most effective with patients with a severe form of an alcohol use disorder. This drug reduces symptoms of long-lasting withdrawal, such as insomnia, anxiety, restlessness, and depression.

3. Disulfiram (Antabuse®) interferes with the breakdown of alcohol, leading to unpleasant reactions if alcohol is consumed, including nausea and irregular heartbeat.

SOURCE: https://www.drugabuse.gov/publications/drugfacts/treatment-approaches-drug-addiction

Because the applicability of adult findings to adolescents is unclear, use of addiction medications for adolescents should proceed with great caution.

Technology

A promising emerging area of treatment is technology-assisted interventions (delivered via computer, Web, text, or smartphone). Technologies can connect adolescents with their peers in real time via secure environments. The benefits of technology-assisted treatment include several user-friendly features, including increased ease of access, enjoyment, and cost-effectiveness (Marsch & Borodovsky, 2016). National data suggest that 95% of teens have access to a smartphone and 89% go online several times daily, typically to interact with peers and receive support (Anderson & Jiang, 2018), making technology-assisted behavior change particularly well suited for adolescents.

Many smartphone applications and other digital mental health products (apps) exist that point individuals to common counseling or stress-reduction techniques to address mental or behavioral problems (particularly for anxiety and depression). Cognitive behavioral principles, meditation, mindfulness, social support through chat rooms, and psychoeducational approaches are commonly offered by these apps. A useful site to shop for such digital products is PsyberGuide (https://psyberguide.org/apps/). A growth area in treatment research is to increase our understanding of how these technology-based models can promote behavior change for youth.

Exercise

Adolescent substance use has been linked to adverse structural and functional brain changes. It is hypothesized that substance use during the teenage years may disrupt the natural brain maturation process in a way that creates a greater "imbalance" between frontal/regulatory (brakes) and cortical-subcortical circuits (gas pedal) regions, thus contributing to further heightened impulsive and reward-driven behaviors.

Physical exercise is known to increase growth of neural connections, and such growth stimulates the brain's reward regions, enhances general brain plasticity, and supports learning and memory. In this light, exercise may help to strengthen the "naïve" or underdeveloped connections between the brain's brake (frontal/regulatory) and gas pedal (cortical-subcortical) circuitry regions, and thus help shape decision making to be less influenced by the imbalance between these two regions.

Recent scientific literature on this topic supports the notion that adolescent physical exercise increases neural activity in a way that helps to modulate this regional brain imbalance. The authors highlight the value of exercise for the prevention and adjunctive treatment of SUD (Nock et al., 2017).

Machine Learning

Machine learning is a branch of artificial intelligence that uses a computer-based approach of data analysis that permits the computer to automatically "learn" without being explicitly programmed. Machine learning is being studied in the treatment field in an effort to predict recovery from substance abuse. The computer is initially programmed ("trained") to identify certain patterns in data from existing databases (e.g., drug treatment outcome data from a large data set). The computer then applies this information to new data (or new cases) in order to make inferences, predictions, or decisions. Machine learning allows for faster and more accurate analysis of massive amounts of data and information than would otherwise be possible.

IMPLEMENTATION

Implementation is defined as delivering an evidence-based treatment program in the same ways it was delivered while it was researched. When implementation fidelity is achieved, treatment quality and effectiveness are optimized. Because rigorous implementation requires financial and staff resources, it can be difficult for treatment programs to deliver treatments with such high standards. Factors found to predict sustainment included the degree of implementation during the initial support period, adequate ongoing funding, infrastructure support, and staff support following the end of funding (Hunter et al., 2014). Common implementation methods include comprehensively training supervisors and counselors about the treatment, conducting regular fidelity checks, and discussing implementation challenges and solutions during supervision.

A superb example of strengthening implementation was conducted by Mark Godley and colleagues with respect to their treatment program, Adolescent-Community Reinforcement Approach (A-CRA) (Godley et al., 2011). The researchers implemented A-CRA across dozens of treatment organizations. Training and certification processes were developed for both clinicians and supervisors. Once supervisors were certified, they then trained their staff. Training for both groups involved reading the A-CRA treatment manual, completing an online quiz on the intervention, and then attending a 3-day training session. The final step in receiving certification required counselors to record actual sessions using A-CRA and uploading digital recordings of those sessions to a secure website to be rated by trained raters using a detailed rating manual (Smith et al., 2007). The clinicians' session recordings needed to receive passing scores on all A-CRA procedures (e.g., achieving an 80% agreement level with expert raters' ratings across all treatment sessions).

Empirical evidence demonstrating the fidelity of the clinician's implementation of evidence-based treatments is less than stellar (Waller & Turner, 2016). Implementation drift is common as many counselors shift away from delivering the treatment components as described in the manual in favor of adjusting and personalizing implementation. The extent to which an evidence-based program delivered with high fidelity yields significantly better outcomes compared to implementation that is weak on fidelity is an ongoing debate in the treatment literature. One focal point of this debate is the issue of treatment tailoring. Tailoring implementation to the unique needs of the youth, including adjusting based on the adolescent's coexisting disorder, is viewed as best practice (National Institute on Drug Abuse, 2014). Such tailoring is encouraged by many evidence-based treatments; treatment manuals often provide guidance in ways to individualize the curriculum based on specific client issues. In this light, fidelity of a treatment programs does not have to be compromised when a counselor strategically applies adaptations.

MINI-REVIEW

- Youth who are using substances may benefit from some type of intervention or treatment response.
- Youth may require multiple interventions and treatments. It is advisable to assign a youth the appropriate level of care that is the least intensive and step up to a more intensive treatment if needed.
- Responses vary by type, setting, and intensity. We describe eight levels of response along a continuum of care, with some of the levels based on the criteria provided by the American Society of Addiction Medicine (ASAM).
- Assessing placement or referral along the continuum of care for an adolescent suspected of drug involvement is complex.

We recommend using the adolescent-specific comprehensive interview, the Comprehensive Adolescent Structured Interview (CASI), to assist with this process.

- Several emerging treatments, which include treatments that are neuroscience based and technology based, are beginning to be evaluated for use with adolescents. Their role in the continuum of care will continue to evolve.

DISCUSSION QUESTIONS

1. What do we know about adolescent brain development that may contribute to instances when an adolescent refuses to get treatment for a substance use disorder?
2. In what ways can parents support recovery for an adolescent during the aftercare period?
3. How would you develop a recovery-oriented system of care (ROSC) that is optimal for an adolescent recovering from a substance use disorder?
4. You are asked to provide expert testimony to a state legislative committee that is considering the plan to stop all public funds for *residential-based* treatment and limit funds only for outpatient treatment for adolescents with a substance use disorder. Your perspective is that such a plan is a bad idea. What points would you make to the legislators that support your view?

FURTHER CURIOSITY AND DIGGING

How much can parents really influence how their kids turn out?

A *Boston Globe* science writer's perspective on this question:

https://www.bostonglobe.com/2020/02/19/magazine/how-much-can-parents-really-control-how-their-kids-turn-out/?outputType=amp&event=event25&__twitter_impression=true

Parents as Interventionists

www.drugfree.org

Principles of Adolescent Substance Use Disorder Treatment

https://www.drugabuse.gov/publications/principles-adolescent-substance-use-disor
der-treatment-research-based-guide/principles-adolescent-substance-use-disorder-
treatment

Digital Products to Promote Mental Health

https://psyberguide.org/apps/

REFERENCES

Anderson, M., & Jiang, J. (2018). Teens, social media & technology 2018. *Pew Research Center, 31*, 1–10.

Andreas, J. B., Pape, H., & Bretteville-Jensen, A. L. (2016). Who are the adolescents saying "No" to cannabis offers. *Drug and Alcohol Dependence, 163*, 64–70.

Bagot, K. S., & Kaminer, Y. (2018). Harm reduction for youth in treatment for substance use disorders: One size does not fit all. *Current Addiction Reports, 5*, 379–385.

Belenko, S., & Logan, T. K. (2003). Delivering more effective treatment to adolescents: Improving the juvenile drug court model. *Journal of Substance Abuse Treatment, 25*, 189–211.

Brown, S. A., McGue, M., Maggs, J., Schulenberg, J., Hingson, R., Swartzwelder, S., Martin, C., Chung, T., Tapert, S. F., Sher, K., Winters, K. C., Lowman, C., & Murphy, S. (2008). A developmental perspective on alcohol and youth ages 16–20. *Pediatrics, 121*, S290–S310.

Clark, D. B., & Winters, K. C. (2002). Measuring risks and outcomes in substance use disorders prevention research. *Journal of Consulting and Clinical Psychology, 70*, 1207–1223.

Coles, A. S., Kozak, K., & George, T. P. (2018). A review of brain stimulation methods to treat substance use disorders. *American Journal on Addictions, 27*, 71–91.

Dodge, K. A., Dishion, T. J., & Lansford, J. E. (Eds.). (2006). *Deviant peer influences in programs for youth: Problems and solutions*. Guilford Press.

Fishman, M. (2019). Placement criteria and treatment planning for adolescents with substance use disorders. In Y. Kaminer & K. C. Winters (Eds.), *Clinical manual of adolescent addictive disorders* (2nd ed., pp. 123–140). American Psychiatric Association.

Galinato, M. H., Lockner, J. W., Fannon-Pavlich, M. J., Sobieraj, J. C., Staples, M. C., Somkuwar, S. S. Ghofranian, A., Chaing, S., Navarro, A. I., Joea, A., & Luikart, B. W. (2018a). A synthetic small-molecule Isoxazole-9 protects against methamphetamine relapse. *Molecular Psychiatry, 23*, 629–638.

Galinato, M. H., Takashima, Y., Fannon, M. J., Quach, L. W., Silva, R. J. M., Mysore, K. K., Terranova, M. J., Dutta, R. R., Ostrom, R. W., Somkuwar, S. S., & Mandyam,

C. D. (2018b). Neurogenesis during abstinence is necessary for context-driven methamphetamine-related memory. *Journal of Neuroscience, 38,* 2029–2042.

Gaume, J., Gmel, G., Faouzi, M., & Daeppen, J. B. (2009). Counselor skill influences outcomes of brief motivational interventions. *Journal of Substance Abuse Treatment, 37,* 151–159.

Godley, S. H., Hedges, K., & Hunter, B. (2011). Gender and racial differences in treatment process and outcome among participants in the adolescent community reinforcement approach. *Psychology of Addictive Behaviors, 25,* 143–154.

Harris, S. K., Woods, E. R., Sherritt, L., Van Hook, S., Boulter, S., Brooks, T., Carey, P., Kossack, R., Kulig, J., & Knight, J. R. (2009). A youth-provider connectedness measure for use in clinical intervention studies. *Journal of Adolescent Health, 44,* S35–S36.

Hayre, R. S., Goulter, N., & Moretti, M. M. (2019). Maltreatment, attachment, and substance use in adolescence: Direct and indirect pathways. *Addictive Behaviors, 90,* 196–203.

Hockenberry, S., & Puzzanchera, C. (2018). *Juvenile court statistics 2016.* National Center for Juvenile Justice.

Hoeve, M., McReynolds, L. S., & Wasserman, G. A. (2014). Service referral for juvenile justice youths: Associations with psychiatric disorder and recidivism. *Administration and Policy in Mental Health, 41,* 379–389.

Hogue, A., Henderson, C. E., Becker, S. J., & Knight, D. K. (2018). Evidence base on outpatient behavioral treatments for adolescent substance use, 2014–2017: Outcomes, treatment delivery, and promising horizons. *Journal of Clinical Child & Adolescent Psychology, 47,* 499–526.

Hogue, A., Henderson, C. E., Ozechowski, T. J., Becker, S. J., & Coatsworth, J. D. (2019). Can the group harm the individual? Reviewing potential iatrogenic effects of group treatment for adolescent substance use. *Clinical Psychology: Science and Practice,* e12307.

Hunter, B. D., Godley, S. H., Hesson-McInnis, M. S., & Roozen, H. G. (2014). Longitudinal change mechanisms for substance use and illegal activity for adolescents in treatment. *Psychology of Addictive Behaviors, 28,* 507–515.

Kirby, K. C., Versek, B., Kerwin, M. E., Meyers, K., Benishek, L. A., Bresani, E., Washio, Y., Arria, A., & Meyers, R. J. (2015). Developing Community Reinforcement and Family Training (CRAFT) for parents of treatment-resistant adolescents. *Journal of Child & Adolescent Substance Abuse, 24,* 155–165.

Levy, S., & Shrier, L. (2015). *Adolescent SBIRT: Toolkit for providers. Massachusetts Department of Public Health.* https://www.mcpap.com/pdf/S2BI%20Toolkit.pdf

Marsch, L. A., & Borodovsky, J. T. (2016). Technology-based interventions for preventing and treating substance use among youth. *Child and Adolescent Psychiatric Clinics, 25,* 755–768.

Mee-Lee, D., Shulman, G. D., Fishman, M., Gastfriend, D., & Miller, M. (2014). *The ASAM criteria: Treatment criteria for addictive, substance-related, and co-occurring conditions* (3rd ed.). The Change Companies.

Meyers, K., McLellan, A. T., Jaeger, J. L. & Pettinati, H. M. (1995). The development of the Comprehensive Addiction Severity Index for Adolescents (CASI-A): An interview for assessing the multiple problems of adolescents. *Journal of Substance Abuse Treatment, 12*, 181–193.

National Center for Health Statistics. (2016). *Health, United States, 2015: With special feature on racial and ethnic health disparities.* Author. https://www.ncbi.nlm.nih.gov/books/NBK367640/

National Institute on Drug Abuse. (2014). *Principles of adolescent substance use disorder treatment: A research-based guide.* NIH Publication Number 14-7953. Author.

Nock, N. L., Minnes, S., & Alberts, J. L. (2017). Neurobiology of substance use in adolescents and potential therapeutic effects of exercise for prevention and treatment of substance use disorders. *Birth Defects Research, 109*, 1711–1729.

Ozechowski, T. J., Becker, S. J., & Hogue, A. (2016). SBIRT-A: Adapting SBIRT to maximize developmental fit for adolescents in primary care. *Journal of Substance Abuse Treatment, 62*, 28–37.

Riggs, P. D., Thompson, L. L., Tapert, S. F., Frascella, J., Mikulich-Gilbertson, S., Dalwani, M., . . . Lohman, M. (2007). Advances in neurobiological research related to interventions in adolescents with substance use disorders: Research to practice. *Drug and Alcohol Dependence, 91*, 306–311.

Rusby, J. C., Light, J. M., Crowley, R., & Westling, E. (2018). Influence of parent–youth relationship, parental monitoring, and parent substance use on adolescent substance use onset. *Journal of Family Psychology, 32*, 310–320.

Scangos, K. W., Makhoul, G. S., Sugrue, L. P., Chang, E. F., & Krystal, A. D. (2021). State-dependent responses to intracranial brain stimulation in a patient with depression. *Nature Medicine, 27*, 229–231.

Smith, J. E., Lundy, S. L., & Gianini, L. (2007). *Community reinforcement approach (CRA) and adolescent community reinforcement approach (A-CRA) coding manual.* University of New Mexico.

Sterling, S., Kline-Simon, A. H., Satre, D. D., Jones, A., Mertens, J., Wong, A., & Weisner, C. (2015). Implementation of screening, brief intervention, and referral to treatment for adolescents in pediatric primary care: A cluster randomized trial. *JAMA Pediatrics, 169*, 1–8.

Substance Abuse and Mental Health Services Administration. (2017). *Key substance use and mental health indicators in the United States: Results from the 2016 National Survey on Drug Use and Health.* Center for Behavioral Health Statistics and Quality, Substance Abuse and Mental Health Services Administration. HHS Publication No. SMA 17-5044, NSDUH Series H-52.

Tanner-Smith, E. E., & Lipsey, M. W. (2015). Brief alcohol interventions for adolescents and young adults: A systematic review and meta-analysis. *Journal of Substance Abuse Treatment, 51*, 1–18.

Teplin, L. A., Abram, K. M., McClelland, G. M., Dulcan, M. K., & Mericle, A. A. (2002). Psychiatric disorders in youth in juvenile detention. *Archives of General Psychiatry, 59*, 1133–1143.

Volkow, N. D., Baler, R. D., Compton, W. M., & Weiss, S. R. (2014). Adverse health effects of marijuana use. *New England Journal of Medicine, 370*, 2219–2227.

Waldron, H. B., & Turner, C. W. (2008). Evidence-based psychosocial treatments for adolescent substance abuse. *Journal of Clinical Child & Adolescent Psychology, 37*, 238–261.

Waller, G., & Turner, H. (2016). Therapist drift redux: Why well-meaning clinicians fail to deliver evidence-based therapy, and how to get back on track. *Behaviour Research and Therapy, 77*, 129–137.

White, C. (2017). Treatment services in the juvenile justice system: Examining the use and funding of services by youth on probation. *Youth Violence and Juvenile Justice, 17*, 62–87.

Winters, K. C. (2016). Adolescent brief interventions. *Journal of Drug Abuse, 2*, 1–3.

Winters, K. C., Botzet, A. M., Stinchfield, R., Gonzalez, R., Finch, A., Piehler, T., Ausherbauer, K., Chalmers, K., & Hemze, A. (2018). Adolescent substance abuse treatment: A review of evidence-based research. In C. Leukefeld, T. Gullotta, & M. Staton Tindall (Eds.), *Adolescent substance abuse: Evidence-based approaches to prevention and treatment* (2nd ed., pp. 141–171). Springer Science+Business Media.

Winters, K. C., & Lee, S. (2008). Likelihood of developing an alcohol and cannabis use disorder during youth: Association with recent use and age. *Drug and Alcohol Dependence, 92*, 239–247.

Winters, K. C., Leitten, W., Wagner, E. F., & O'Leary Tevyaw, T. (2007). Use of brief interventions in a middle and high school setting. *Journal of School Health, 77*, 196–206.

Zajac, K., Drazdowski, T. K., & Sheidow, A. J. (2019). Management of youth with substance use disorders in the juvenile justice system. In Y. Kaminer & K. C. Winters (Eds.), *Clinical manual of adolescent addictive disorders* (2nd ed., pp. 521–542). American Psychiatric Association.

Cognitive Behavior and Dialectic Behavior Therapies

INTRODUCTION

The next four chapters focus on the most prominent and distinct treatment approaches for adolescents with substance use and coexisting disorders. We discuss in this chapter cognitive behavioral therapy approaches, including dialectical behavior therapy, a type of cognitive therapy. In subsequent chapters we discuss motivational enhancement therapy (Chapter 11), family-based approaches (Chapter 12), and 12-Step therapy (Chapter 13).

Whereas all of these strategies are suitable for youth suspected of substance use, there are two features common to all of these approaches—each is *evidence-based* and each incorporates elements of *behavioral therapy principles* (Winters et al., 2018). These treatment strategies have been scientifically tested and found to be effective in the treatment of adolescents with a substance use disorder (SUD). And regardless of treatment philosophy, these effective approaches consist of some type behavioral therapy; treatment goals include at least some focus on changing the adolescent's behavior to promote health. Also, these approaches are showing promise in treating adolescents with an SUD and co-occurring disorder (Bender et al., 2006; Hogue et al., 2018; Winters et al., 2018).

In the prior chapter, we briefly described a handful of emerging, nonbehavioral treatments for adolescent SUD. These strategies are not yet widely accepted in the field and are still in their "preliminary evidence phase." This includes medications to assist adolescents in achieving abstinence; none are approved yet by the U.S. Food and Drug Administration (FDA) for adolescents, but controlled trials are being conducted and in the near future there may be medication-assisted options for adolescents.

The authors recognize that when an adolescent with an SUD receives treatment, it is likely the "end of the beginning" of what can be a complex and extended recovery process (Fishman, 2019). As discussed in Chapter 9, a treatment episode is best viewed as part of a continuum of care. This continuum includes support in the community after treatment, which may include aftercare services provided by the treatment program, self-help group participation, and other recovery support programs.

COGNITIVE BEHAVIORAL THERAPY (CBT)

CBT strategies take the view that clinical problems, such as SUD and other behavioral problems, are learned behaviors. These learned behaviors are presumed to be initiated and maintained by environmental factors, and thus the therapy approaches are derived from this line of thinking. CBT is a well-established approach as a stand-alone treatment, but there are some indications that the combination of CBT with motivational interventions may be more effective than just CBT (Hogue et al., 2018).

A combined CBT and motivational interviewing (MI) protocol was used in the Cannabis Youth Treatment (CYT) study, a well-known randomized field experiment of 600 adolescents. This study compared five various combinations of CBT/MI across four sites (Dennis et al., 2004). Variations were generally based on the number sessions and differences in types of CBT. All five interventions produced similarly significant reductions in cannabis use and negative consequences of use from pretreatment to the 3-month follow-up, and these reductions were sustained through the 12-month follow-up. Also, changes in marijuana use were accompanied by some improvement in psychosocial problems.

CBT approaches are organized around three learning principles that are typically combined into a multicomponent program: classical conditioning, operant conditioning, and social learning theory. These basic principles are described below.

Pavlov's original research on dogs had more to with eating than the nature of conditioned behavior. He and his colleagues originally were studying how eating and salivary, gastric, and pancreatic secretions were influenced by eating. Pavlov used a "fake" feeding design that would trick the dog into thinking it is eating food. He would remove a dog's esophagus and create an opening in the animal's throat for the food to fall out and never reach the dog's stomach. He would measure the quantity and chemical properties of the various secretions, a body of work that won him the 1904 Nobel Prize in Physiology or Medicine.

As often happens in science, discovery goes down unexpected paths. The emerging Pavlovian science of understanding human behavior dwarfed his original study of dog secretions.

From Pavlov's Nobel address: "Essentially, only one thing in life is of real interest to us—our psychical experience. Its mechanism, however, was and still is shrouded in profound obscurity. All human resources—art, religion, literature, philosophy, and the historical sciences—all have joined in the attempt to throw light upon this darkness. But humanity has at its disposal yet another powerful resource—natural science with its strict objective methods."

SOURCE: Michael Spector https://www.newyorker.com/magazine/2014/11/24/drool

Classical Conditioning

Eminent psychologist John Watson, building on the observations by a Russian physiologist Pavlov, proposed that new learned behavior simply involves two stimuli that are linked (Watson, 1913). When a stimulus in the environment is first experienced, an unlearned response or behavior is produced (i.e., unconditioned). An example: A song is heard for the first time and it elicits a favorable reaction in the person. A conditioned response or behavior occurs when the stimulus and unconditioned response are associated with another stimulus. Subsequently, that stimulus can produce the favorable reaction in the absence of the original stimulus. To extend our example: If there was a person present when the song was originally heard, when the individual meets that person later the same favorable feelings will be elicited. The conditioned or new response is the post-conditioning pleasant feeling for the person in new situations.

Operant Conditioning

Skinner further described operant learning as a function of different patterns (or schedules) of reinforcement. These schedules affect the speed of learning the new behavior and how resistant the new behavior is to elimination or extinction. The distinct learning schedules are the following (Ferster & Skinner, 1957):

1. Continuous reinforcement: The individual is positively reinforced every time a specific behavior occurs.
2. Fixed ratio reinforcement: The behavior is reinforced only after the behavior occurs a specified number of times (e.g., a reinforcement is given after a fixed number of times the behavior as occurred).
3. Fixed interval reinforcement: Behavior reinforcement is given after a fixed time interval (e.g., reinforcement always delivered after 1 hour).
4. Variable ratio and variable interval reinforcements. Behaviors are reinforced after a variable number of times or a variable time interval. These latter two schedules produce the fastest and strongest response rate and are the most resistant to extinction.

Operant conditioning is a learning method that occurs on the basis of consequences—either rewards or punishments—for behavior (Skinner, 1938). The new behavior is conditioned to the extent that the individual makes an association between a particular behavior and a consequence. Skinner viewed classical conditioning as too simplistic to explain complex human behavior. He believed that the best way to understand behavior is to look at the consequence (outcome) of an individual's actions. In this light, behavior that is reinforced tends to be repeated (i.e., strengthened). Reinforcement can be the addition of something pleasant or the removal of an unpleasant reinforce. Behavior that is not reinforced tends to be eliminated or extinguished (i.e., weakened), which can include punishment, that is, the introduction of an aversive event.

Social Cognitive Learning

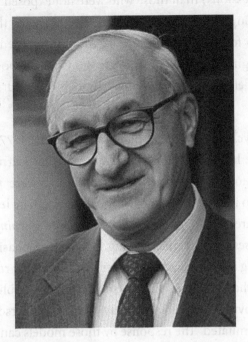

Influential social learning theorist, Albert Bandura, Ph.D. (1925—2021).
Photo courtesy of Albert Bandura.

Albert Bandura studied children's behavior after they watched a human adult model act aggressively toward a Bobo doll, a doll-like toy with a rounded bottom and low center of mass that rocks back to an upright position after it has been knocked down. In one variation of his experiment, he measured the children's behavior after seeing the human model get rewarded, get punished, or experience no consequence for physically abusing the Bobo doll. Bandura's social learning theory indicates that people learn social behavior by being rewarded or punished (operant conditioning), but they can also learn from watching somebody else being rewarded or punished (observational learning). In the "punishment" version of the experiment, Bandura observed that the children exposed to the aggressive model were more likely to pursue physically aggressive behavior (e.g., imitative physical aggressions) than those who were not exposed to the aggressive model. Boys exhibited more aggressive behavior than girls, and Bandura also found that children are more influenced by same-sex models (e.g., girls exhibited more aggression when exposed to aggressive girls models than aggressive male models) (Bandura, 1977).

The famous psychologist Albert Bandura (Bandura, 1977) advanced the social cognitive learning theory. His view was that learning theories of classical conditioning and operant conditioning were valid, but they lacked these two important elements: 1) behavior can be learned from the environment through the process of *observational learning,* and 2) *active cognitive processes* support this learning. Bandura emphasized that observational learning is focused on the power that influential role models have on a person's behaviors. Role models, such as parents, siblings, peers, and co-workers, provide examples of behavior that are personally incorporated and later imitated. The response by those models can strengthen the person's behavior when its reinforced or weaken the behavior if it's not reinforced. Moreover, how a person thinks about their behavior also shapes the learning of new behaviors. Individuals do not automatically observe the behavior of a model and imitate it; observational learning occurs with cognitive processes at work. Thus, mediating cognitive processes affects whether a person imitates behaviors, and if so, if the "modeled" behavior is adjusted. An important cognitive factor highlighted by Bandura is willpower—that is, the motivation of the person to behavior in a certain way.

Limitations to These Principles

These three learning theories emphasize the importance of the environment, the influence of other people, and cognitive processes. Each has its strengths and, as a group, provide valuable insights into the nature of learned behavior. But the complexity of human behavior may not be fully captured by learning theories. The underpinnings of how human behavior is learned is quite complex and involves the interaction between nature (biology) and nurture (environment).

COGNITIVE BEHAVIORAL THERAPY FOR SUBSTANCE USE DISORDERS

The limitations of learning theories to fully explain the origins of behavior do not mean that these principles cannot be useful when changing or modifying a person's use of substances. CBT approaches have a long-standing place as a valid counseling tool to help an adolescent with a substance use problem.

There is a subtype of CBT referred to as rational emotive behavior therapy (REBT). Developed by the American psychologist Albert Ellis, this approach actively aims to resolve the client's emotional and behavioral problems by targeting underlying beliefs. REBT presumes that clients have erroneous or "irrational" beliefs about situations related to one's life, and that these beliefs are the root cause of the distress and problems. Ellis (2003) suggested a handful of core irrational beliefs or philosophies that are all too common among people. Here is one such example: *I absolutely MUST, under practically all conditions and at all times, perform well (or outstandingly well) and win the approval (or complete love) of significant others. If I fail in these important—and sacred—respects, that is awful and I am a bad, incompetent, unworthy person, who will probably always fail and deserves to suffer.*

A central theme of CBT is that settings, situations, or states serve as potential "triggers" for the adolescent's initial substance use and, for some, progression to an SUD, and the client is taught to identify these contextual factors (e.g., Marlatt & Gordon, 1985). Thus, substance use is viewed as a behavior that follows antecedents (i.e., triggers) and that lead to immediate reinforcement (e.g., intoxicating effects) but which eventually lead to negative consequences (e.g., social consequences; addiction). Triggers can come in various forms, such as internal sources (when feeling bored or anxious; to forget trauma) and external sources (e.g., social situation; listening to music; presence of a peer). In order to change the "target" behavior that is elicited by the trigger, the counselor's task is to help the client understand the relationship between the trigger and subsequent behavior.

In this light, the counselor conducts a *functional analysis* in order to identify the client's triggers. A functional analysis is conducted with the patient in order to identify contextual factors, such as the settings, situations, or states, which may serve as potential "triggers" for abuse (Witkiewitz & Marlatt, 2004). The counselor makes note of these and seeks to establish which trigger or triggers are the most salient for the client in order to increase insight and awareness so that the client is aware of the effect that these factors have on drug use. As the client becomes more familiar with these outside factors, they will learn that they can control something that can help prevent or better manage the negative behavior.

The second core CBT principle is to address these "antecedents" underlying the behavior that must be changed. Specifically, CBT strategies teach the client 1) strategies to resist the triggers that are eliciting the negative behaviors, 2) to identify alternative reinforcers that compete with drug use (Higgins et al., 1994), and 3) based on the social learning model, to respond to influences from environmental events (e.g., peer influences) that can shape one's behavior (Bandura, 1986).

Specific CBT Strategies to Address Substance Abuse

Therapy sessions of CBT characteristically include the following strategies: modeling, behavior rehearsal, feedback, and homework assignments. In applying them, it is important to take into account the age and developmental level of the adolescent. Younger adolescents (e.g., ages 12–15) will likely need more basic social and coping skills training than older adolescents.

Modeling. Modeling is a therapeutic method whereby the client learns new coping skills by imitating the therapist or another person, such as a parent or a peer. A CBT therapist will typically use the therapy session as an opportunity for the adolescent to observe the therapist role play the desired behavior (verbal or nonverbal), followed by engaging the client to practice the target new responses. For an adolescent receiving drug treatment, modeling often targets effective verbal responses to use in social situations where there is pressure to use drugs. Effective behavioral modeling in a clinical setting is optimized when these four components are practiced (Bandura, 1975).

1. **Attention**: The client must watch and pay attention to the behavior being modeled.
2. **Retention**: The client must remember the behavior well enough to recreate it.
3. **Reproduction**: The client must physically or verbally recreate the actions observed in step 1.
4. **Reinforcement**: The client's modeled behavior must be rewarded by the therapist.

Behavioral rehearsal. This therapy technique involves practicing and imagining behaviors, responses, and social skills in order to prepare for when they will be used in the environment. Behavioral rehearsal in the context of therapy is similar to actors rehearsing for a play by practicing their lines and stage actions as if they were performing before a live audience. A client's behavioral rehearsal is similar—they rehearse and practice behaviors and responses, such as social skills, in order to be ready to use these behaviors in real situations. The therapist's task to facilitate behavioral rehearsal can involve having the client imagine themselves in a social setting and picture how they would perform the desired behaviors and responses. Also, the therapist can use role playing in order for the client to practice these behaviors in the clinical setting.

Feedback. Feedback is used by the therapist to support skill acquisition in a nonthreatening and meaningful way. As we discuss in the motivational enhancement therapy chapter (see Chapter 11), feedback includes providing the client with information and constructive criticism about what the client is doing well. Feedback can also include reflecting statements ("I hear you say that this behavior skill may be difficult to use with your friends"). Feedback is aimed at making the client feel less anxious and promoting the learning of new skills.

Action plan. Referred to in some writings as homework, this component is key to CBT. Action plans are to be developed collaboratively between the client and therapist, and examples include rehearsing new skills, practicing coping strategies, and restructuring negative or maladaptive cognitions. Homework assignments should be related to a specific goal and be relevant, meaningful, and practical and supported by in-session rehearsal. Also, there should be a discussion about how to address possible barriers to completion.

Research on action plans in therapy has revealed some meaningful results that can be understood collectively through a procedure called *meta-analysis.* A meta-analysis is a statistical summary of a body of research. A recent met-analysis by Kazantzis and colleagues (2010) examined 14 controlled studies that directly compared treatment outcomes for clients assigned to psychotherapy with or without homework. The data favored the homework conditions, with the average client in the homework group reporting better outcomes than about 70% of those in the no-homework conditions.

Why does CBT work? Coping with situations that might trigger a relapse has been identified as a significant reason for why CBT is effective (Myers et al., 1993). More specifically, coping skills are used to address social pressures to use substances and to bolster ways to utilize social supports for help and advice (Myers et al., 1993). A comprehensive review also found that CBT increases motivation to reduce substance use, increases affect regulation, and increases self-efficacy to reduce use (Black & Chung, 2014). Regarding the latter factor, self-efficacy (or self-confidence) is the perception that a person can accomplish what they set out to achieve, including the ability to resist substance use in potential high-risk situations (Burleson & Kaminer, 2005).

Contingency Management

Contingence management (CM) is a well-researched type of CBT. When applied to substance abuse, the CM approach is based on the scientific principles and conceptual framework of behavior analysis and behavioral pharmacology (Higgins et al., 1994). In this light, the use of substances is considered a special case of operant behavior maintained by the reinforcing effects when drugs are used. Tangible rewards contingent on desired behavior (e.g., abstinence) are provided to the client. CM procedures can use a variety of reinforcers, many of which are commonly used in, or readily adaptable to, standard clinic settings for adolescents. Experts have identified the key ingredients to effective CM, which we summarize in Box 10.1.

One limitation to CM is that, ideologically, some clinicians and administrators do not favor the idea of "paying a client to remain abstinent." As expected, public opinion may also hold the same view. Another barrier to implementing CM is the concern about its cost.

But are these concerns fair? If CM increases favorable outcome, including eliciting greater abstinence rates, everyone benefits. And many CM incentives are low cost (e.g., $10 coupon), and there are indications that CM increases attendance in community adolescent SUD treatment programs (Branson et al., 2012). With increased attendance, there is an increase in clinical billing; such extra billing revenue is likely to offset the costs of implementing the CM program (Lott & Jencius, 2009).

BOX 10.1

RECOMMENDED DESIGN AND IMPLEMENTATION FEATURES
OF CONTINGENCE MANAGEMENT (CM) FOR ADOLESCENTS
(STANGER ET AL., 2016)

1. Target the most important behaviors to be changed. Choose ones that can be quantified objectively and occur frequently. Examples are substance use abstinence, treatment attendance, and avoiding drug-using social situations.
2. Choose a reinforcer and specify its magnitude. Vouchers and cash are desirable reinforcers by adolescents and acceptable to staff. Payments can be made in a variety of ways, including remotely by staff on reloadable credit cards.
3. Negotiate with the client a time-limited and relatively simple behavioral contract. Be specific regarding the targeted behavior, monitoring procedures (e.g., drug urinalysis), and reinforcement schedule. Keep the contract straightforward so that staff can apply the system consistently and adolescent clients can understand it.
4. Monitor the compliance with the contract to ensure that it is consistently implemented by both staff and clients.
5. Improve and adjust the CM procedures as needed by keeping records, consulting with staff, and receiving feedback from clients regarding the contract's strengths and weaknesses.

Adolescent Community Reinforcement's (ACRA's) relative effectiveness compared to that of other CBT-based approaches was further highlighted in a recent review of treatment approaches to address adolescent drug abuse (Winters et al., 2018). The authors conclude that contingency management is a key component to ACRA's success.

CM has produced impressive outcomes in controlled adult studies (Stitzer & Petry, 2015), and there are some studies now with adolescents that affirm its effectiveness with this age group (Randall, 2017; Stanger et al., 2016). Typically, in adolescent CM studies, the strategy is to re-arrange the adolescent's environment so that drug use and abstinence are readily detected, drug abstinence is positively reinforced, and drug use results in an immediate loss of reinforcement. Also, other behaviors to reinforce drug abstinence can be rewarded, such as compliance with the treatment plan and changes in behaviors that promote a healthy lifestyle. CM-based interventions have shown strong effects as part of other evidence-based strategies, such as Multi-Systemic Therapy (MST; Henggeler, 2017) and the Adolescent Community Reinforcement approach (ACRA; Godley et al., 2014).

Emerging examples of CM. One example of a new CM-based approach for adolescents is a *home-based incentive program* that includes involvement from parents (Stanger et al., 2015). Home-based CM involves teaching parents to develop and monitor a CM contract that specifies positive and negative consequences to be implemented on a regular basis (e.g., weekly) contingent on target behaviors, such as abstinence. An important component is to include the adolescent's input on selecting rewards.

An interesting variant of implementing a low-cost incentive program is the *fishbowl drawing* procedure. Developed by Petry and Martin (2002), this procedure involves a drawing bowl with numerous slips of paper that vary in magnitude of the prize (e.g., some slips as low as a $1 and some as high as $20). Clients get to draw from the bowl, contingent on meeting their contract goal. Extra draws are earned for each consecutive week the adolescent attends treatment or has continuous abstinence.

It can be expected that *remotely delivered* CM strategies will grow in popularity. Bickel and colleagues (Koffarnus et al., 2018) have tested such an approach with adults and found impressive outcomes. CM clients were equipped with a Soberlink breathalyzer (see Figure 10.1), which is designed for remote verification of the identity of the user and remote monitoring of alcohol abstinence. The contingent reward was based on the results of the breathalyzer. This digital component of this CM program reduced staff and client and burden, and those in the CM breathalyzer condition had significantly higher abstinence rates compared to the non-CM group.

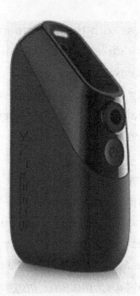

Figure 10.1 Soberlink breathalyser designed for remote verification of the identity of the user, and remote monitoring of abstinence.
SOURCE: Soberlink.

DIALECTICAL BEHAVIOR THERAPY

Introduction

Dialectical behavior therapy (DBT) was created by psychologist Marsha Linehan in an effort to ease the acute suffering of her female patients diagnosed with borderline personality disorder (BPD; see Chapter 7). (DBT's application has been extended to treat patients with PTSD; also see Chapter 7.) The term *dialectical* refers to the Buddhist concept of opposing forces, or in this case, the opposite pulls of change and acceptance. DBT therapists guide clients in making changes that will help in reaching personal goals, with the understanding and acceptance that change is a constant in life and everything is interconnected.

Dr. Linehan saw a disparity of services to serve those patients with a BPD, and she learned through research that CBT alone was not sufficient (Dimeff & Koerner, 2007; Linehan, 1993). In 1993, she published the text and workbook for this approach, *Cognitive Behavioral Treatment of Borderline Personality Disorder and Skills Training Manual for Treating Borderline Personality Disorder*. Since that time, DBT has been gaining popularity across the United States and internationally. Linehan (personal communication, 2013) stated, "There is continuous research being completed to support its [DBT's] efficacy; it [DBT] is very applicable across many different settings due to its flexibility and practicality for many disorders across the life span."

In a survey study of 2,278 therapists trained in DBT by Linehan's training organization, Behavioral Tech, DeGiorgio et al. (2010) reported the frequent use of eclectic approaches in therapy. Furthermore, research documented an increase in the effective use of adaptations or assimilated elements of DBT in practice. Researchers theorized that DBT is appealing to therapists who vary in theoretical orientation because DBT itself is a combination of many different approaches. This study also supported extensive literature that DBT is effective with individuals with BPD, but more important is the fact that DBT is still employed by therapists who modify DBT to fit the population they serve.

Core Skills

DBT has four core skills that are taught in skills labs to therapy participants: mindfulness, distress tolerance, emotion regulation, and interpersonal effectiveness.

Mindfulness. Mindfulness has Buddhist roots. It is the practice of being single-minded. It is a practice of self-awareness. The goal is for clients to become aware of their thoughts, feelings, and reactions. Examples of this are increased awareness of body movements, such as breathing, and increased awareness of what is happening in the environment (Dimeff & Koerner, 2007; Linehan, 1993). The practice helps clients observe the world in a nonjudgmental manner.

Distress tolerance. Distress tolerance is a set of skills that are developed to replace unhealthy ways of coping with unpleasant situations or

concerns. The premise is that it is almost impossible to give up one behavior without replacing it with another. The goal is for each person to have
many different skills to choose from and to try as many as needed until
the crisis or unpleasant emotion has passed (Dimeff & Koerner, 2007;
Linehan, 1993).

Emotion regulation. Emotion regulation involves clients' learning
about their emotions and vulnerabilities when they experience extreme
emotions. Most importantly, once emotions are better understood, they
are easier to manage. Understanding the impact of emotions on their
thoughts and behaviors empowers individuals so that emotions do not
run their lives and they feel more in control (Dimeff & Koerner, 2007;
Linehan, 1993).

Interpersonal effectiveness. Interpersonal effectiveness is the ability to
interact with others, all different kinds of people, in a productive way. It
also works to increase personal effectiveness in significant relationships
that are close or important without placing too much emphasis on oneself
or the other person; it assists in providing skills to balance relationships
(Dimeff & Koerner, 2007; Linehan, 1993).

Adaptation of Dialectic Behavior Therapy for Adolescents

Adolescent DBT programs use the same four core principles as adult
programs—mindfulness, distress tolerance, emotion regulation, interpersonal effectiveness. Also, a fifth principle, of walking the middle path, and
other features of DBT are tailored for adolescents. One key adolescent feature is that DBT with adolescents requires significant parental involvement
(Benham, 2012; Dimeff & Koerner, 2007). Miller and colleagues (Miller
et al., 2000) went further in their work to describe the use of DBT with
adolescents. They aligned some of the developmental issues of adolescents
with the concepts of DBT; Table 10.1 illustrates their assertions.

Walking the middle path. Walking the middle path involves finding
a balance of acceptance and change (Christensen et al., 2009; Dimeff
& Koerner, 2007). Walking the middle path is a fifth skill module that

Table 10.1 DIALECTICAL BEHAVIOR THERAPY FOR
ADOLESCENTS' PROBLEMS AND SKILLS

Problems	Skills
Confusion about yourself	MINDFULNESS
	wise mind
	observe
	describe
	participate
	don't judge
	stay focused
	do what works
Impulsivity	DISTRESS TOLERANCE
	distract (ACCEPTS)
	(Activities, Contributing, Comparisons, Emotions, Pushing Away, Thoughts, Sensations)
	self-soothe
	pros and cons
	radical acceptance
Emotional instability	EMOTION REGULATION
	reduce vulnerability (PLEASE)
	(treat Physical illness, balance Eating, Avoid mood-altering drugs, balance Sleep, Exercise)
	build mastery
	building positive experiences
	act opposite
Interpersonal problems	INTERPERSONAL EFFECTIVENESS
	cheerleading statements
	improving the relationship (GIVE)
	(be Gentle, act Interested, Validate, use an Easy manner)
	getting what you want (DEARMAN)
	(Describe, Express, Assert, Reinforce, take hold of your Mind, appear confident, Negotiate)
	keeping your self-respect (FAST)
	(be Fair, no Apologies, Stick to values, be Truthful)

focuses on teaching adolescents and their parents the concepts of dialectics, validation, and behavioral therapy, with specific emphasis on the relationship between parents and teens. Because these relationships can be very problematic and stressful, parents and children are often locked in power struggles that can be overcome by learning the concepts of dialectics, validation, and reinforcement.

Parental involvement. As a part of the program, parents are asked to attend a DBT skills lecture once a week. These sessions help parents be more involved in their child's care and be a part of the treatment team (Goldstein et al., 2007; Miller et al., 2007). In addition to the parent skills lectures, non-DBT family therapy is also required. The goals of family therapy are a combination of individual and family needs but also include six overarching goals:

1. Educate family members to gain an understanding that their adolescent family member is vulnerable to emotional dysregulation.
2. Begin to view problems as systemic, and identify ways family members may be contributing to the problem.
3. Improve communication in the family as a whole.
4. Develop parenting skills needed to work with an adolescent with a co-occurring disorder.
5. Increase the family's and adolescent's support network.
6. Reduce aggressive and/or violent interactions (Dimeff & Koerner, 2007).

In addition, therapists adapting DBT to adolescents incorporate specific techniques that are more developmentally appropriate and appealing to the adolescent intensive outpatient program attendee. Three commonly used techniques are discussed below.

Behavior chain analysis. DBT emphasizes healthy coping and decision making. When a serious problem behavior occurs, a behavior chain analysis is conducted to explore the events that led up to the problem behavior and to explore alternatives to the decisions that lead up to the

DBT Chain Analysis

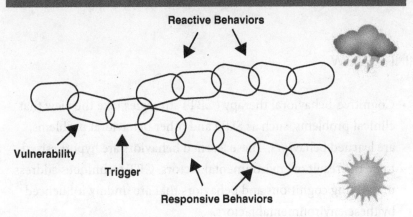

Figure 10.2 Behavior chain analysis.
© 2002, Marcia Linehan. Graphic by Jaelline Jaffe, PhD.

problematic behavior (Goldstein et al., 2007) (see Figure 10.2). The purpose of the analysis is to prepare the youth for the next challenging decision. When a challenging decision or situation arises, the adolescent can reflect on the behavior analysis to provide a road map for healthier decision making.

DEAR MAN. The DEAR MAN technique illustrates the importance of basic communication skills, especially when adolescents experience difficulty or frustration. DEAR MAN is an acronym that stands for describe, express, assert, reinforce, mindful, appear confident, and negotiate (Dimeff & Koerner, 2007; Linehan, 1993). This technique is helpful when adolescents need to ask for what they need or when they need to say no. The DEAR MAN technique is a component of interpersonal effectiveness (Dimeff & Koerner, 2007; Linehan, 1993).

Radical acceptance. The DBT skill of radical acceptance is covered as a component of distress tolerance. Radical acceptance is an important concept for the developmental stage of adolescence as well as for those who have an SUD. Radical acceptance teaches acceptance of life situations even when they involve a painful or difficult situation. According to this principle, suffering about difficult situations lasts longer when they are not accepted (Dimeff & Koerner, 2007; Linehan, 1993).

MINI-REVIEW

- Cognitive-behavioral therapy (CBT) strategies take the view that clinical problems, such as SUD and other behavioral problems, are learned behaviors. These learned behaviors are hypothesized to be the result of environmental factors. CBT techniques address underlying cognitions and behaviors that are unduly influenced by these environmental factors.
- CBT approaches are organized around three learning principles that are typically combined into a multicomponent program: classical conditioning (the role of environmental stimuli that contribute to behaviors), operant conditioning (how rewards and punishment influence behaviors), and social learning theory (the power that influential role models have on a person's behaviors).
- A central theme of CBT when applied to address an SUD is that the adolescent's settings, situations, or internal emotional states serve as potential "triggers" for the person's initial substance use and, for some, progression to a substance use disorder.
- Dialectical behavior therapy (DBT), originally developed by Marsha Linehan to treat her female patients diagnosed with borderline personality disorder, focuses on client skills for identifying and transforming negative thinking patterns and learning ways to effectively cope with stress and to regulate emotions.
- DBT consists of the following core skills when applied to adolescents: mindfulness, distress tolerance, emotion regulation, interpersonal effectiveness, and walking the middle path.
- Also important with adolescents receiving DBT is parent involvement. Parents are taught skills related to supporting the adolescent, improving parent–adolescent communication, and enhancing the family support network.

DISCUSSION POINTS

1. Classical conditioning can occur in the classroom, and this phenomenon can be a deterrent or an asset to learning. Discuss examples of both.

    Also, how does operant conditioning occur in the classroom? What are examples of reinforcers? What are examples of non-reinforcers (punishments)?

2. Discuss how social learning influences occur during adolescence and ways in which these influences have an impact on a teenager's life.

3. Discuss common triggers for an adolescent's substance use. Compare and contrast triggers associated with first starting to use and those that maintain use. Then compare and contrast triggers for alcohol and cannabis use.

4. Compare counseling a 12-year-old versus a 17-year-old when using CBT techniques. What adjustments would be needed when applying the strategies listed in the chapter? Would any of them be more or less useful to apply for the younger teen? The older teen?

5. Including a "fun" component to a CBT-based action plan may promote compliance by the teenager. What are some ways that the homework assignments can have a fun angle for them?

6. Discuss the four core skills of DBT pertaining to adolescents (mindfulness, distress tolerance, emotion regulation, and interpersonal effectiveness) in light of adolescent development discussed in Chapter 2 and Chapter 3. How do these core skills support adolescent social development? How do they support adolescent brain development?

FURTHER CURIOSITY AND DIGGING

More about Cognitive Behavior Therapy

American Psychological Association. (2017). *What is cognitive behavioral therapy?* https://www.apa.org/ptsd-guideline/patients-and-families/cognitive-behavioral

Bobo Doll Experiment

https://www.khanacademy.org/test-prep/mcat/behavior/theories-personality/v/observational-learning

Dialectic Behavior Therapy

There are several YouTube talks by Marsha Linehan about DBT:

Linehan, M. (2017). *Strategies for emotion regulation*. [Video]. YouTube. https://www.youtube.com/watch?v=lXFYV8L3sHQ

Linehan, M. (2017). *How she learned radical acceptance*. [Video]. YouTube. https://www.youtube.com/watch?v=OTG7YEWkJFI

Linehan, M. (2017). *How she came to develop dialectical behavior therapy (DBT)*. [Video]. YouTube. https://www.youtube.com/watch?v=bULL3sSc_-I

Mindfulness for Teens

http://mindfulnessforteens.com/

REFERENCES

Bandura, A. (1975). Analysis of modeling processes. *School Psychology Digest, 4*, 4–10.

Bandura, A. (1977). *Social learning theory*. Prentice Hall.

Bandura, A. (1986). *Social foundations of thought and action: A social cognitive theory*. Prentice Hall.

Benham, D. K. (2012). Extending an adult DBT program to adolescent clients: Adapting dialectical behavior therapy for younger clients and parents proves helpful. *Behavioral Healthcare, 32*, 24–26.

Bender, K., Springer, D. W., & Kim, J. S. (2006). Treatment effectiveness with dually diagnosed adolescents: A systematic review. *Brief Treatment and Crisis Intervention, 6*(3), 177–205.

Black, J. J., & Chung, T. (2014). Mechanisms of change in adolescent substance use treatment: How does treatment work?. *Substance Abuse, 35*, 344–351.

Branson, C. E., Barbuti, A. M., Clemmey, P., Herman, L., & Bhutia, P. (2012). A pilot study of low-cost contingency management to increase attendance in an adolescent substance abuse program. *American Journal on Addictions, 21*, 126–129.

Burleson, J. A., & Kaminer, Y. (2005). Self-efficacy as a predictor of treatment outcome in adolescent substance use disorders. *Addictive Behavior, 30*, 1751–1764.

Christensen, K., Riddoch, G. N., & Huber, J. E. (2009). *Dialectical behavior therapy skills: 101 mindfulness exercises and other fun activities for children and adolescents*. Author House.

DeGiorgio, K. E., Glass, C. R., & Arnkoff, D. B. (2010). Therapists use of DBT: A survey study of clinical practice. *Cognitive and Behavioral Practice, 17*, 213–221.

Dennis, M., Godley, S. H., Diamond, G., Tims, F. M., Babor, T., Donaldson, J., . . . Hamilton, N. (2004). The Cannabis Youth Treatment (CYT) study: Main findings from two randomized trials. *Journal of Substance Abuse Treatment, 27*, 197–213.

Dimeff, L. A., & Koerner, K. (2007). *Dialectical behavior therapy in clinical practice*. Guilford Press.

Ellis, A. (2003). Early theories and practices of rational emotive behavior theory and how they have been augmented and revised during the last three decades. *Journal of Rational-Emotive & Cognitive-Behavior Therapy, 21*, 219–240.

Ferster, C. B., & Skinner, B. F. (1957). *Schedules of reinforcement*. Appleton-Century-Crofts.

Fishman, M. (2019). Placement criteria and treatment planning for adolescents with substance use disorders. In Y. Kaminer & K. C. Winters (Eds.), *Clinical manual of adolescent addictive disorders* (2nd ed., pp. 123–140). American Psychiatric Association.

Godley, M. D., Godley, S. H., Dennis, M. L., Funk, R. R., Passetti, L. L., & Petry, N. M. (2014). A randomized trial of assertive continuing care and contingency management for adolescents with substance use disorders. *Journal of Consulting and Clinical Psychology, 82*, 40–51.

Goldstein, T. R., Axelson, D. A., Birmaher, B., & Brent, D. A. (2007). Dialectical behavior therapy for adolescents with bipolar disorder: A 1-year open trial. *Journal American Academy of Child and Adolescent Psychiatry, 46*, 820–830.

Henggeler, S. W. (2017). Multisystemic therapy. The Encyclopedia of Juvenile Delinquency and *Justice*, 1–5. https://doi.org/10.1002/9781118524275.ejdj0048

Higgins, S. T., Budney, A. J., & Bickel, W. K. (1994). Applying behavioral concepts and principles to the treatment of cocaine dependence. *Drug and Alcohol Dependence 34*, 87–97.

Hogue, A., Henderson, C. E., Becker, S. J., & Knight, D. K. (2018). Evidence base on outpatient behavioral treatments for adolescent substance use, 2014–2017: Outcomes, treatment delivery, and promising horizons. *Journal of Clinical Child & Adolescent Psychology, 47*, 499–526.

Kazantzis, N., Whittington, C., & Dattilio, F. (2010). Meta-analysis of homework effects in cognitive and behavioral therapy: A replication and extension. *Clinical Psychology: Science and Practice, 17*, 144–156.

Koffarnus, M. N., Bickel, W. K., & Kablinger, A. S. (2018). Remote alcohol monitoring to facilitate incentive-based treatment for alcohol use disorder: A randomized trial. *Alcoholism: Clinical and Experimental Research, 42*, 2423–2431.

Linehan, M. (1993). *Cognitive behavioral treatment of borderline personality disorder*. Guilford Press.

Lott, D. C., & Jencius, S. (2009). Effectiveness of very low-cost contingency management in a community adolescent treatment program. *Drug and Alcohol Dependence, 102*, 162–165.

Marlatt, G. A., & Gordon, J. R. (1985). *Relapse prevention*. Guilford Press.

Miller, A. L., Rathus, J. H., DuBose, A. P., Dexter-Mazza, E. T., & Goldklang, A. R. (2007). Dialectical behavior therapy for adolescents. In L. A. Dimeff & K. Koerner (Eds.), *Dialectical behavior therapy in clinical practice: Applications across disorders and settings* (pp. 245–263). Guilford Press.

Miller, A. L., Wyman, S. E., Huppert, J. D., Glassman, S. L., & Rathus, J. H. (2000). Analysis of behavioral skills utilized by suicidal adolescents receiving dialectical behavior therapy. *Cognitive and Behavioral Practice, 7*, 183–187.

Myers, M. G., Brown, S., & Mott, V. (1993). Coping as a predictor of adolescent substance abuse treatment outcome. *Journal of Substance Abuse*, 5, 15–29.

Petry, N. M., & Martin, B. (2002). Low-cost contingency management for treating cocaine- and opioid-abusing methadone patients. *Journal of Consulting and Clinical Psychology*, 70, 398–405.

Randall, J. (2017). Challenges and possible solutions for implementing contingency management for adolescent substance use disorder in community-based settings *Journal of Child & Adolescent Substance Abuse*, 26, 332–337.

Skinner, B. F. (1938). *The behavior of organisms: An experimental analysis.* Appleton-Century.

Stanger, C., Lansing, A. H., & Budney, A. J. (2016). Advances in research on contingency management for adolescent substance use. *Child and Adolescent Psychiatry Clinics of North America*, 25, 645–659.

Stanger, C., Ryan, S. R., Scherer, E. A., Norton, G. E., & Budney, A. J. (2015). Clinic-and home-based contingency management plus parent training for adolescent cannabis use disorders. *Journal of the American Academy of Child & Adolescent Psychiatry*, 54, 445–453.

Stitzer, M., & Petry, N. (2015). Contingency management. In M. Galanter & K. T. Brady (Eds.), *The American publishing textbook of substance abuse treatment* (5th ed., pp. 423–439). American Psychiatric Publishing Inc.

Watson, J. B. (1913). Psychology as the behaviorist views it. *Psychological Review*, 20, 158–177.

Winters, K. C., Botzet, A. M., Stinchfield, R., Gonzalez, R., Finch, A., Piehler, T., Ausherbauer, K., Chalmers, K., & Hemze, A. (2018). Adolescent substance abuse treatment: A review of evidence-based research. In C. Leukefeld, T. Gullotta, & M. Staton Tindall (Eds.), *Adolescent substance abuse: Evidence-based approaches to prevention and treatment* (2nd ed., pp. 141–171). Springer Science+Business Media.

Witkiewitz, K., & Marlatt, G. A. (2004). Relapse prevention for alcohol and drug problems: That was Zen, this is Tao. *American Psychologist*, 59, 224–235.

Motivational Enhancement Treatment

INTRODUCTION

Most adolescents with a drug problem do not readily come to this conclusion, even in the face of experiencing many negative consequences linked to their drug use. As we noted in Chapter 9, it is estimated that only about 10% of adolescents with a substance use disorder (SUD) have access to formal treatment (Substance Abuse and Mental Health Services Administration, 2017). Moreover, it is rare for an adolescent to think they need treatment. This frustrating situation often leads to less-than-ideal circumstances in an effort to get an adolescent into treatment (e.g., use of coercion or deception; treatment mandated by the courts).

Thus, counseling and treatment approaches that promote motivation to change are very relevant. An approach that has been at the forefront in the addiction field for decades is motivational enhancement therapy (MET) and related strategies. MET as a counseling strategy helps a client to address their reluctance about participating in counseling and making a commitment to change. The ease and adaptability of this counseling style have demonstrated its usefulness when working with adolescents (Naar-King & Suarez, 2011). An MET therapist uses a client-centered, nonconfrontational style in assisting the youth to explore different facets of their use patterns. Adolescents are encouraged to examine the pros and cons of their use and to create goals to help them achieve a healthier lifestyle. The therapist provides personalized feedback and respects the youth's freedom of choice regarding their own behavior. MET is typically delivered in conjunction with other treatment approaches; it would be rare to find a treatment program or counselor that does not use MET techniques. It is generally accepted that all models or approaches of adolescent drug treatment include to some degree components of MET. It is used as a prelude to more intense treatment, in combination with other therapies, and as a stand-alone therapy.

The length of MET varies considerably. At one end there is a version that is a brief, 15-minute conversation. This form would typically use just motivational interviewing techniques and focus on improving the adolescent's recognition that drug use is unhealthy, and briefly discuss ways to reduce or stop use. Longer versions have been developed that consist of two to three 1-hour sessions. MET has also been adapted for use in family systems therapy, called systemic-motivational therapy, which focuses on relational issues affecting SUD. These longer programs more thoroughly delve into psychological and social factors that appear to drive the teenager's drug use, and both short- and long-term plans for change are discussed.

STAGE OF CHANGE THEORY

The theoretical underpinnings of MET is the transtheoretical Stage of Change (SOC) model. Developed by Prochaska and DiClemente in the late 1970s (Prochaska et al., 1992), this model posits that the behavioral health change process involves progress through six stages of

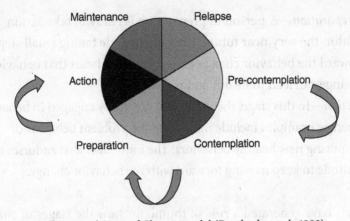

Figure 11.1 Transtheoretical Stage of Change model (Prochaska et al., 1992).

change: precontemplation, contemplation, preparation, action, relapse, and maintenance (see Figure 11.1).

The model was originally conceptualized as an explanation of stages common to smoking cessation behavior, but subsequent research has shown this pattern of change across numerous health behaviors (Prochaska & Velicer, 1997). The model evolved on the basis of this common observation: Successful quitting of smoking rarely occurred unless a person was ready to do so (action), and prior to that, the smoker typically experienced various level of ambivalence (precontemplation and contemplation). Following is a definition of each stage of change.

1. *Precontemplation*—An individual in this stage typically shows the following features: unawareness that their behavior is a problem; underappreciation of the pros of changing their behavior; low emphasis on the cons of changing behavior; and no intention to make changes in the foreseeable future.
2. *Contemplation*—In this stage, the person begins to show signs that behavior change will occur in the foreseeable future. Although some ambivalence is present, positive signs of future behavior change include recognition that the unhealthy behavior may be creating problems, and a more balanced perception of the pros and cons of changing the behavior.

3. *Preparation*—A person in preparation is ready to take action within the very near future. Changes include taking small steps toward the behavior change and a change of heart that behavior change can lead to health and well-being.

4. *Action*—In this stage, the individual is actively engaged in behavior change; examples include modifying the problem behavior or acquiring new healthy behaviors. The individual also endorses an attitude to keep moving forward with the behavior change.

Experts have generated a rule of thumb for how the stages of change are distributed for populations with health risk behaviors: 40% in precontemplation, 40% in contemplation, and 20% in preparation (Prochaska & Velicer, 1997). This implies that many people engage in unhealthy behaviors but are not ready to change. Think of an example in your life. Do you have a "bad habit" that you have eventually changed? What was your experience like during precontemplation, contemplation, and preparation?

5. *Relapse*—The relapse stage occurs when a person fails to continue the behavior change and returns to the unhealthy habits. To resume involvement in the action stage, a person often revisits the contemplation and precontemplation stages.

6. *Maintenance*—Maintaining behavior change over an extended period is what defines this stage. An individual in this stage also shows intent to prevent relapsing back to their unhealthy habits and a desire to not return to their unhealthy behaviors.

Stage of Change and Treatment

Applied research has demonstrated dramatic improvements in recruitment, retention, and progress using stage-matched interventions and proactive recruitment procedures. *Stage-matching* means that, based on where the client is located in the SOC, the counseling approach will vary accordingly—all with the intent to move the person to the next stage of change and, subsequently, completely through the model to the maintenance stage, which is the ideal stage of behavior change.

In Chapter 9 we discussed the Screening, Brief Intervention and Referral Treatment (SBIRT) approach. One major reason for the development of the SBIRT model is to provide guidance on how to clinically address the fact that people vary in their stage in terms of motivation to change health behaviors.

The SOC model provides a general road map for how to adjust the clinical task in order to match the client's level of motivation to change. This notion of "stage-adjusting" is important to the behavior change process. Imagine two examples, one at each end of the "ready to change" spectrum.

Case 1: An adolescent has been coerced by her parents to seek counseling. She does not think she has a drug use problem, has no interest in counseling, and is intent on making this experience go as quickly as possible. Within this context, the counselor can reasonably assume that the client is in precontemplation. The counselor's strategy would *not* be to quickly establish the adolescent's goals for behavior change; doing so would be premature. Rather, the counselor should focus on motivating the client to think about change and, if this is successful, move to establish goals.

Case 2: A teenager has insight that he has a drug problem and goes to the school counselor to seek help. He fully acknowledges that he has to make some changes in his life. In this instance, the counselor would not need to devote time to improving his motivation to change. Rather, she should reward him for seeking help and discuss how to seek his goals and strategies to deal with any barriers that he may face when working on his goals.

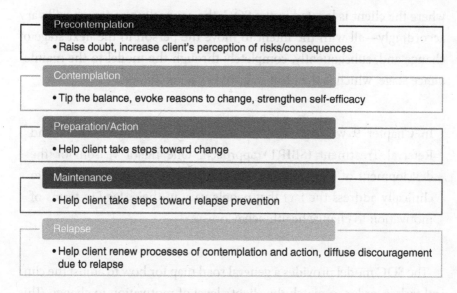

Precontemplation
- Raise doubt, increase client's perception of risks/consequences

Contemplation
- Tip the balance, evoke reasons to change, strengthen self-efficacy

Preparation/Action
- Help client take steps toward change

Maintenance
- Help client take steps toward relapse prevention

Relapse
- Help client renew processes of contemplation and action, diffuse discouragement due to relapse

Figure 11.2 Stage of change and counselor's tasks.

Provided in Figure 11.2 is a brief description of the counselor's task, based on what stage of change the client is positioned.

Assessing Stage of Change

Adapting treatment on the basis of the client's SOC status requires assessing their current status in the SOC at the outset of treatment.

Provided in Table 11.1 is a list of well-researched assessment measures to assess a client's SOC, some of which have been developed for adolescents.

Limitations of the SOC Model

Despite its many benefits, experts have noted several limitations of the SOC model. Measuring a client's location in the model can be problematic; many individuals report a combination of attitudes about change and cannot be reliably labeled with a single stage. One assumption of the model is that clients make logical plans in their decisions and choose

Table 11.1 Psychometrically Sound Assessment Tools to Assess a
Client's Stage of Change

Instrument	Intended Sample	Format	Source
Problem Recognition Questionnaire	Adolescents	24 items; 3 scales	Cady et al., 1996
SOCRATES	Adults	19 items; 3 scales (version 8)	https://casaa.unm.edu/ inst/SOCRATESv8.pdf
Readiness to Change Ruler	Adolescents and adults	3 items	Zimmerman et al., 2000

realistic goals; this is not always true, particularly for adolescent clients. Finally, the model does not account for the social context of the client, such as socioeconomic status, community standards, and age.

MOTIVATIONAL INTERVIEWING

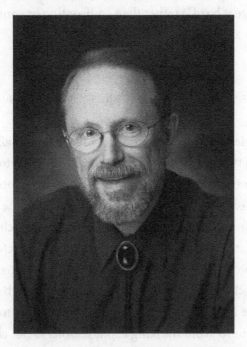

William Miller, Ph.D. (1947–), the pioneering psychologist who advanced the use of motivational interviewing to address addictive behaviors.
Photo courtesy of William Miller.

The clinical application of MET is organized around motivational interviewing (MI). The origins of MI can be traced to Carl Rogers' counseling approaches from the 1950s. The Rogerian approach was revised by William Miller in the early 1980s to more specifically deal with problem drinking (Miller, 1983). Miller sought to offer an alternative to the confrontational style often practiced by counselors with alcoholics. He developed an intuitive approach to address resistance and denial in clients via a motivational process that combined principles based on Carl Rogers' work and on the SOC model posited by Prochaska and colleagues (Prochaska et al., 1992). The main components of MI include an initial assessment of the adolescent's motivation to participate in counseling, followed by interviewing techniques in which the therapist uses feedback to help the adolescent think about change and eventually make a commitment to change. A key goal for the counselor is to elicit "change talk" from the teenager—that is, expressions of intentions to change behavior in the desired direction. If the adolescent resists willingness to engage and to build a plan for change, the therapist responds with empathy ("I understand that change is hard") rather than confronting or contradicting them. Provided below are details of the core elements of MI.

Basic Elements and Features of Motivational Interviewing

MI is a goal-oriented treatment practice that intentionally encourages a collaboration between the client and therapist in order to strengthen the client's motivation and commitment to achieve goals. As noted above, MI is primarily based on a Rogerian counseling approach and the SOC theory, yet it also borrows from humanistic therapy and positive psychology. Together, the patient and interviewer use reasons for change, directed by the client, to address ambivalence and turn the desired goal into realistic changes (Miller & Rollnick, 2012). Client ambivalence serves as a barrier to change; MI strategies are used to bring the client's attitude closer to thinking about realistic goals and to avoid thinking about reasons to not change (Miller & Rollnick, 2012).

The counselor uses MI skills and techniques to help the client increase their awareness that current use of drugs is unhealthy, to reduce hesitation to change, and to settle on ways to make real change. For adolescents, the goal is often to become drug-free, but change may also take the form of harm- or risk-reduction (e.g., reduce intensity of drug use; no use before or during school; avoid driving while intoxicated).

MI involves the counselor and the client progressing along four overlapping processes: 1) engaging (building a therapeutic relationship between counselor and client); 2) focusing (maintaining a specific direction in discussing behavior change [change talk]); 3) evoking (eliciting the client's own motivations for change); and 4) planning (developing a commitment to change and establishing a plan of action).

OARS. The core MI interviewing skills have been summarized by the acronym OARS (Miller & Rollnick, 2012), which we summarize below.

O = Open questions. Open questions are the opposite of closed questions. Closed questions typically elicit a limited response such as "yes" or "no. Open questions invite the client to provide details or to "tell their story" without leading them in a specific direction. This type of questions is an excellent way to get a conversation going. Of course, any user of open questions must be willing to be a good listener.

The following examples provide a contrast between open and closed questions for the same topic. Which type of question is likely to yield richer information?

(Closed) Did you have a good relationship with your parents?

(Open) What can you tell me about your relationship with your parents?

A = Affirmations. Affirmations are genuine and realistic statements and discussions that recognize and support the client's assets and strengths, as well as promote goals and behaviors that lead in the direction of positive change. Affirmations build confidence in an adolescent's ability to achieve their goals. Examples of affirming responses are the following:

> I appreciate that you are willing to spend time with me to talk about what is going on in your life.
>
> I can understand that using drugs helps to relax you.
>
> Our discussion of changes you may make indicate that you are thinking about your health.

R = Reflective listening. Reflecting listening refers to the counselor reflecting back what is said by the client. This skill is viewed as vital for building trust between the counselor and the client and for promoting motivation to change. Poor reflective listening would involve misinterpreting what is said, assuming incorrectly a client's motives or needs, and giving a different interpretation to what the words mean. To hone this skill, experts encourage learning to *think* reflectively. That is, consider what the client's thoughts are that underlie what they are saying. Also important with reflective listening is to respect the person's point of view. With adolescent clients, there may be a tendency to show disapproval of the teen's behavior. But a reflective listener can acknowledge a client's' point of view without approving it. There are three basic levels of reflective listening:

1. Repeating or rephrasing: The counselor repeats or substitutes synonyms or phrases, and stays close to what the speaker has said: "So you are telling me that you are here because you were told by others to attend."
2. Paraphrasing: The counselor restates the meaning and content from the client's statements: "It sounds like you are not interested in stopping all drinking at this time."
3. Reflection of feeling: The most complicated type of reflective listening, reflection of feeling, requires that the counselor emphasize the importance of communication by using empathy and recognizing the client's emotions and feelings: "I can see this

is important to you—you do not want to make changes that may interfere with your friendships."

S = Summarize. Effective use of summaries occurs throughout the counseling, with particular application at transition points or to facilitate a new direction in the session. Examples include summarizing after there has been a lengthy discussion about a particular topic, or when it is an opportune time to discuss behavior change goals. Summarizing helps to ensure that there is clear communication between the counselor and client. Miller and Rollnick (2012) have identified seven elements that comprise good use of summarizing.

1. Begin with a statement indicating you are making a summary. Examples include: "Let's review what we have talked about. This is what I understand we have talked about. What have I missed?"
2. Give special attention to "change statements." These statements by the client suggest or indicate a willingness to change. The more these statements are verbalized, the better. Types of change statements are problem recognition ("I can see that my drug use has upset others"), intent to change ("It makes sense that I work toward reducing my drug use"), and specific plans to change ("Okay, I am going to try this plan").
3. Recognize ambivalence. An adolescent client will likely express ambivalence throughout the counseling session. It is useful to include both sides of their thoughts in the summary statement: "I can see that you have on one hand thought about your situation this way. On the other hand, there is this point of view that we have talked about."
4. Include information in summary statements from other sources. Sources include your own clinical experience, research knowledge, and significant others of the client.
5. Be concise. Distill the information into clear and concise statements.

6. Provide an invitation for the adolescent to contribute to the summarizing: "Did I miss anything? What would you like to add or change?"

7. Consider using the summarizing process to further encourage change. The client's responses to your summary statements may provide additional indications to promote planning or engaging in behavior change.

Use of MET in Brief Interventions

As noted above, MET is typically delivered in conjunction with other treatment approaches, and this is no exception with respect to its use in a brief intervention (BI). We discussed BIs in Chapter 9 as a component of the Screening, Brief Intervention, and Referral to Treatment (SBIRT) model. To summarize: BIs, which can range from a brief conversion of 15 minutes to a small handful of sessions (Winters et al., 2018), typically consist of educational services that aim to help the client increase motivation to change and to make some concrete plans to reduce or stop drug use. Forms of BIs include interventions in school health clinics, as a diversion program in the juvenile justice system, intervention used in pediatric clinics and emergency departments, and as a bridge for those seeking comprehensive treatment but on a waiting list (National Institute on Drug Abuse, 2014). Most BIs described in the literature are administered in a standard face-to-face format, yet computerized, self-administered versions are also available (Cunningham et al., 2009). BIs are becoming an attractive therapeutic approach because of cost-containment policies of managed care and because their features, many of which are MET based, are "adolescent-friendly" (e.g., the number of therapeutic contacts is brief; the approach is developmentally fitting given that many drug-abusing youth are not "career" drug abusers; adolescents are likely to be very receptive to person-centered change strategies). To further support the use of BIs for adolescents, drug use by adolescents spans a wide range in severity, in terms of length of use and quantity and frequency of use, which leads to varying severity of resulting negative psychosocial consequences and impairment. As we noted in Chapter 5, an appreciable percentage of drug-using adolescents are experiencing problems at a mild-to-moderate level, which many experts count as the "sweet spot" for use of a BI (e.g., Winters, 2016).

For readers interested in the use of motivational interviewing skills within an SBIRT model for adolescents, following is a battery of observational videos from the Boston University School of Public Health BNI-ART Institute:

Rapport: SBIRT for alcohol/drugs with adolescents www.youtube.com/watch?v=v3_uxCpZ7wg

Pros & Cons: SBIRT for alcohol/drugs with adolescents www.youtube.com/watch?v=dLGYfADKYJo

Feedback: SBIRT for alcohol/drugs with adolescents www.youtube.com/watch?v=h5bpAvmjrcs

Readiness Rules: SBIRT for alcohol/drugs with adolescents www.youtube.com/watch?v=oVVociJ0P8o

Action Plan: SBIRT for alcohol/drugs with adolescents www.youtube.com/watch?v=dqOs5N4QPNw

Summary and Thanks: SBIRT for alcohol/drugs with adolescents www.youtube.com/watch?v=WKVPZUtWXME

There is a relatively recent movement for BIs to be part of the multicomponent clinical model SBIRT (Vendetti et al., 2017; Winters, 2016). This model posits that a clinical service for a teenager suspected of drug use should include a coordinated screening. If the adolescent has a score in the mild-to-moderate range, a BI is applied, and at its conclusion, if more services are needed, the adolescent is referred for more treatment.

There is growing support for the efficacy of BIs, based on findings from several published meta-analyses or literature reviews of this model for adolescents (e.g., Carney & Myers, 2012; Tanner- Smith & Lipsey, 2015). These meta-analyses concur that, despite some exceptions (e.g., Haller et al., 2014), the efficacy of BI is generally encouraging. These findings have occurred in multiple settings, including schools (e.g., Winters et al., 2014), juvenile offender settings (e.g., Dembo et al., 2014), primary care (e.g., Levy & Knight, 2008), and emergency departments (e.g., Monti et al., 1999). Of note is that typically BIs significantly outperform control or comparison conditions (Winters, 2016).

Case Vignettes of Motivational Interviewing in a Brief Intervention

Andria is a 15-year-old girl being seen by her pediatrician for a school physical exam. She answers "no" to all three of the opening questions about substance use: "Have you ever drunk alcohol?" "Have you ever used marijuana?" "Have you ever used any other drug not prescribed by a doctor to get high?" However, she admits that her parents have expressed concern about her possible use of alcohol. Dr. Anderson says, "It is great that you have made some good decisions in your choice not to use alcohol or other drugs and alcohol. I hope you feel that it is important to keep this up. But tell me more about why you think your parents are concerned about alcohol drinking." Andria responds that her parents believe her friends drink too often and that she has attended many drinking parties. Effective use of MI by Dr. Anderson would include him showing an understanding of Andria's views about her parents and engaging her with ways to discuss this issue with her parents and encourage her to use strategies to avoid peer pressure to drink.

Jorge is a 16-year-old boy who comes to the office after injuring his ankle at football practice. During the exam, the team physician administers a brief, self-report substance use screen, a procedure required by the school when a student receives health care in the school. The young man says that he has been drunk on several occasions, but not at the time of this injury. He has never used other drugs and his score on a screening tool is 0. Dr. Miller says, "I can appreciate that you may do some drinking as teenager. But it seems that when you drink you do so heavily. I am concerned about this because drinking like that can do some serious damage to your developing brain. At your age, your brain is still maturing. I would recommend that you wait until you are older to drink. What do you think about the idea of not drinking alcohol at all until you are age 21?" Dr. Miller spends the next 5 minutes asking Jorge about the pros of drinking and the cons of drinking, and seeks to move him to a greater appreciation of the cons of drinking.

Katie is a 17-year-old young woman who comes to the school health clinic with flu-like symptoms. On a routine screening, she reveals that she smokes marijuana on a fairly regular basis. She has the maximum score on the screening questionnaire and indicates that she has smoked marijuana on a nearly weekly basis for over a year. The school counselor further asks about the typical setting and peers that are linked to her use. The discussion moves to the decisional balance exercise. Katie can only offer a single con of using marijuana—her parents would be upset if they knew she used. After talking more about the issue of her parents, the counselor asks Katie about how using might be affecting her grades. "Tell me your thoughts about using marijuana and its possible impact on your school-work." Katie shows some insight as she admits that using gets in the way with school, and her grades have dropped some in the past year. The counselor praises her by saying, "I am impressed that you are thinking about this important issue. I know many students want to do well in school, and you apparently are one of them. May I make a suggestion?" ("Yes" is offered by Katie.) "I would like for us to meet a couple of times over the next 2 weeks for about 45 minutes each time and we can talk more about these issues. I am not going to tell you what to do about your health. It will be your decision if you want to make any changes. Would that be okay?" Katie decides this is an acceptable plan and the two agree on the date of their first appointment.

MET and Engaging Families in the Treatment Process

Parents and other family members can provide vital support to the adolescent's efforts toward behavior change. In addition to providing moral and emotional support, parents are also important by supporting the client's goals, encouraging effective communication in the household, and providing practical support, such as paying the treatment bill and making appointments. Family-based strategies specifically addressing adolescent drug abuse are common to the field (see Chapter 12 for a full discussion of family therapy). Family-based treatment approaches highlight the need to engage the family, including parents, siblings, and sometimes peers, in the adolescent's treatment. Thus, involving the family can be particularly important, as the adolescent will often be living with at least one parent and be subject to the parent's controls, rules, and/or supports.

A prominent example of an effective way to engage entire families *into treatment* is an intervention called Strategic Structural Systems Engagement (SSSE; Szapocznik et al., 1990). SSSE is based on the premise that the same dysfunctional family interaction pattern that has contributed to and maintained the adolescent's drug use will be a major barrier to family engagement in treatment. The goal of SSSE is to begin the work of diagnosing, joining, and restructuring the family with the very first contact, thereby facilitating the engagement of the entire family into therapy. The basic elements of SSSE consist of strategies applied to convince the parent(s) to attend the intake appointment (via joining; establishing alliances; using negotiating and reframing strategies), as well as techniques to promote eventual treatment engagement and participation by all family members (via joining all family members; conducting out-of-office visits to family members or significant others who were critical of the therapy process).

Parents as a motivating agent to promote adolescent treatment (CRAFT). Community Reinforcement and Family Training (CRAFT) was designed to address the challenge of convincing a reticent person to seek treatment (Kirby et al., 2015; Meyers & Smith, 1997). Based on the operant-based fundamentals of behavioral psychology, CRAFT purposely does not pressure reluctant individuals to attend treatment. Rather, this program takes a more indirect route. It involves a trained therapist teaching a concerned significant other (CSO) to change the home environment of the treatmentambivalent individual to both reward behaviors that promote the individual being drug-free and withholding rewards when the individual is using drugs (Meyers & Smith, 1997). Let us consider how this would work with a reticent adolescent and the parent being the CSO. Assume the adolescent spends a lot of time playing video games. The parent would discuss with the teenager the importance of being drug-free and that access to video game playing would be contingent on achieving that goal. The message would include some variation of this sentence: "I wanted to let you know that it is very important to me that you are free of drugs while you are growing as a teenager. So what if we agree on a plan: I will let you play your video games for a reasonable amount of time, after your homework is done, and during your free time. In return you, from now on, do not use alcohol or other drugs. But the video games will be taken away if you cannot abide by this." It is critical that the parent follow through with the plan to permit the reward or remove the reward, based on the adolescent's behavior.

Use of Reinforcements in MET

Several incentive-based approaches for adolescents have been developed and researched with an eye toward promoting treatment engagement. Incentive-based strategies can be a stand-alone treatment or integrated into the variety of other treatment approaches that are becoming the mainstay to address adolescent drug abuse (e.g., any MET approach, cognitive behavioral therapy [CBT], family therapy) (Hogue et al., 2018).

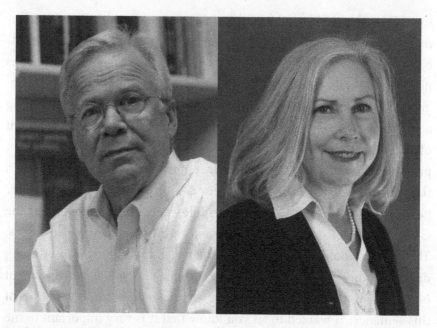

Psychologists Susan and Mark Godley, co-authors of the eminent community-based contingency management approaches to address adolescent substance abuse. Photos courtesy of Chestnut Health Systems.

The most prominent example is contingency management (CM), which encourages behavior change by providing adolescents with immediate rewards contingent on positive changes in behavior, such as negative urine tests or meeting treatment goals. This approach is based on the operant conditioning principle that the use of consequences can modify behavior. Rewards are often in the form of award prizes (e.g., dollar prizes; coupons for the adolescent's favorite store) (Sindelar et al., 2007). There are two noteworthy variations of CM. The community reinforcement plus vouchers approach (CRA) involves the use of vouchers to reward treatment compliance and abstinence, frequent and random urine screens to detect drug use, and several tools to support successful recovery (e.g., functional analyses to identify triggers for drug use; self-management plans to address identified triggers; and the development of drug avoidance skills). A modified version of CRA is ACRA; this program has several features that are intended for adolescents (Godley et al., 2014). A significant adjustment is the participation of the parent/caregiver. In addition to the individual adolescent sessions, the parent attends four sessions—two devoted to parenting practices alone, and two sessions with both the parent and adolescent. The parent sessions focus on basic skills pertaining to communication and problem-solving; the joint sessions focus on what the adolescent has learned in their individual sessions. An extension to A-CRA is the home-based continuing care-approach to support long-term recovery, called Assertive Continuing Care (ACC) (Godley et al., 2007).

Case Illustration of a Two-Session MET

Below we provide a case vignette of a therapist who applied MET when counseling Annette, a young woman with a drug problem. The counselor uses MI and CBT throughout the sessions. This case is a compilation of several real clients. There are two discussion questions provided at the end.

Background. Annette is a 17-year-old female who is a junior in high school. She is an average-performing student (her grades are mostly B's and C's), has a few close school friends, and has not had any in-school behavior problems. She was referred to a school counselor because a teacher caught her with a small amount of marijuana.

The assessment indicated that Annette is a weekly marijuana smoker, with some use occurring on school days, and that she recently experienced a significant life stress event. Her father passed away about a year ago and the adjustment for her and the relationship with her mother (she is an only child) have been difficult. Annette admits that she started smoking marijuana about 2 years ago and has increased her use since her father's death.

Session 1. The counselor was careful to ask open-ended questions regarding whether or not Annette saw her marijuana use as a problem. Annette said the teacher overreacted and that her use of marijuana was nothing to worry about. "I use with my friends and do not see any problems with it." She further mentioned that she has never tried to quit or thought much about any change in her use of marijuana. During these first few minutes of the session, Annette's attitude was moderately defiant; she had a challenging tone and reminded the counselor that she was not interested in "any of this counseling thing."

The counselor reassured Annette that she has a right to make her own decisions, that no one was going to tell her what to do, but was hoping the two could discuss what is going on in her life, including marijuana use. "What if we begin with a simple exercise. Here are few questions about your use of marijuana. Is this ok?" Annette reluctantly agreed, so the counselor engaged her in a "decisional balance" exercise. It begins with, "What are some of the benefits of your use of marijuana?" She identified the social benefits, particularly when she is using with her boyfriend. The boyfriend is 18 years old and apparently has a steady supply of marijuana. Additionally, Annette indicated that smoking helps her to relax.

Despite Annette not initially identifying any negatives consequences of using marijuana, the counselor continued to probe. "Almost everything a person does has both negative and positive effects," the counselor said. Annette admitted that using marijuana and providing it to others, including the boyfriend, was upsetting to her mother. "And my Dad would be very mad at me if he knew about this."

The counselor asked her if there was anything else she could think of. With some probing by the counselor, Annette admitted that if she continued to use, she may have trouble getting passing grades in school. She was getting C's, and was growing less and less interested in school. She said that her mother did not seem to care all that much that she was bringing home a report card with mostly C's.

Next the counselor summarized the results from the decisional balance exercise. Annette saw the benefits of use outweighing any negative consequences. "Annette, here is a 10-point scale to look at. This is a gauge to see how ready you are at this time to reduce your use of marijuana. A "1" means you are not ready at all; a "10" means you are very ready to change. Where along this scale would you place yourself? She chose a "2" on this Readiness to Change scale, indicating a low level of motivation to change (precontemplation stage).

The session next moved to goal-setting. Given Annette's low interest in discussing marijuana use, the counselor focused on the issue about Annette's relatively poor grades and growing disinterest in school, including how her deceased father would have been upset by her poor school performance. The counselor guided the conversation along the lines that marijuana use can contribute to lower school achievement. "What do you think about this possibility: "Your grades are suffering because of your marijuana use," the counselor posed. This open-ended question was followed by Annette admitting that she often used marijuana before school but not during school. The counselor steered Annette into an expanded discussion about how her use of marijuana still could be impacting school performance because she is high during school. The counselor said, "You seem to be saying that being high while in school does not affect your learning. Everything I know about marijuana indicates the opposite. In what way would being high during school *not interfere* with learning?"

Consider this counselor's statements: "You seem to be saying that being high while in school does not affect your learning. Everything I know about marijuana indicates the opposite. In what way would being high during school *not interfere* with learning?"

The motivational interviewing strategy used by the counselor here is called *developing discrepancy*. This method involves the therapist directing attention toward the discrepancy between an individual's desired state of being and that individual's actual state of being. The therapist helps the client to focus their attention on how current behavior differs from ideal or desired behavior. Discrepancy is initially highlighted when the therapist raises the client's awareness of the negative personal, social, or health consequences of using substances, and then leveraging this discussion to help the client rethink the consequences of continuing to use substances.

Annette admitted that she may be showing bad judgment in using before school and instead of doing homework. The counselor asked Annette, "Would you like to do anything about this?" With some reluctance, Annette hinted that it might be a good idea to not use before school. This suggests Annette had moved from precontemplation to the next stage—contemplation. "But quitting use altogether is not something that interests me," she said. The counselor proceeded to negotiate with Annette the goal of not using before school for all of the school days from now until the next session. They also discussed the advantages of waiting to use until after homework was done if use was going to occur. Keep in mind that this harm reduction goal is somewhat controversial, given that Annette is a minor and is using an illegal substance. The counselor is following motivational enhancement principles by not pushing for abstinence right now, given Annette's resistance.

As a final exercise in the session, the counselor probed what barriers Annette might face with this goal. She admitted to this possible issue: It has been the habit for her and boyfriend to use marijuana together before school. This led to a discussion about strategies. Suggestions included *what to say* to the boyfriend ("It's okay, you go ahead and use; I don't want to right now"), *preplanning* (telling him beforehand that she didn't want to use every day before school), and *using humor* ("You know why it's called 'dope'"?).

Annette agreed, somewhat reluctantly, to meet with the counselor again in 10 days to discuss how things had progressed.

Session 2. The session began with some small talk, and then the counselor moved into a discussion about how it went for Annette with the behavior change goal. "I was a bit surprised. It was not all that difficult to not use before school," Annette said. She further admitted that she felt satisfaction for showing some self-control, a point that the counselor reinforced. "You are pleased that you could achieve something that earlier you thought might be tough to do." Also, Annette admitted that schoolwork seemed easier. These positive experiences were reflected by the fact Annette now placed herself at the number "5" on the Readiness to Change Scale, which is up from the number 2 that she recorded during the first session. The counselor once again reflected back to Annette this good news.

The counselor took advantage of this modest improvement in the positive direction and encouraged Annette to think about more meaningful changes regarding marijuana use. This suggestion elicited only a moderate response. "What would need to change in your life for you to stop using marijuana?" the counselor asked. Annette did not have much of an answer. Concerned that the session momentum was going downhill, the counselor shifted the discussion. "Would it be okay if we talk about other parts of your life? How are things going at home?" Annette quickly took this opportunity to describe a challenging picture about the relationship with her mother. The counselor used open-ended questions to get details. Annette described these home issues: her mother is still in grief over the loss of her husband; Annette is concerned that if her mother knew about the marijuana use there would be conflicts; and her mother is not pleased with the boyfriend. The counselor encouraged Annette to think about what she would like to do with the relationship with the mother. It was decided that Annette would now work on three additional goals: 1) to spend at least a few minutes each day engaging with her mother in small talk; 2) to look for and respond to signs that her mother would benefit from extra support from Annette; 3) to think more about her relationship with the boyfriend. Annette and the counselor discussed specific behavioral steps and strategies to address each goal, including keeping notes of the pros and cons of her relationship with the boyfriend.

Finally, it was agreed that the two would meet again. Annette offered that meeting in a month would be okay. The counselor reminded Annette that her friends can be a source of support, and to not rule out that her mother may appreciate the opportunity to provide advice and support. The counselor was impressed that Annette finished the session by talking about how her mother is a good person to confide in and that she also has a couple girlfriends with whom she is close.

MINI-REVIEW

- The counseling and treatment approach that promotes motivation to change is motivational enhancement therapy (MET) and related strategies. MET is a counseling strategy that helps a client to address their reluctance about participating in counseling and making a commitment to change.
- MET is typically delivered in conjunction with other treatment approaches; it would be rare to find a treatment program or counselor nowadays that does not use MET techniques.
- The theoretical underpinning of MET is the transtheoretical Stage of Change (SOC) model. This model posits that the behavioral health change process involves progress through six stages of

change: precontemplation, contemplation, preparation, action, relapse, and maintenance.

- The clinical application of MET is organized around motivational interviewing (MI). The main elements of MI include an initial assessment of the adolescent's motivation to participate in counseling, followed by interviewing techniques in which the therapist uses feedback to help elicit "change talk" from the youth and eventually have them make a commitment to change.
- MET has also been integrated into family therapy and contingency management strategies.

DISCUSSION POINTS

1. What habits have you had where you were probably "stuck" in precontemplation for quite some time?
2. For a habit that you changed, describe what you did in the preparation and action phases.
3. Discuss this controversy about contingency management: It is a counseling approach that involves paying a person to get healthy.
4. Discuss the following questions concerning the two-session Annette case vignette:
   a. Identify examples in Session 1 where Annette is in the precontemplation stage.
   b. What did you like about the way the counselor handled the two sessions?
   c. What did you not like about the way the counselor handled the two sessions?

FURTHER CURIOSITY AND DIGGING

More about Motivation

Pink, D. (2009). *The puzzle of motivation*. [Video]. TedGlobal. https://www.ted.com/talks/dan_pink_the_puzzle_of_motivation/transcript?language=en

More about Motivational Interviewing

Adolescent SBIRT: www.sbirt.webs.com/webinars

Matulich, B. (2013). *Motivational interviewing: An introduction.* [Video] YouTube. https://www.youtube.com/watch?v=s3MCJZ7OGRk

Motivational interviewing: Adolescent follow up on positive alcohol screen. [Video]. YouTube. Produced by HealthTeamWorks [nonprofit]. www.youtube.com/watch?v=JZrYk86EDlQ

Community Reinforcement and Family Training (CRAFT): https://motivationandcha nge.com/outpatient-treatment/for-families/craft-overview/

References

Cady, M., Winters, K. C., Jordan, D. A., Solberg, K. R., & Stinchfield, R. D. (1996). Measuring treatment readiness for adolescent drug abusers. *Journal of Child and Adolescent Substance Abuse, 5,* 73–91.

Carney, T., & Myers, B. (2012). Effectiveness of early interventions for substance-using adolescents: Findings from a systematic review and meta-analysis. *Substance Abuse Treatment, Prevention, and Policy, 7,* 1–15.

Cunningham, R. M., Walton, M. A., Goldstein, A., Chermack, S. T., Shope, J. T., Raymond Bingham, C., . . . Blow, F. C. (2009). Three-month follow-up of brief computerized and therapist interventions for alcohol and violence among teens. *Academic Emergency Medicine, 16,* 1193–1207.

Dembo, R., Briones-Robinson, R., Wareham, J., Schmeidler, J., Winters, K. C., Barrett, K., Ungaro, R., Karas, L., & Belenko, S. (2014). Impact of brief intervention services on drug-using, truant youth arrest charges over time. *Journal of Child & Adolescent Substance Abuse, 23,* 375–388.

Godley, M. D., Godley, S. H., Dennis, M. L., Funk, R. R., & Passetti, L. L. (2007). The effect of assertive continuing care on continuing care linkage, adherence and abstinence following residential treatment for adolescents with substance use disorders. *Addiction, 102,* 81–93.

Godley, S. H., Smith, J. E., Passetti, L. L., & Subramaniam, G. (2014). The Adolescent Community Reinforcement Approach (A-CRA) as a model paradigm for the management of adolescents with substance use disorders and co-occurring psychiatric disorders. *Substance Abuse, 35,* 352–363.

Haller, D. M., Meynard, A., Lefebvre, D., Ukoumunne, O. C., Narring, F., & Broers, B. (2014). Effectiveness of training family physicians to deliver a brief intervention to address excessive substance use among young patients: A cluster randomized controlled trial. *CMAJ, 186,* E263–E272.

Hogue, A., Henderson, C. E., Becker, S. J., & Knight, D. K. (2018). Evidence base on outpatient behavioral treatments for adolescent substance use, 2014–2017: Outcomes, treatment delivery, and promising horizons. *Journal of Clinical Child & Adolescent Psychology, 47,* 499–526.

Kirby, K. C., Versek, B., Kerwin, M. E., Meyers, K., Benishek, L. A., Bresani, E., . . . Meyers, R. J. (2015). Developing Community Reinforcement and Family Training (CRAFT) for parents of treatment-resistant adolescents. *Journal of Child & Adolescent Substance Abuse, 24,* 155–165.

Levy, S., & Knight, J. R. (2008). Screening, brief intervention, and referral to treatment for adolescents. *Journal of Addiction Medicine, 2,* 215–221.

Meyers, R. J., & Smith, J. E. (1997). Getting off the fence: Procedures to engage treatment-resistant drinkers. *Journal of Substance Abuse Treatment, 14,* 467–472.

Miller, W. R. (1983). Motivational interviewing with problem drinkers. *Behavioural Psychotherapy, 11,* 147–172.

Miller, W. R., & Rollnick, S. (2012). *Motivational interviewing: Helping people change.* Guilford Press.

Monti, P. M., Colby, S. M., Barnett, N. P., Spirito, A., Rohsenow, D. J., Myers, M., . . . Lewander, W. (1999). Brief intervention for harm reduction with alcohol-positive older adolescents in a hospital emergency department. *Journal of Consulting and Clinical Psychology, 67,* 989–994.

Naar-King, S., & Suarez, M. (2011). *Motivational interviewing with adolescents and young adults.* Guilford Press.

National Institute on Drug Abuse. (2014). *Principles of adolescent substance use disorder treatment: A research-based guide.* NIH Publication Number 14-7953.

Prochaska, J. O., DiClemente, C. C., & Norcross, J. C. (1992). In search of how people change: Applications to the addictive behaviors. *American Psychologist, 47,* 1102–1114.

Prochaska, J. O., & Velicer, W. F. (1997). The transtheoretical model of health behavior change. *American Journal of Health Promotion, 12,* 38–48.

Sindelar, J., Elbel, B., & Petry, N. M. (2007). What do we get for our money? Cost-effectiveness of adding contingency management. *Addiction, 102,* 309–316.

Substance Abuse and Mental Health Services Administration. (2017). *Key substance use and mental health indicators in the United States: Results from the 2016 National Survey on Drug Use and Health.* Center for Behavioral Health Statistics and Quality, Substance Abuse and Mental Health Services Administration. HHS Publication No. SMA 17-5044, NSDUH Series H-52.

Szapocznik, J., Perez-Vidal, A., Hervis, O. E., Brickman, A. L., & Kurtines, W. M. (1990). Innovations in family therapy: Strategies for overcoming resistance to treatment. In R. A. Wells & V. J. Giannetti (Eds.), *Handbook of brief psychotherapies* (pp. 93–114). Plenum.

Tanner-Smith, E. E., & Lipsey, M. W. (2015). Brief alcohol interventions for adolescents and young adults: A systematic review and meta-analysis. *Journal of Substance Abuse Treatment, 51,* 1–18.

Vendetti, J., Gmyrek, A., Damon, D., Singh, M., McRee, B., & Del Boca, F. (2017). Screening, brief intervention and referral to treatment (SBIRT): Implementation barriers, facilitators and model migration. *Addiction, 112,* 23–33.

Winters, K. C. (2016). Adolescent brief interventions. *Journal of Drug Abuse, 2,* 1–3.

Winters, K. C., Botzet, A. M., Stinchfield, R., Gonzalez, R., Finch, A., Piehler, T., Ausherbauer, K., Chalmers, K., & Hemze, A. (2018). Adolescent substance abuse treatment: A review of evidence-based research. In C. Leukefeld, T. Gullotta, & M. Staton Tindall (Eds.), *Adolescent substance abuse: Evidence-based approaches to prevention and treatment* (2nd ed., pp. 141–171). Springer Science+Business Media.

Winters, K. C., Lee, S., Botzet, A., Fahnhorst, T., & Nicholson, A. (2014). One-year outcomes of a brief intervention for drug abusing adolescents. *Psychology of Addictive Behaviors, 28,* 464–474.

Zimmerman, G. L., Olsen, C. G., & Bosworth, M. F. (2000). A "stages of change" approach to helping patients change behavior. *American Family Physician, 61,* 1409–1416.

Family-Based Treatments

INTRODUCTION

The aim of family therapies for adolescents with a substance abuse problem is to address what is presumed to be family risk factors that are main contributors to the problem. These factors include poor family communication, lack of or weak effective parenting practices, and poor family connectedness. Thus, the core underlying premise of family therapy is that the family unit has a significant and long-lasting influence on the adolescent and their behavior (Bobek et al., 2019).

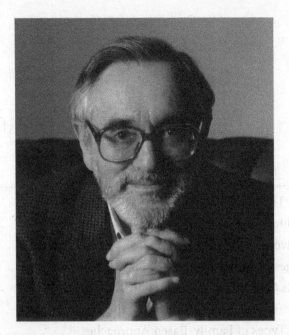

The scholarly origins of the multisystem approach to family theory can be traced to the Argentinian family therapist, Salvador Minuchin (Minuchin, 1974).
Photo courtesy of Minuchin Center for the Family.

Family therapy is often cited as a multisystem approach. What is meant by that? Any multisystem therapy approach assumes that behavior change for the client requires that the therapist address several "spheres" or sources of influence of the adolescent's behavior. With respect to family therapy, not only are family factors targeted, but also considered are influences from peers, school, local community, and other family members (e.g., siblings).

Whereas family therapy approaches consist of involving family members (typically at least one parent or guardian and the adolescent), therapy can be can be enhanced if siblings and other adult household members are included. Also, it is common to mix in a handful of sessions or partial sessions with just the adolescent alone or with a parent alone.

As we describe in detail below, some family therapies were designed to specifically address adolescent substance abuse, whereas others were originally designed for addressing broad youth problem behaviors but have proved effective with issues associated with substance abuse. Also, treatment strategies discussed earlier (e.g., cognitive behavioral therapy in Chapter 10 and motivational enhancement therapy in Chapter 11) are typically integrated into family-based treatment.

EFFECTIVENESS OF FAMILY THERAPY

Family therapy approaches have consistently been associated with favorable outcomes. Of significance are the findings from a recent comprehensive review of adolescent drug abuse treatment approaches (Hogue et al., 2018) in which five major categories of family therapies are discussed: behavioral, systems, functional, ecological, and educational, as defined by Becker and Curry (2008). These labels are based on the degree to which the focus of therapy is within the system of the family. Family treatment approaches were rated as superior to all other models in addressing adolescent drug abuse. Ecological family therapy stood out as the category most supported by evidence (Hogue et al., 2018). (We discuss below the primary family-based approaches.)

Ecological family therapy originated from therapeutic work with substance-abusing adolescents who had run away from home. The target of this model's therapeutic techniques are family interaction patterns, with a consideration of how individual, interpersonal, and environment contextual factors impact family interactions. Therapy techniques include reframing, relabeling, communication skills training, and conflict resolution (Hogue et al., 2018).

Also, family therapy approaches are very effective for adolescents with externalizing problems, such as oppositional defiant disorder and conduct disorder (McCart & Sheidow, 2016). And how do they fare with internalizing disorders, such as depression and anxiety? Family therapies also are quite effective with this domain (Hogue & Liddle, 2009). (For more about internalizing and externalizing disorders, see Chapters 6 and 7, respectively.)

CHANGES IN THE FAMILY IN THE UNITED STATES

Family therapists are faced with unique challenges resulting from the fact the family structure in the United States today does not resemble what was typical decades back. Issues pertaining to obtaining approval for therapy for the adolescent and who is involved in counseling may be complicated by the presence of a nontraditional nuclear family situation. Also, family therapy goals can be compounded when parents are in discord, are separated, or have joint custody.

To put these challenges in historical context, we take a brief look at the American family today. In terms of parenthood, the relative frequency of divorce, remarriage, and cohabitation has led to a decline in the two-biological parent household. And the size of families is smaller, due to the rise in single-parent households and the trend that Americans are having fewer children.

The role of women in the family has seen dramatic changes. Nearly 4 in 10 births occur to women who are single or living with a nonmarital partner (Thomas, 2020). Another major shift in recent years is that more mothers have entered the labor force and some are the *primary* breadwinners in their families (Pew Research Center, 2015).

These trends mean that currently there is no standard family structure in the United States. Just about 50 years ago, nearly 75% of all children in America were being raised together by two married parents in their first marriage. A 2018 survey indicated that almost a quarter of U.S. children under the age of 18 live with one parent and no other adults (23%), which is more than three times the share of children around the world who do (7%).

This changing landscape of the family unit is displayed in Figure 12.1 (Pew Research Center, 2022). The diversity rates of living arrangements for youth now include higher historical rates of two parents in remarriage, cohabiting parents, and single parents. Moreover, many youth are raised in family structures that change during their at-home years, given the greater prevalence of remarriage and (nonmarital) recoupling in the United States. A 2014 report by the U.S. Census indicated that, over a 3-year period, about 30% of children younger than 6 years of age had experienced a major change in their family or household structure, in the form

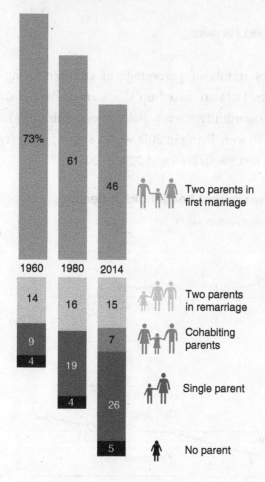

For children, growing diversity in family living arrangements

% of children living with...

73% | 61 | 46 — Two parents in first marriage

1960 | 1980 | 2014

14 | 16 | 15 — Two parents in remarriage

9 | | 7 — Cohabiting parents

4 | 19 | 26 — Single parent

| 4 | 5 — No parent

Note: Based on children under 18. Data regarding cohabitation are not available for 1960 and 1980; in those years, children with cohabiting parents are included in "one parent." For 2014, the total share of children living with two married parents is 62% after rounding. Figures do not add up to 100% due to rounding.

Source: Pew Research Center analysis of 1960 and 1980 decennial census and 2014 American Community Survey (IPUMS)

PEW RESEARCH CENTER

Figure 12.1 Percent of children living in various family arrangements.
SOURCE: "Parenting in America." Pew Research Center, Washington, D.C. (DECEMBER 17, 2015). https://www.pewsocialtrends.org/2015/12/17/parenting-in-america/

of either parental divorce, separation, marriage, cohabitation, or death (Pew Research Center, 2015).

Single and Blended Families

Figure 12.2 shows trends of percentage of children living with one, two, or no parents. Data are based on U.S. Census Bureau data and the 2014 American Community Survey. Fully one-fourth (26%) of children younger than age 18 were living in 2014 with a single parent (typically the mother), up from just 9% in 1960 and 22% in 2000.

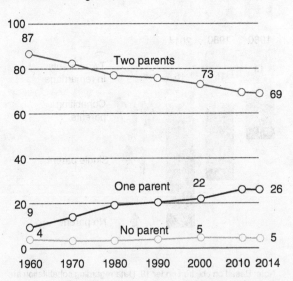

The two-parent household in decline

% of children living with...

Note: Based on children under 18. From 1990–2014, a child living with cohabiting parents is counted as living with two parents. Prior to 1990 cohabiting parents are included in "one parent."

Source: Pew Research Center analysis of 1960–2000 Decennial Census and 2010 and 2014 American Community Survey (IPUMS)

PEW RESEARCH CENTER

Figure 12.2 Percent of children living in households with two, one or no parents. SOURCE: "Parenting in America." Pew Research Center, Washington, D.C. (DECEMBER 17, 2015). https://www.pewsocialtrends.org/2015/12/17/parenting-in-america/

Another perspective is that the 2020 U.S. Census Bureau data indicate that 65% of children are living in a household with two parents married to each other; by contrast, the percentage in 1960 was 88% (U.S. Census, 2021).

PARENTS CAN STILL BE INFLUENTIAL TO THEIR TEENAGER

A core assumption of family therapy is that parents are an important "change agent" in the family and continue to exert influence on their adolescent, despite parents' tendency to not believe they are influential. This parental attitude is understandable given the psychological forces of individuation and separation during adolescence (see Chapter 2). Parental awareness of their teenager's displays of autonomy may discourage their confidence in having influence in their son's or daughters' life and their willingness to try to exert influence (Steinberg & Morris, 2001). Yet parents can be a vehicle for change with respect to their teenager's drug use and other behaviors (Botzet et al., 2019; Jackson, 2002; Winters et al., 2015). Experts have identified four reasons for such optimism.

The Kosterman et al. study (2016) has an interesting contemporary angle: It examined parents' reactions to marijuana legalization and changes in attitudes and behaviors over time. Data were from about 400 parents in Washington State who were interviewed 15 times between 1985 and 2014. Adult nonmedical marijuana use was legalized in Washington in 2012 and retail outlets opened in 2014. Results showed the following: (a) one-third of parents incorrectly believed the legal age of nonmedical marijuana use to be 18 (it is 21); (b) over time there was a significant increase in approval of adult marijuana use and decrease in perceived harm of regular use; (c) there was wide opposition to adolescent use and use around one's children; and (d) substantial increases in frequency of use and marijuana use disorder occurred among parents who used. The authors concluded that, despite increased acceptance and frequency of adult use and some misperceptions about cannabis laws, parents remain opposed to adolescent cannabis use.

1. The great majority of parents overwhelmingly *disapprove* of drug use by their children (Jackson, 2002; Kosterman et al., 2016). Thus, motivating parents to help with addressing a drug problem in their teenager is often not a challenge for the therapist.

Protective *drug use* socialization is defined as specific activities by parents that instill and reinforce attitudinal and behavioral norms against any underage use of alcohol and other drugs (save for sipping alcohol at a religious service, which is excluded from the definition of drug use). Following is a list of some protective steps for parents.

1. Reduce parental complacency about any level of drug use during childhood.
2. Parents have defined and communicated family rules and expectations regarding substance use.
3. Parents monitor affiliation with peers who are known to be drug users.
4. The child has no access to alcohol of other drugs in the home.
5. Parents cease involving children in adult alcohol use (e.g., by asking them to fetch or pour drinks).

2. Parents have a *major role in providing protective socialization* during the childhood years, and this continues into adolescence (e.g., Barnes et al., 2006). Parents have ongoing access to the teenager, which promotes continuous influences, multiple teachable moments in various real-world situations, and numerous opportunities to enforce family norms and expectations. Studies have shown that strong parent–adolescent bonds reduce the likelihood of adolescent drug use (Burdzovic

Andreas et al., 2016). Also, most adolescents continue to be receptive to parental influences pertaining to value-type issues, such as attitudes and expectations about personal drug use (Jackson, 2002).

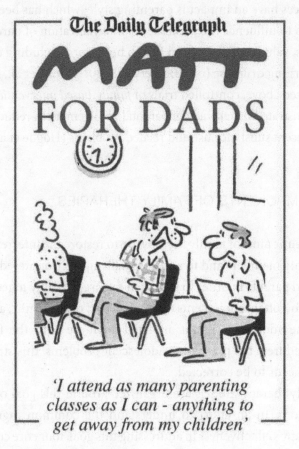

'I attend as many parenting classes as I can - anything to get away from my children'

© Matt/Telegraph Media Group Limited

3. *Parenting practices* also have an impact. Such practices that promote desired behaviors by the adolescent include setting clear expectations, implementing high-level monitoring, reinforcing appropriate behavior, communicating to the child the risks of drug use, supporting drug use resistance behaviors by the child, and communicating a no-tolerance attitude toward drug

use (Clark & Winters, 2002). And parents can use multiple approaches and strategies to influence their child, including experiences, communication, rule setting, norm setting, discipline, monitoring, and role modeling (Dishion et al., 2003). An important mechanism by which effective parenting practices have an impact is parenting style, which has been shown to influence the adolescent's internalization of parents' beliefs, values, attitudes, and health behaviors, including those concerning drug use (e.g., Botzet et al., 2019; Stone et al., 2012).

4. As noted above, controlled trials of *family-based interventions* have demonstrated the efficacy of parental involvement in reducing adolescent substance use and related problems (Hogue et al., 2018).

CORE COMPONENTS OF FAMILY THERAPIES

The therapeutic aims of family therapy are to restore the interrelationships among family members and to address challenges encountered by the adolescent and parents in order to maintain a sense of family togetherness or cohesion. Too often, adolescents do not feel part of the family, and parents feel that the adolescent is not affiliated anymore with the family. For therapy to address the presenting adolescent problems, this strain within the family needs to be corrected.

All family therapy models are organized around this goal of repairing family discord. In an effort to understand the common ingredients of family therapy's effectiveness in addressing this goal, four core components have been identified (Bobek et al., 2019). We summarize these four components below.

Family Engagement

Family engagement begins with attendance but must go deeper by virtue of both the connectedness that is developed between the therapist and all family members and supporting a climate in therapy where all participants are invested in the treatment goals. Some family therapy models contend that family engagement is the most important component to treatment success, thus family therapists should receive intensive training in skills in building alliances among the adolescent and parents and strategies to establish therapist credibility (Santisteban et al., 1996). Skills in motivational interviewing are now viewed as essential (see Chapter 11). Barriers to engagement are viewed as normative and not to be considered as "resistance." To optimize family engagement when treating an adolescent with a substance use disorder (SUD), the therapist seeks to convince family members that therapy is a benefit to not only the adolescent but also to family relationships.

Relational Reframing

The main point of this feature is to steer the view by the adolescent and parents that the nature of the problem and the solutions to them are based on the interrelationships among family members. Such reframing of the situation is intended to move attention and blame away from the adolescent and instead move the focus onto the family system. It is important, however, not to merely shift blame to parents but to emphasize how they are a source of positive change. Counseling techniques that support relational reframing techniques include keeping a focus on how family members relate to each other, educating them on behaviors that are developmentally normative during adolescence (e.g., taking risks), and encouraging family members to focus on the positives of family life and each member's strengths and assets. Consistent with motivational enhancement techniques, negative behaviors by a family member are not to be viewed as pathological but rather are reframed by the counselor as a reaction to a situation that has a functional value for the person. Also, relational reframing interventions are not a one-way focus on the adolescent; the counselor also attends to the behaviors and cognitions of the parents. This therapy technique, which can lead to parental resistance given the mindset that it is the adolescent with the main problem, requires the counselor to convince the family that a family-wide response is needed. An underlying premise of family therapy is that, as one member of a family makes positive changes, others will make similar changes. Common discussions and exercises to promote reframing are to target underlying expectations about family roles and behaviors and family rules.

Family Behavior Change

This component consists of the specific therapeutic strategies to promote learning or reinforcing skills that will move the family toward improved relationships. As noted above, skills are taught from the framework that all family members, not just the adolescent, are the target for behavior change. Skills and topics focus on communication (e.g., setting behavior expectations, limit setting, and collaborative conflict resolution), family activities, and family rules (e.g., rules about substance use). The counselor can work with the whole family at once, meet with individuals, or combine these approaches. Homework assignments are used to encourage family members to practice the skills in the family and at home.

Experts are beginning to appreciate the value of teaching parents motivational interviewing (MI) skills. Consider the parallels between a client who is not very motivated to make behavior changes and an adolescent who is showing defiance against and resistance to parental influence. One of the book's authors (Winters) introduced MI skills in a recent parenting class he taught. They were introduced to a parent version of OARS; see below.

Open questions = Stay away from questions that are closed-ended. Begin open-ended question with "Why" or "What" or "Tell me more."

Affirmations = Be as positive as you can. Discuss your teenager's successes as much a possible; instill positivity and hope.

Reflective listening = Place a high priority on being a good listener, even when the conversation is tense. Allow the teenager to talk.

Summary reflections = Often provide brief summaries of what your teenager has said. Doing so instills confidence in your teenager that you are listening and understanding their point of view (even if you disagree).

Family Restructuring

This component addresses the nature of family interrelationships. The task of the therapist is to motivate family members to see the importance of changing underlying assumptions and behaviors about family life. This can include changes in attachment among family members. An example is a parent and adolescent who have developed a habit of interacting only when there is a conflict about the adolescent's behavior. Moving this interpersonal dynamic from a negative path to a more positive one involves educating the family members of this unhealthy cycle, highlighting existing strengths in the family that need greater focus, and working with them about new interaction practices.

MAJOR TYPES OF FAMILY-BASED APPROACHES

Family-based treatments for adolescent substance abuse have been studied for decades. The first rigorous research published in a peer-reviewed journal was the work by James Alexander and colleagues (Klein et al., 1977). Adolescents in the juvenile justice system ($N = 86$) were randomly assigned to one of four treatment conditions: no treatment controls, a client-centered family approach, an eclectic-dynamic approach, and a behaviorally oriented short-term family systems approach. The family systems approach, when compared to the other conditions, produced a significantly better reduction in subsequent court contacts over a 3 year-follow-up period.

Family-based treatments vary in the extent to which their focus is within the family system or outside of it (Becker & Curry, 2008). Behavioral and educational types focus more on outside the family (e.g., family rules and expectations; how the family spends time together) using behavioral therapy principles (see Chapter 10), whereas system, functional, and ecological types focus more on the inside of the family (e.g., interrelationships among family members; family member roles). There are a handful of "brand name" family therapies specifically designed to treat adolescent substance abuse. The four prominent ones are reviewed below (listed alphabetically).

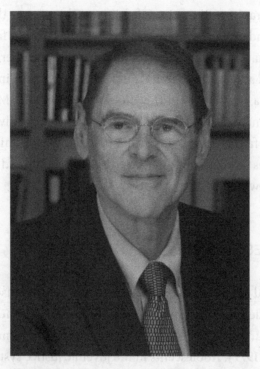

José Szapocznik, Ph.D., the developer of brief strategic family therapy (BSFT). Photo courtesy of José Szapocznik.

Brief Strategic Family Therapy (BSFT)

BSFT, designed to address drug abuse as well as delinquency, includes traditional models of structural family therapy and strategic family therapy (Szapocznik et al., 2103). As a system-focused program, BSFT views the adolescent's problem behaviors as originating from unhealthy family alliances, maladaptive family interactions, and poor parenting practices. Sessions are conducted at locations that are convenient to the family, including the family's home. The counselor's main task is to identify the nature of the maladaptive interactions in the family and assist in changing them in order to support a healthy family climate. BSFT has been tested with one efficacy study and one effectiveness study; both provided support that BSFT is an effective program with adolescents (Szapocznik et al., 2013).

Treatment outcome studies can be distinguished on the basis of either an efficacy or effectiveness study. An *efficacy study* occurs under ideal and controlled circumstances that are designed and controlled by the researcher. An *effectiveness study* refers to researching how a treatment performs under "real-world" conditions. Most outcome studies in the research literature are efficacy studies.

Functional Family Therapy (FFT)

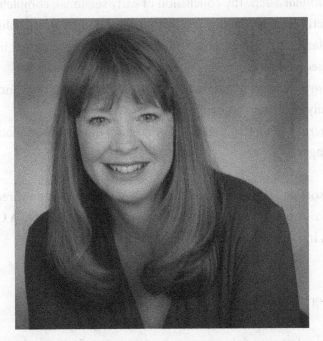

Holly Waldron, Ph.D., and colleagues developed functional family therapy (FFT). Photo courtesy of Holly Waldron.

FFT was originally designed to treat adolescents with oppositional defiant and conduct disorders (see Chapter 7) and related disruptive behaviors. Later it was revised to be applied for youth with an SUD (Waldron et al., 2013). Consistent with a functional family approach, FFT views adolescent substance abuse as developing in the context of maladaptive family relationships. Thus, FFT targets the entire family and requires participation by all family members in the home. The goal of therapy is to improve family communication and interactions (Waldron et al., 2013). Intensity varies according to the severity of the case; as few as eight sessions can be sufficient for mild cases and up to 30 sessions over several months may be needed for more difficult and complex family situations. The five distinct phases of FFT and their respective goal are indicated below:

1. *Engagement:* (pre-intervention); maximize family initial expectation of positive change
2. *Motivation:* (early sessions); create a motivational context for long-term change
3. *Relational assets:* (by conclusion of early sessions); complete a functional assessment (see Chapter 10) of family relationships to clarify therapeutic entry points for changing behaviors in subsequent phases
4. *Behavior change:* (middle sessions); facilitate individual and family relationship changes
5. *Generalization:* (later sessions); maintain individual and family changes

FFT is associated with very high engagement rates. Based on three efficacy studies, for the most part, FFT was equivalent or superior to a CBT-only approach in reducing substance use (Waldron et al., 2013).

Multidimensional Family Therapy (MDFT)

MDFT, as a hybrid of the systems and functional approaches, employs a developmental model which assumes that individual, family, and community risk and resiliency factors determine the adolescent's developmental trajectory, including substance abuse (Liddle, 2013). Treatment focuses on the adolescent and the adolescent–parent relationship, with a consideration of social and contextual factors. Because substance abuse coexists with other behavior disorders, MDFT also addresses delinquency, aggressive behaviors, and emotional distress.

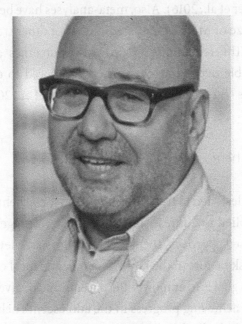

The primary developer of multidimensional family therapy (MDFT) is Howard Liddle, Ph.D.
Photo courtesy of Howard Liddle.

The therapist's responsibilities include creating the conditions that motivate youth and parents for behavior change, promoting a working relationship among family members, and individualizing treatment goals based on the strengths of family members.

A reminder: A *meta-analysis* is a statistical analysis that combines the results of multiple scientific studies that address the same research question. By combining the results of multiple individual studies, a meta-analysis integrates the results to find general trends across the studies.

MDFT has been tested in several randomized control trials (RCTs). In a review by Walther and colleagues (2016), RCTs were described that compared MDFT to cognitive behavioral therapy (CBT) and motivational enhancement therapy (MET). A consistent trend in the results was that MDFT showed comparatively superior outcomes on cannabis use for younger adolescents and those with a more serious substance abuse problem (Walther et al., 2016). Also, meta-analyses have been used to evaluate the effect size of MDFT compared to that of other treatment models (Liddle, 2016). The reductions in drug use outcomes associated with MDFT are durable over time, even when compared to other evidence-based treatments (e.g., CBT) (Liddle, 2013; Liddle et al., 2018).

Multisystemic Therapy (MST)

MST, originally designed to treat adolescent antisocial behaviors, has been adapted and applied to address substance abuse (Henggeler et al., 1992). As a systems-based approach, the target behaviors are viewed as resulting from multiple risk factors in the family, school, and local community. The counselor's main goal is to empower the parents or caregivers to be a major change agent for achieving progress in the adolescent's behaviors. Specific MST features include the following: services are typically delivered in the family's home; sessions can extend over the course of several months and total approximately 60 hours of counseling; and clinical services are provided on a 24-hour/7-day/week on-call schedule.

A unique benefit of family-based treatment is the possibility that the *siblings* of the target adolescent may be positively affected. In trials of both MST and FFT, the research teams found decreases in drug use among both the target youth and the siblings in the family (Henggeler & Schaeffer, 2016; Waldron et al., 2013). This finding supports the cost-effectiveness of family approaches, given that siblings may also reap benefits.

MST has been tested with RCTs. Findings support the view that MST has a favorable impact on delinquency behaviors and drug use (van der Stouwe et al., 2014). An adaptation of MST, coined multisystemic therapy–substance abuse (MST-SA), was tested in a juvenile drug court and found to be effective (Henggeler et al., 2006; Letourneau et al., 2013).

Of note is a unique comparison of family therapy with another approach. Azrin and colleagues (Azrin et al., 2001) randomly assigned youth with an SUD and comorbid conduct disorder to either individual cognitive therapy or family behavioral therapy. At post-treatment and at 6-month follow-up, both groups showed equal improvement in terms of drugs use and conduct problems.

MINI-REVIEW

- Family therapies for adolescents with a substance abuse problem presume that family risk factors are the main contributor to the adolescent's problem. In that light, the teen's substance abuse problem is a consequence of a larger problem. Family risk factors that are attended to in treatment typically center on poor family communication, lack of or weak effective parenting practices, and poor family connectedness.
- Currently there is no standard family structure in the United States, given changes with respect to parenthood, the relative frequency of divorce, remarriage, and cohabitation, and the greater role of women in the workforce. Historically, the size of families is smaller than in previous decades, and there is a rise in single-parent households. This changing landscape of the family unit can pose unique challenges when conducting family therapy.
- Parents continue to exert an influence on a teenager's values and behaviors and thus are vital change agents within the family therapy model.

- Core components of family therapy are the following: family engagement (the connectedness between the therapist and all family members); relational reframing (educating family members that the interrelationships among them are the source of and solutions to the adolescent's SUD); family behavior change (specific therapeutic tools that promote improved relationships among family members); and family restructuring (motivating family members to see the importance of changing underlying assumptions and behaviors about family life).
- Brief strategic family therapy, functional family therapy, multidimensional family therapy, and multisystemic therapy are four prominent and well-researched family therapy approaches used to address adolescent drug abuse.
- Whereas no formal comparison between the four approaches has been conducted, literature reviews and meta-analyses, for the most part, point to family therapy as comparatively superior to non-family therapy strategies to address adolescents with an SUD.

DISCUSSION POINTS

1. A consideration when treating an adolescent is if they have siblings. It can be expected that an older sibling will have more influence than a younger sibling on the target adolescent. What do you think are the reasons for this?

2. As noted in the chapter, there are protective steps that parents can take in an effort to prevent adolescent substance use (the list is repeated below). Name and discuss *additional* parenting protective steps.
   a. Reduce parental complacency about any level of drug use during childhood.
   b. Parents have defined and communicated family rules and expectations regarding substance use.

    c. Parents monitor affiliation with peers who are known to be drug users.

    d. The child has no access to alcohol of other drugs in the home.

    e. Parents cease involving children in adult alcohol use (e.g., by asking them to fetch or pour drinks).

3. Discuss how motivational interviewing strategies can be used by a counselor to work with family resistance.

4. One theme in family therapy is to discuss if the family has regular family meetings and, if so, whether family rules about substance use have been discussed. Imagine you are working with a family that does not have regular family meetings. What specific tips would you offer to help a family plan for and conduct such meetings?

5. Evidenced-based treatments are first studied in a very controlled research context (efficacy studies). But the use of treatments in a naturalistic, non-research setting is not the same as its use in an efficacy trial. Discuss how implementing a family treatment in a naturalistic setting can be different from its use in a research study.

FURTHER CURIOSITY AND DIGGING

More about Family Therapy

Robinson, E., Power, L., & Allan, D. (2010). What works with adolescents? Family connections and involvement in interventions for adolescent problem behaviours. https://aifs.gov.au/cfca/publications/what-works-adolescents-family-connections-and-involvem

More about Multisystemic Therapy

Multisystemic therapy. [Video]. YouTube. https://www.youtube.com/watch?v=Hqqv DPQqxK0

More about Multidimensional Family Therapy Case Presentation (2 parts)

Multidimensional family therapy (2 of 2). [Video]. YouTube. https://www.youtube.com/ watch?v=YzjGqlPlU-g

REFERENCES

Azrin, N. H., Donohue, B., Teichner, G. A., Crum, T., Howell, J., & DeCato, L. A. (2001). A controlled evaluation and description of individual-cognitive problem solving and family-behavior therapies in dually-diagnosed conduct-disordered and substance-dependent youth. *Journal of Child & Adolescent Substance Abuse*, *11*(1), 1–43.

Barnes, G. M., Hoffman, J. H., Welte, J. W., Farrell, M. P., & Dintcheff, B. A. (2006). Effects of parental monitoring and peer deviance on substance use and delinquency. *Journal of Marriage and Family*, *68*, 1084–1104.

Becker, S. J., & Curry, J. F. (2008). Outpatient interventions for adolescent substance abuse: A quality of evidence review. *Journal of Consulting and Clinical Psychology*, *76*, 531–534.

Bobek, M., Godly, S. H., & Hogue, A. (2019). Family and community-based therapies. In Y. Kaminer & K. C. Winters (Eds.), *Clinical manual of adolescent addictive disorders* (2nd ed., pp. 301–318). American Psychiatric Association.

Botzet, A. M., Dittel, C., Birkeland, R., Lee, S., Grabowski, J., & Winters, K. C. (2019). Parents as interventionists: Addressing adolescent substance use. *Journal of Substance Abuse Treatment*, *99*, 124–133.

Burdzovic Andreas, J. B., Pape, H., & Bretteville-Jensen, A. L. (2016). Who are the adolescents saying "No" to cannabis offers. *Drug and Alcohol Dependence*, *163*, 64–70.

Clark, D. B., & Winters, K. C. (2002). Measuring risks and outcomes in substance use disorders prevention research. *Journal of Consulting and Clinical Psychology*, *70*, 1207–1223.

Dishion, T. J., Nelson, S. E., & Kavanagh, K. (2003). The family check-up with high-risk young adolescents: Preventing early-onset substance use by parent monitoring. *Behavior Therapy*, *34*, 553–571.

Henggeler, S. W., Halliday-Boykins, C. A., Cunningham, P. B., Randall, J., Shapiro, S. B., & Chapman, J. E. (2006). Juvenile drug court: Enhancing outcomes by integrating evidence-based treatments. *Journal of Consulting and Clinical Psychology*, *74*, 42–54.

Henggeler, S. W., Melton, G. B., & Smith, L. A. (1992). Family preservation using multisystemic therapy: An effective alternative to incarcerating serious juvenile offenders. *Journal of Consulting and Clinical Psychology*, *60*, 953–961.

Henggeler, S. W., & Schaeffer, C. M. (2016). Multisystemic therapy: Clinical overview, outcomes, and implementation research. *Family Process*, *55*(3), 514–528.

Hogue, A., Henderson, C. E., Becker, S. J., & Knight, D. K. (2018). Evidence base on outpatient behavioral treatments for adolescent substance use, 2014–2017: Outcomes, treatment delivery, and promising horizons. *Journal of Clinical Child & Adolescent Psychology*, *47*, 499–526.

Hogue, A., & Liddle, H. A. (2009). Family-based treatment for adolescent substance abuse: Controlled trials and new horizons in services research. *Journal of Family Therapy*, *31*, 126–154.

Jackson, C. (2002). Perceived legitimacy of parental authority and tobacco and alcohol use during early adolescence. *Journal of Adolescent Health*, *31*, 425–432.

Klein, N. C., Alexander, J. F., & Parsons, B. V. (1977). Impact of family systems intervention on recidivism and sibling delinquency: A model of primary prevention and program evaluation. *Journal of Consulting and Clinical Psychology, 45*, 469–474.

Kosterman, R., Bailey, J. A., Guttmannova, K., Jones, T. M., Eisenberg, N., Hill, K. G., & Hawkins, J. D. (2016). Marijuana legalization and parents' attitudes, use, and parenting in Washington State. *Journal of Adolescent Health, 59*, 450–456.

Letourneau, E. J., Henggeler, S. W., McCart, M. R., Borduin, C. M., Schewe, P. A., & Armstrong, K. S. (2013). Two-year follow-up of a randomized effectiveness trial evaluating MST for juveniles who sexually offend. *Journal of Family Psychology, 27*, 978–985.

Liddle, H. A. (2013). Multidimensional family therapy for adolescent substance abuse: A developmental approach. In P. Miller (Ed.), *Interventions for addiction: Comprehensive addictive behaviors and disorders* (pp. 87–96). Academic Press.

Liddle, H. A., Dakof, G. A., Rowe, C. L., Henderson, C., Greenbaum, P., Wang, W., & Alberga, L. (2018). Multidimensional family therapy as a community-based alternative to residential treatment for adolescents with substance use and co-occurring mental health disorders. *Journal of Substance Abuse Treatment, 90*, 47–56.

McCart, M. R., & Sheidow, A. J. (2016). Evidence-based psychosocial treatments for adolescents with disruptive behavior. *Journal of Clinical Child & Adolescent Psychology, 45*, 529–563.

Minuchin, S. (1974). *Families and family therapy.* Harvard University Press.

Pew Research Center. (2015, December 17). *1. The American family today.* https://www.pewsocialtrends.org/2015/12/17/1-the-american-family-today/

Pew Research Center. (2022, March 22). *Household structure and family roles.* https://www.pewresearch.org/topics/household-and-family-structure/

Santisteban, D. A., Szapocznik, J., Perez-Vidal, A., Kurtines, W. M., Murray, E. J., & LaPerriere, A. (1996). Efficacy of intervention for engaging youth and families into treatment and some variables that may contribute to differential effectiveness. *Journal of Family Psychology, 10*, 35–44.

Steinberg, L., & Morris, A. S. (2001). Adolescent development. *Annual Review of Psychology, 52*, 83–110.

Stone, A. L., Becker, L. G., Huber, A. M., & Catalano, R. F. (2012). Review of risk and protective factors of substance use and problem use in emerging adulthood. *Addictive Behaviors, 37*, 747–775.

Szapocznik, J., Muir, J. A., & Schwartz, S. J. (2013). Brief strategic family therapy for adolescent drug abuse: Treatment and implementation. In P. Miller (Ed.), *Interventions for addiction: Comprehensive addictive behaviors and disorders* (pp. 97–108). Academic Press.

Thomas, D. (2020, April 10). As family structures change in U.S., a growing share of Americans say it makes no difference. Pew Research Center. https://www.pewresearch.org/fact-tank/2020/04/10/as-family-structures-change-in-u-s-a-growing-share-of-americans-say-it-makes-no-difference/

U.S. Census. (2021). *Historical living arrangements of children.* https://www.census.gov/data/tables/time-series/demo/families/children.html

van der Stouwe, T., Asscher, J. J., Stams, G. J. J., Deković, M., & van der Laan, P. H. (2014). The effectiveness of multisystemic therapy (MST): A meta-analysis. *Clinical Psychology Review, 34*, 468–481.

Waldron, H. B., Brody, J. L., Robbins, M. S., & Alexander, J. F. (2013). Functional family therapy for adolescent substance use disorders. In P. Miller (Ed.), *Interventions for addiction: Comprehensive addictive behaviors and disorders* (pp. 109–116). Academic Press.

Walther, L., Gantner, A., Heinz, A., & Majic, T. (2016). Evidence-based treatment options in cannabis dependency. *Deutsches Ärzteblatt International, 113*, 653–659. doi:10.3238/arztebl.2016.0653

Winters, K. C., Botzet, A., Dittel, C., Fahnhorst, T., & Nicholson, A. (2015). Can parents provide brief intervention services to their drug-abusing teenager? *Journal of Child & Adolescent Substance Abuse, 24*, 134–141.

12-Step-Based Treatment

INTRODUCTION

Twelve-step programs for adolescents involve having adolescents work on specific steps toward recovery, attendance at self-support groups (Alcoholic Anonymous [AA] and Narcotics Anonymous [NA]), and obtaining the assistance of a sponsor, who is another person in recovery from substance use problems. Each of the 12 steps (detailed below), which are geared toward living day-to-day without the need for drugs, has a spiritual principle behind it. Whereas it is generally accepted that the 12-step philosophy is the most commonly applied treatment strategy in the United States for *adults* with a substance use disorder (SUD), its application in adolescent treatment programs is more complicated. A national study of *adolescent-specific* treatment facilities conducted by Knudsen et al. (2008) found only 7% of programs based their treatment *solely on* a 12-step model.

The Minnesota Model, also known as the *abstinence model*, of addiction treatment was created in a Minnesota-based state mental hospital in the 1950s by two individuals, one of whom was to become a psychologist and the other a psychiatrist. Neither of these young men had prior experience treating persons with a substance use disorder.

There were two key elements of this novel approach at the time to treating addiction. One was to blend professional and trained non-professional (recovering) staff around the principles of Alcoholics Anonymous. There was an individualized treatment plan with active family involvement in a 28-day inpatient setting and participation in Alcoholics Anonymous both during and after treatment. The second major element was educating patients and family members that addiction is a chronic disorder.

The model spread from its early days to a small not-for-profit organization called the Hazelden Foundation and then throughout the country.

SOURCE: Anderson et al. (1999).

Formal treatment programs organized around the 12 steps, often referred to as the "Minnesota Model," consist of lectures, assignments including 12-step work (e.g., reading assignments from the *Big Books* of AA/NA), a therapeutic milieu, attendance at AA/NA meetings, family therapy, counseling and recreational activities, and, perhaps most important, group work. The focus of groups is psychoeducational in nature, providing information on the 12-step principles and personal testimonies about the negative effects of substance use, expressing and clarifying feelings, and sharing strategies of dealing with common problems of adolescence. In years past, quasi-professional staff conducted the counseling. Such traditions have been replaced; staff now consist of certified clinicians and other licensed, trained service providers. Also a thing of the past is the traditional residential-based program of 28 days. The more common settings are day programs or outpatient programs.

But the overwhelming majority of treatment programs utilize the basic principles of AA as a *component* of their treatment approach, and most programs refer their adolescent clients to a drug-free, community mutual-help organization, such as AA, NA, or Marijuana Anonymous (MA). One study found that 84% of programs reported linking youth to community AA/NA groups at discharge (Sussman, 2010).

RELEVANCE TO ADOLESCENTS

Developmentally adjusted 12-step programs and self-help support groups can support an adolescent's recovery. But the applicability of the 12-step method for youth has been questioned because of limitations in developmentally appropriate content. Adolescence is a time of establishing a personal identity and independence from authority figures, developmental milestones that can be inconsistent with the main tenants of AA of acceptance and surrender. Youth are less likely to be as interested in spiritual ideas and less inclined to connect to the overt religious language in the 12 steps than are adults. As we discuss in more detail below, most mutual self-help programs in the community are mainly composed of adults. It is estimated that only 2% of participants in self-help groups are under the age of 21 (Young, 2012), which creates barriers for adolescents, as they may struggle to relate to older group members (Kelly & Urbanoski, 2012). It comes as no surprise, then, that efforts to adapt 12-step treatment for adolescents are important. Current adaptations of this approach include the Minnesota Model treatment approach for adolescents (Anderson et al., 1999) and Jaffe's (1990) developmentally appropriate modifications of the first five steps of a 12-step program (described below).

Admittedly, the language and terminology of this treatment approach may not be particularly youth-friendly. Also, the coercive approaches of the 1990s, including programs like Scared Straight, were often falsely aligned with 12-step recovery. Yet many of the strategies of our present-day evidence-based treatments are reflected in the 12-step treatment modality. An empathetic nonconfrontational approach using feedback and an emphasis on individual responsibility are fundamental strategies of motivational interviewing, and these themes are inherent to 12-step treatment as well. Cognitive behavioral therapy (CBT) strategies, such as the use of distraction and calling one's sponsor to deal with thoughts and urges of using, are integral parts of a 12-step program.

Do you have to be religious in order to benefit from the 12-step approach? Experts say no.

It is true that the 12 steps were originally based on the principles of a spiritual organization, values, and the role of religion decades ago.

Today, the term "Higher Power" is used rather than "God" in order to be more relevant to a wide group of people. A Higher Power can be nature, the universe, fate, karma, your support system, the recovery group itself, or anything of a personal nature.

A recent systematic review of the mechanisms of behavior change through which AA has been shown to work revealed that AA enhances abstinence self-efficacy and active coping efforts. AA also works through maintaining and enhancing motivation for abstinence within a supportive peer recovery context (Kelly et al., 2009)—all purported mechanisms of commonly used CBT. There are parallels to contingency management (CM) as well: A common feature of a 12-step approach is to award reinforcers in the form of chips for periods of sober time, and AA meetings and sponsor relationships contain large amounts of positive reinforcement. Parenting management techniques and family issues are part of Alanon and Alateen. Finally, the Higher Power concepts of 12-step recovery are contained in mindfulness-based treatment for chronic disorders—dialectical behavior therapy. Thus, although the language may differ, underneath 12-step methods there are elements of many commonly used contemporary treatments (McCrady, 1994).

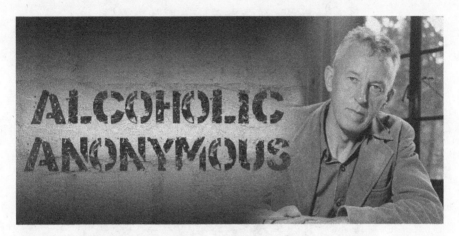

Bill Wilson, one of the co-founders of Alcoholics Anonymous.
Image design courtesy of True Behavioral Health, Newport Beach, CA, USA.

HISTORICAL CONTEXT

The history of the 12-step recovery approach can be traced to the development of Alcoholics Anonymous in 1935, and by a New York stockbroker, Bill Wilson ("Bill W"). Bill was attending meetings of the Oxford Group in an attempt to stop drinking and live a better life. The Oxford Group attempted to practice a simple Christianity without a denomination (Anderson et al., 1999). The group's philosophy was centered around these themes: surrendering one's will to God; taking a personal inventory of one's moral thinking and behavior; confessing past crimes; making amends; and helping others. During Bill W.'s fourth hospitalization for alcoholism treatment, while experiencing distressing alcohol withdrawal, he continued to attend the Oxford Group meetings. He soon realized that his contributions in the group meetings and trying to help other alcoholics was uplifting and helped him to not drink.

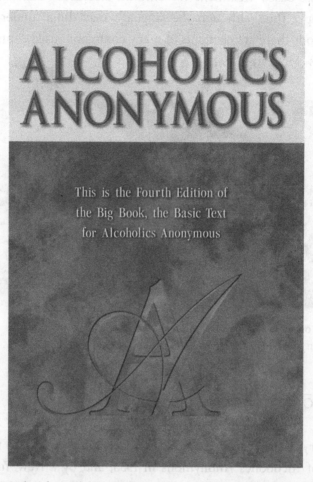

ALCOHOLICS
ANONYMOUS

This is the Fourth Edition of
the Big Book, the Basic Text
for Alcoholics Anonymous

The publication that changed the conversation about alcoholism and popularized the 12-step model of recovery is known as the *Big Book of Alcoholics Anonymous*. Bill W., the core founder of Alcoholics Anonymous, and many other individuals as part of the AA movement, authored the book. It is considered the seminal textbook on the 12-step recovery program.

In 1935, while still struggling with alcoholism and on a business trip in Akron, Ohio, Bill W. met Dr. Robert Smith ("Dr. Bob"), an alcoholic physician, who was also dealing with his drinking problem. Both agreed the Oxford Group methods had many strengths, but they felt something was missing. They spent several hours discussing their plight. This unique evening of "sharing" between two struggling alcoholics seeking a better path toward health led to a shift from the Oxford Group to a new organization, devoted solely to the recovery from alcoholism. The basic themes from that evening became the basic tenets of AA. This grass roots, community-based, peer-run recovery strategy has been extended to other drug addictions (e.g., NA, MA), other behavioral addictions (e.g., Overeaters Anonymous; Sex and Love Addicts Anonymous; Gamblers Anonymous) and to support the significant others of an addicted person (e.g., Alanon; Alateen) (Kelly & Yeterian, 2011).

ELEMENTS OF 12-STEP TREATMENT AND ADJUSTMENTS FOR ADOLESCENTS

12 Steps

The 12 steps (Alcoholics Anonymous, 1976) are a set of guiding principles that provide a framework of behavior change in order for the person to reach sobriety. The original 12 steps are indicated below.

Step 1: We admitted we were powerless over alcohol—that our lives had become unmanageable.

Step 2: Came to believe that a Power greater than ourselves could restore us to sanity.

Step 3: Made a decision to turn our will and our lives over to the care of God *as we understood Him*.

Step 4: Made a searching and fearless moral inventory of ourselves.

Step 5: Admitted to God, to ourselves, and to another human being the exact nature of our wrongs.

Step 6: Were entirely ready to have God remove all these defects of character.

Step 7: Humbly asked Him to remove our shortcomings.

Step 8: Made a list of all persons we had harmed, and became willing to make amends to them all.

Step 9: Made direct amends to such people wherever possible, except when to do so would injure them or others.

Step 10: Continued to take personal inventory and when we were wrong promptly admitted it.

Step 11: Sought through prayer and meditation to improve our conscious contact with God, *as we understood Him*, praying only for knowledge of His will for us and the power to carry that out.

Step 12: Having had a spiritual awakening as the result of these Steps, we tried to carry this message to alcoholics, and to practice these principles in all our affairs.

Adjustments for Adolescents

The principles of each of the 12 steps can be further adjusted to be more meaningful for an adolescent (see Table 13.1). The steps vary as to their respective therapeutic goal (Kelly & Yeterian, 2011). For example, one set of steps is aimed at supporting the adolescent's self-esteem and self-efficacy (or self-accomplishment) (Steps 1, 2, 3, 9 and 12); another set pertains to the therapy goal of increasing the adolescent's insight that a substance use problem exists and that there are factors contributing to it (Steps 4 and 5).

The Importance of Steps 1–5

The first five steps are typically addressed with adolescents during the primary treatment experience. These five steps are the following: (1) admitting that you are powerless over the addictive substance and that it has made life unmanageable, (2) believing that a power greater than yourself could restore you to health, (3) making a decision to turn your will over to a higher power as you interpret it to be, (4) taking a moral inventory of

Table 13.1 THEMES AND INTERPRETATIONS OF THE 12 STEPS FOR ADOLESCENTS
(ADAPTED FROM KELLY & YETERIAN, 2011)

12 Steps	Theme	Interpretation for Adolescents
1. We admitted we were powerless over our addiction—that our lives had become unmanageable.	Honesty	Substance use is causing me problems.
2. Came to believe that a Power greater than ourselves could restore us to sanity.	Open-mindedness	Change can be made, and help and support are available.
3. Made a decision to turn our will and our lives over to the care of God as we understood Him.	Willingness	I commit to get help and accept support.
4. Made a searching and fearless moral inventory of ourselves.	Self-assessment and appraisal	Insight will be sought about what troubles me and why.
5. Admitted to God, to ourselves, and to another human being the exact nature of our wrongs.	Self-forgiveness; accurate self-appraisal	I openly and honestly discuss issues that are bothering me with trusted people.
6. Were entirely ready to have God remove all these defects of character.	Readiness to change	Necessary changes will be made.
7. Humbly asked Him to remove our shortcomings.	Humility/accurate appraisal	Necessary changes will continue to be made and refined.
8. Made a list of all persons we had harmed and became willing to make amends to them all.	Taking responsibility and forgiveness of self/others	Sources of guilt and shame are mended, including relationships.

(continued)

Table 13.1 CONTINUED

12 Steps	Theme	Interpretation for Adolescents
9. Made direct amends to such people wherever possible, except when to do so would injure them or others.	Restitution to others	Making ammends includes talking with key people.
10. Continued to take personal inventory and when we were wrong, promptly admitted it.	Emotional balance	Maintain a path of self-examination and correcting mistakes.
11. Sought through prayer and meditation to improve our conscious contact with God, as we understood Him, praying only for knowledge of His will for us and the power to carry that out.	Connectedness and emotional balance	Maintain healthy relationships.
12. Have had a spiritual awakening as the result of these steps, we tried to carry this message to addicts and to practice these principles in all our affairs.	Helping others achieve recovery	Stay on course with recovery goals; continue to seek help from your support network; provide support for others.

yourself, and (5) admitting to yourself and to others the nature of your wrongs. It is expected that the teenager will address the remaining seven steps during aftercare.

Jaffe (1990) developed a workbook format in which the descriptions of the first five steps are modified in order to make them easier to understand for the adolescent. In this format, the adolescent writes answers to specific questions for each step, which are then reviewed by the counselor and can be presented as part of group therapy. Provided below is a brief overview of the workbook's instructions for each step (Jaffe, 1990).

Jaffe notes that admitting powerlessness is not to be construed as meaning weakness. It means asking for help. This may seem a contrarian notion, but the idea is that when you can admit that you don't have power (or full power), it can be easier to ask for help (power) from others.

1. *We admitted we were powerless over alcohol—that our lives had become unmanageable.* The workbook instructs the adolescents to examine in detail the negative consequences of their alcohol and drug use. Various issues are explored, such as the ways that drug and alcohol use puts their own and others' lives in danger and the effects it has on family, school, work, mood, and self-esteem. The major goal is to accurately appraise whether drugs and alcohol are destroying their lives such that they need to stop use in order to make their lives better. Because adolescents often desire to feel powerful, the workbook emphasizes that by abstaining from alcohol and drugs the individual becomes more empowered to have greater confidence and control in their life. Although many adult programs emphasize the concept of surrendering and admitting one is an addict, these tend to be not as useful for adolescents. Rather, enhancing power by doing what one needs to do (i.e., stop using alcohol and drugs) is emphasized.

In addition to Jaffe's 1990 workbook, he developed another workbook in 2001, the *Adolescent Substance Abuse Intervention Workbook* (Jaffe, 2001; Jaffe et al., 2008). This workbook modified the first step to concretely guide the adolescent to explore how 12 areas of the adolescent's life may have been negatively affected by alcohol or drugs. This helps the adolescent move from pre-contemplation to contemplation according to the stages of change (Prochaska et al., 1992). This workbook becomes the basis for a 2-hour intervention: one hour to complete the questions and checklists, and another hour to present this to a group or counselor.

In addition to using the strategies of motivational enhancement therapy, completing this intervention also corresponds to working the first step of AA/NA.

2. *We came to believe that a power greater than ourselves could restore us to sanity.* This step is approached in the adolescent workbook by recognizing that the first higher power in a child's life is the person who raised them. For many drug-abusing or drug-addicted adolescents, their parental figures were neglectful or abusive. Mourning—eliciting the pain and sadness caused by the disappointments of their childhood higher powers—enables them to begin to develop a sense of something positive in the universe that they can turn to for help. The concept of a higher power is not a religious belief but a spiritual feeling that one can trust something positive (i.e., the group, another person, nature, etc.) to take care of those aspects of one's life that one cannot control: One needs to have trust in the stability of the world and realize that one controls one's own behavior but not what others say or do. For many adolescents, the concrete positive feeling of their relationships with other members becomes their 12-step higher power.

3. *We made a decision to turn our will and our lives over to the care of God as we understood Him.* The adolescent workbook presents an interpretation of this step that involves having the adolescents make a decision to commit themselves to working the steps and having a positive spiritual power. The teenagers are helped to recognize that they had turned over their lives to alcohol and drugs. Now they are being asked to turn their lives over to a positive program.

4. *We made a searching and fearless moral inventory of ourselves.* The workbook instructs the adolescents to answer numerous detailed questions covering all aspects of their childhood and present life.

5. *We admitted to God, to ourselves, and to another human being the exact nature of our wrongs.* At this point the adolescents discuss their inventories with a counselor or their sponsor.

The extent and nature of the influence of deviant peers on youth behavior during group therapy is debated among experts. There is one school of thought that naturally occurring peer interactions during group-based interventions may exacerbate deviant attitudes and behavior among others (e.g., increased substance use, behavior and legal problems). This problem may be most serious when the composition of a group includes deviant youth and youth with less delinquency. Another point of view is that group composition in terms of conduct disorder symptoms is *not* associated with worse outcomes, the logic being that there may be a slight *advantage* for youth with high conduct disorder to be included in groups with fewer symptoms.

There can be a risk in support-group settings that the conversation among adolescents can turn to talk that extolls the perceived benefits of drug use. This is called the *contagion effect* (Dishion & Dodge, 2005). Group leaders need to be aware of such a possibility and be ready to direct the discussion in more positive directions, if necessary.

MUTUAL SELF-HELP

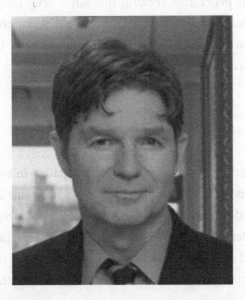

John Kelly, Ph.D., the leading researcher of mutual self-help for adolescents. Photo courtesy of John Kelly.

Relapse is common among adolescents when treatment ends (Dennis et al., 2004; Winters et al., 2018). To help extend the benefits of professional interventions, many adolescent treatment programs refer clients to community-based, mutual self-help recovery groups, such as AA and NA (Kelly et al., 2019). As noted above, referral to AA/NA groups following adolescent SUD treatment appears to be the norm, irrespective of the theoretical orientation of the program in which adolescents received treatment. Such recovery programs stress the participant's acceptance that life has become unmanageable, that abstinence from drug use is needed, and that will power alone cannot overcome the problem. Participation in self-help, recovery support services can reinforce a drug-free lifestyle and other goals made during treatment. Self-help groups are free of charge. Community AA/NA meetings focus on continued work with the 12 steps under supervision by counselors of treatment programs or a person in recovery (Knudsen et al., 2008). Participants meet in a group with others in recovery, once a week or more, sharing their experiences, offering mutual encouragement, and reinforcing the fundamental principles of the 12 steps (e.g., long- term recovery involves a process of spiritual renewal).

An additional benefit of mutual-help programs for adolescents is that they provide the opportunity for the young person to develop new friendships with peers also seeking the same drug-free lifestyle (Kelly et al., 2019). Doing so is important, given that a major contributor to relapse is when an adolescent continues to affiliate with their substance-using friends (Brown et al., 2005).

Role of a Sponsor

An important and necessary element of participating in an AA-based self-help group is having a sponsor. A *sponsor* is a long-standing member of the group who develops a special supportive relationship with the new member in order to help the individual stay sober and to encourage "working" the 12 steps. The responsibility of the sponsor includes making frequent contacts via telephone and e-mail/text and having frequent

individual meetings with the adolescent. Ideally, a sponsor for an adolescent is close in age to them; there is a growing trend of young adults
who have been a long-standing members of the group to be sponsors for
a recovering adolescent.

Age Barrier to 12-Step Participation

Despite the promising aspects of 12-step mutual-help groups, young
people face barriers to participation in these groups (Kelly et al., 2019).
One major issue is the lack of same-aged members. Only 2% of AA
members are younger than 21 years of age, and only 11% are under age
30 (Alcoholics Anonymous, 2008). A similar problem is with NA membership; about 1% are under age 21, and 11% are age 21 to 30 (Narcotics
Anonymous, 2015). The lack of age similarity may mean adolescents, who
typically have a shorter drug use history and fewer negative consequences
than older individuals in membership groups, might find it difficult to feel
comfortable in a typical AA or NA meeting. Indirect evidence for this issue
of age discrepancy is provided by Kelly and colleagues, who found that
adolescents who attended 12-step meetings that included some similar-
aged youth had better attendance and reported superior post-treatment
substance use outcomes when compared to youth attending adult-only
meetings (Kelly et al., 2019). Whereas large metropolitan areas have AA
or NA meetings labeled as "Young People's" meetings, their availability is
quite variable.

Other Considerations When Referring Youth to 12-Step Groups

Passetti and Godley (2008) studied the referral practices pertaining to over
1,600 adolescents by 28 clinicians at eight different treatment programs.
Clinicians reported that referring an adolescent to 12-step meetings was
significantly based on two main factors: severity of the substance use
and related problems, and whether the adolescent was developmentally

mature enough to understand 12-step concepts such as "powerlessness."
With respect to severity of problems, the thinking is that the 12-step recovery model was developed as a treatment for severe-end substance
use problems that reflect dependence or addiction. It is not good clinical
practice for youth with a lower-end severity of substance use problems
(e.g., abusive-like involvement with substances) to prescribe to AA/NA
participation.

Young adolescents, with their developmental lack of introspection and
less serious alcohol and drug involvement, are usually more appropriate
for family therapy treatments. The issue of adolescent maturity is important given that 12-step recovery requires the ability to understand program concepts that may not resonate with many adolescents. Counselors
can emphasize to the teenager that 12-step groups involve sharing
experiences and positive relationships, and "higher power" can be personally internalized as the feeling of not being alone and seeking emotional
support from others (Kelly et al., 2008).

There are other factors to consider when referring adolescents to 12-step
groups, as suggested by experts (e.g., Jaffe, 2001; Passetti & White, 2008).

1. Attending 12-step meetings can be a negative experience. Whereas
   professionally led adolescent substance abuse therapy groups
   will optimize safety (Burleson et al., 2006), 12-step meetings that
   are open and peer-led may consist of attendees who are fulfilling
   parole requirements with no interest in recovery. Thus, the group
   environment may not be supportive of therapeutic goals.

2. As noted above, connecting adolescent clients to a group with
   a significant number of other adolescents and young adults
   improves attendance and outcome (Kelly et al., 2019).

3. Meetings are led by nonprofessionals and are open to anyone
   with a desire to stop using alcohol or drugs, thus, local meetings
   can vary with respect to their interpersonal climate and cultural
   orientation. Adolescents may need to "shop" to find a meeting
   that is a good fit.

4. The referring clinicians should assess the sponsor assigned to their client, to evaluate the sponsor's recovery history, stability, and appropriateness to work with adolescents.

Twelve-Step Facilitation (TSF)

A hybrid of the 12-step approach is "twelve-step facilitation" (TSF). TSF is used to systematically educate patients about the nature, purpose, and scope of mutual self-help groups, such as AA and NA, and to encourage, facilitate, and monitor participation in them over time. This strategy can be easily delivered as an outpatient program, either in a group or individual format. The only RCT of a TSF for adolescents found that over a 6-month follow period, compared to the non-TSF group, youth in the TSF condition had double the rate of 12-step participation and significantly greater outcomes in terms of continuous abstinence and fewer substance use–related negative consequences (Kelly et al., 2017).

EFFECTIVENESS

The extent and rigor of evidence regarding the 12-step approach for adolescents are narrower than in the adult literature (see Kelly et al., 2020 for a review of the AA outcome literature for adults). Based on a synthesis of several literature reviews (Jaffee & Kelly, 2011; Kelly et al., 2010, 2019; Winters et al., 2018), we provide a summary of the main findings on the effectiveness of 12-step programs for adolescents.

A *randomized controlled trial* (RCT) is a study in which participants are allocated at random (by chance alone) to receive one of several clinical interventions. Each of the study participants has an equal chance to be allocated to the interventions. The only expected difference between the control and experimental groups in an RCT is the outcome variable being studied.

Usually one or more of the interventions are the "target" groups, and one is a comparison or control group. A comparison group typically is standard practice; a no-treatment control group can be no intervention at all or a group that receives a placebo condition (e.g., a sham intervention or a "sugar pill"). As best as possible, the participants are not informed by the study administrators whether they have been assigned to a target or a placebo group.

A recent literature review of 12-step-based treatment studies that addressed *adult* alcohol use disorder concluded that manualized 12-step based interventions usually produced higher rates of continuous abstinence from alcohol than the other established treatments, and non-manualized versions of 12-step interventions were comparable to the other treatments (Kelly et al., 2020).

1. The majority of research findings are based on observational or naturalistic studies—that is, youth are not randomly assigned to treatment but rather are followed after receiving 12-step treatment, to assess outcome (e.g., Winters et al., 2000). In some instances, outcomes for those who completed treatment are compared to outcomes for those who did not (non-completers), which is an important comparison given that if treatment is effective, completers are expected to show more favorable outcome. To date, no randomized controlled trials (RCTs) among adolescent samples exist that directly compare 12-step treatment as a primary or index treatment approach against other treatment approaches (e.g., family-based, motivational enhancement, CBT). Thus, the comparative effectiveness of 12-step programs for adolescents among other approaches is not known. Nonetheless, observational studies show that benefits

are obtained by youth who receive 12-step treatment, in terms of reduced substance use and improvements on psychosocial functioning.

2. When participation in 12-step-based, mutual self-help groups occurs, meaningful benefits for youth are typical: The greater the attendance, the better the outcome. An 8-year follow-up study found that, on average, youth gained 2 days of abstinence for each AA or NA meeting attended, over and above all other factors associated with better outcomes (Kelly et al., 2008).

3. Increased attendance in mutual self-help is more likely when the age composition of a meeting includes many young people. This age issue contributes to the recovering youth finding suitable social networks that are conducive to and supportive of recovery.

4. Similar to adult studies, another benefit for youth by participating in the 12-step approach is that it reduces health care costs.

PEER SUPPORT AND RECOVERY HIGH SCHOOLS AS AFTERCARE

Developing new, sober peer groups is a vital yet challenging feature of the recovery process for adolescents after treatment. Peer recovery support and recovery high schools (RHS) are two types of services in the community that can promote the goal of living a drug-free lifestyle.

Peer Support

The strong association between favorable outcome and participation in pro-social activities is highlighted by the importance of peer support. Adolescents who can avoid the pull from delinquent peers but can affiliate more with peers who have outside pro-social interests such as music, art, or sports will increase the likelihood of promoting their own health and well-being. Support from peers can be informal and may originate from connecting to peers that the youth met at a local self-help group or by establishing new friends at school. A growing trend is to train young adults to be a peer recovery coach (sometimes referred to as *peer mentoring*). Coaching focuses on supporting the assets and strengths of a person and providing personal expertise in the keys to successful recovery. Using features of motivational interviewing, a peer coach asks questions, expresses empathy, focuses on helping the person establish and achieve healthy goals, and encourages the youth to take the lead in addressing their own recovery needs.

Recovery High Schools (RHS)

One aim of a recovery high schools (RHS), by providing a supportive educational and therapeutic environment, is to increase recovery and reduce school failure or dropout rates. A recent study (Weimer et al., 2019) compared substance use and educational outcomes for adolescents who had received specialty SUD treatment; 143 who enrolled in an RHS were compared to 117 who enrolled in a non-RHS school. The RHS students were compared to the non-RHS students at the 12-month follow-up period. The RHS students had significantly less substance use and a significantly higher rate of high school graduation.

A major challenge for recovering youth is to prevent the school social environment from contributing to a relapse. Given that the traditional high school in the United States has many students who drink or use other drugs, the school setting may undermine treatment effects. As noted by recovery experts, the "school sits at the heart of the threat of relapse and other unhealthy and maladaptive behaviors" (Winters et al., 2018, p. 159).

Yet schools can be an environment with multiple opportunities to provide assets and promote recovery. On an informal level, this may take the form of peers taking the initiative to support their friend's recovery goals or a school counselor offering advice. A more systematic approach is provided by RHS. This type of school is an alternative high school option (or an insert program in a traditional school) that provides supportive services for students recovering from an SUD. RHS require that students be drug-free and maintain a program of recovery (Finch et al., 2014). Most, though not all, schools are based in the 12-step model of recovery, are typically staffed by a teacher who also is a certified chemical dependency counselor, and have close affiliations with local drug treatment programs. These schools provide a range of academic and therapeutic services for students. A portion of the school day is devoted to group therapy, and students typically receive remedial educational services and counseling for co-occurring behavioral problems (Finch et al., 2014). About 100 RHS have operated since 1979, and according to the Association of Recovery Schools, as of 2020 there are currently 42 RHS in 16 states (https://reco veryschools.org/).

SELF-HELP ALTERNATIVES TO THE 12-STEP APPROACH

Many national groups offer a self-help alternative to the 12-step approach. These groups have characteristics that are similar to the 12 steps: emphasis on internal control; guidelines for dealing with triggers of substance; the goal is abstinence (with one exception). But they differ in that they are secular and focus on current issues and do not dwell on past behaviors. The 12-step alternatives listed below are in order of date of establishment (in parentheses)

1. Women for Sobriety (1976): The focus of this program is on positive thinking, personal responsibility, and embracing the future.
2. Secular Organizations for Sobriety (SOS) (1985): SOS provides several strategies to achieve and maintain abstinence from substances, as well as to address other behavioral addictions (e.g., food addiction, problem gambling).

3. Self-Management and Recovery Training (SMART Recovery) (1994): This program emphasizes strategies to cope with urges and cravings, based on cognitive behavioral therapy and motivational interviewing.

4. Moderation Management (1994): This program is designed for those who are concerned that their drinking is a problem but want to moderate it before it gets out of control. Guidelines of moderate drinking are taught.

5. LifeRing Secular Recovery (2001): The focus of this recovery program is on the three S's: sober, secular, and self-directed.

6. The Wellbriety Movement (2015): this American Indian/ Alaska Native movement carries the message of cultural knowledge about recovery for tribal individuals, families, and communities.

MINI-REVIEW

- Twelve-step treatment and mutual help organizations, such as AA and NA, are a common element in the treatment and recovery of adolescents with an SUD. Adapting the 12 steps for youth is recommended; these adaptations can retain the core step concepts and yet provide a more amenable version for teenagers.

- There is a growing descriptive research base supporting the efficacy of 12-step programs. Whereas the there are no random assignment studies of 12-step treatment when delivered in a residential setting, 12-step facilitation as an outpatient program has shown promise when studied with controlled conditions.

- AA/NA self-help groups are free community resources that are widely available in most parts of the country and have no restriction on length of participation. The longer and more intensive the participation, the more likely the person will remain in recovery. Participation is more likely when the age composition of a meeting includes many young people.

- Peer support groups and recovery high schools offer paths for youth in recovery to develop new, sober peer groups.
- Several self-help alternatives to the 12-step model exist; one common feature among them is that they take a secular approach.

DISCUSSION POINTS

1. What counseling strategies can be used when conducting group therapy with teenagers to reduce the possible problem of the "contagion effect"—that is, the possibility that delinquent group members will negatively influence the less delinquent members?
2. Outcome studies that compare the treatment completer group with the non-completer group generally show better outcomes for the completer group. What are some reasons for this?
3. Twelve-step proponents make the case that youth participating in a 12-step program will reduce future health costs for the person receiving that treatment. In what ways can health costs be reduced?
4. Discuss why self-help alternatives to the 12-step approach may be better for some youth. And how might they be worse?

FURTHER CURIOSITY AND DIGGING

Descriptions of Two Prominent 12-Step Programs for Adolescents

Hazelden Center for Youth and Families: https://www.hazeldenbettyford.org/locations/plymouth

Caron Treatment Center: https://www.caron.org/locations/caron-pennsylvania

More on Alcoholics Anonymous

Glaser, G. (2015). *The irrationality of Alcoholics Anonymous.* https://www.theatlantic.com/magazine/archive/2015/04/the-irrationality-of-alcoholics-anonymous/386255/

Treatment and Recovery

Partnership to End Addiction. (2022). *Keeping your child healthy following treatment.* https://drugfree.org/parent-blog/steps-to-take-before-son-or-daughter-returns-from-addiction-treatment/

More About Peer Support Programs

Substance Abuse and Mental Health Services Administration. (2022). *Peers.* https://www.samhsa.gov/brss-tacs/recovery-support-tools/peers

REFERENCES

Alcoholics Anonymous. (1976). *Alcoholics Anonymous* (3rd ed.). Alcoholics Anonymous World Services.

Anderson, D. J., McGovern, J. P., & DuPont, R. L. (1999). The origins of the Minnesota Model of addiction treatment—a first person account. *Journal of Addictive Diseases, 18,* 107–114.

Brown, S. A., Anderson, K. G., Ramo, D. E., & Tomlinson, K. L. (2005). Treatment of adolescent alcohol-related problems. In M. Galanter, C. Lowman, G. M. Boyd, V. B. Faden, E. Witt, & D. Lagressa (Eds.), *Recent developments in alcoholism* (pp. 327–348). Springer.

Burleson, J. A., Kaminer, Y., & Dennis, M. L. (2006). Absence of iatrogenic or contagion effects in adolescent group therapy: Findings from the Cannabis Youth Treatment (CYT) Study. *American Journal on Addictions, 15*(Suppl. 1), 4–15.

Dennis, M., Godley, S. H., Diamond, G., Tims, F. M., Babor, T., Donaldson, J., . . . Hamilton, N. (2004). The Cannabis Youth Treatment (CYT) Study: Main findings from two randomized trials. *Journal of Substance Abuse Treatment, 27,* 197–213.

Dishion, T. J., & Dodge, K. A. (2005). Peer contagion in interventions for children and adolescents: Moving towards an understanding of the ecology and dynamics of change. *Journal of Abnormal Child Psychology, 33,* 395–400.

Finch, A. J., Moberg, D. P., & Krupp, A. L. (2014). Continuing care in high schools: A descriptive study of recovery high school programs. *Journal of Child & Adolescent Substance Abuse, 23,* 116–129.

Jaffe, S. L. (1990). *Step workbook for adolescent chemical dependency recovery: A guide to the first five steps.* American Psychiatric Association Publishing.

Jaffe, S. L. (2001). *Adolescent substance abuse intervention workbook.* American Psychiatric Association Publishing.

Jaffe, S. L., Allen, S., Fernandez, M., & Winters, K. C. (2008). Pilot study of a two-hour workbook intervention for juvenile delinquents with substance abuse. Unpublished report.

Jaffe, S. L., & Kelly, J. F. (2011). Twelve-step mutual-help programs for adolescents. In Y. Kaminer & K. C. Winters (Eds.), *Clinical manual of adolescent substance abuse treatment* (pp. 269–282). American Psychiatric Publishing, Inc.

Kelly, J. F., Abry, A. W., & Fallah-Sohey, N. (2019). Twelve-step and mutual-self-help. In Y. Kaminer & K. C. Winters (Eds.), *Clinical manual of adolescent addictive disorders* (2nd ed., pp. 319–348). American Psychiatric Association.

Kelly, J. F., Abry, A., Ferri, M., & Humphreys, K. (2020). Alcoholics Anonymous and 12-step facilitation treatments for alcohol use disorder: A distillation of a 2020 Cochrane Review for clinicians and policy makers. *Alcohol and Alcoholism, 55,* 641–651.

Kelly, J. F., Brown, S. A., Abrantes, A., Kahler, C. W., & Myers, M. (2008). Social recovery model: An 8-year investigation of adolescent 12-step group involvement following inpatient treatment. *Alcoholism: Clinical and Experimental Research, 32,* 1468-1478.

Kelly, J. F., Dow, S. J., Yeterian, J. D., & Kahler, C. W. (2010). Can 12-step group participation strengthen and extend the benefits of adolescent addiction treatment? A prospective analysis. *Drug and Alcohol Dependence, 110,* 117–125.

Kelly, J. F., Kaminer, Y., Kahler, C. W., Hoeppner, B., Yeterian, J., Cristello, J. V., & Timko, C. (2017). A pilot randomized clinical trial testing integrated 12-step facilitation (ITSF) treatment for adolescent substance use disorder. *Addiction, 112,* 2155–2166.

Kelly, J. F., Magill, M., & Stout, R.L. (2009). How do people recover from alcohol dependence? A systematic review of the research on mechanisms of behavior change in Alcoholics Anonymous. *Addiction Research & Theory, 17,* 236–259.

Kelly, J. F, & Urbanoski, K. (2012). Youth recovery contexts: The incremental effects of 12-step attendance and involvement on adolescent outpatient outcomes. *Alcoholism, Clinical and Experimental Research, 36,* 1219–1229.

Kelly, J. F., & Yeterian, J.D. (2011). The role of mutual-help groups in extending the framework of treatment. *Alcohol Research & Health, 33,* 350–355.

Knudsen, H. K., Ducharme, L. J., Roman, P. M., & Johnson, J. A. (2008). *Service delivery and use of evidence-based treatment practices in adolescent substance abuse treatment settings: Project report.* University of Georgia.

McCrady, B. S. (1994). Alcoholics Anonymous and behavior therapy: Can habits be treated as diseases? Can diseases be treated as habits? *Journal of Consulting and Clinical Psychology, 62,* 1159–1166.

Narcotics Anonymous World Services. (2015). *Narcotics Anonymous 2015 membership survey.* https://www.na.org/admin/include/spaw2/uploads/pdf/pr/MembershipSurvey 2016.pdf

Passetti, L. L., & Godley, S. H. (2008). Adolescent substance abuse treatment clinician's self-help meeting referral practices and adolescent attendance rates. *Journal of Psychoactive Drugs, 40,* 30–40.

Passetti, L. L., & White, W. L. (2008). Recovery support meetings for youths: Considerations when referring young people to 12-step and alternative groups. *Journal of Groups in Addiction & Recovery, 2,* 97–121.

Prochaska, J. O., DiClemente, C. C., & Norcross, J. C. (1992). In search of how people change: Applications to the addictive behaviors. *American Psychologist, 47,* 1102–1114.

Sussman, S. (2010). A review of Alcoholics Anonymous/Narcotics Anonymous programs for teens. *Evaluation & the Health Professions, 33,* 26–55.

Weimer, D. L., Moberg, D. P., French, F., Tanner-Smith, E. E., & Finch, A. J. (2019). Net benefits of recovery high schools: Higher cost but increased sobriety and increased probability of high school graduation. *Journal of Mental Health Policy and Economics*, *22*, 109–120.

Winters, K. C., Botzet, A. M., Stinchfield, R., Gonzalez, R., Finch, A., Piehler, T., Ausherbauer, K., Chalmers, K., & Hemze, A. (2018). Adolescent substance abuse treatment: A review of evidence-based research. In C. Leukefeld, T. Gullotta, & M. Staton Tindall (Eds.), *Adolescent substance abuse: Evidence-based approaches to prevention and treatment* (2nd ed., pp. 141–171). Springer Science+Business Media.

Winters, K. C., Stinchfield, R. D., Opland, E., Weller, C., & Latimer, W. W. (2000). The effectiveness of the Minnesota Model approach in the treatment of adolescent drug abusers. *Addiction*, *95*, 601–612.

Young, L. B. (2012). Alcoholics Anonymous sponsorship: Characteristics of sponsored and sponsoring members. *Alcoholism Treatment Quarterly*, *30*, 52–66.

CHAPTER 2

1. Environmental factors have a negligible influence on the way a teen physically develops. True **False**
2. The stages of sexual maturation in adolescents are known as the Tanner stages. **True** False
3. The two puberty hormones that likely affect the developing brain are testosterone and dopamine. True **False**
4. The authors base their description of psychosocial development on the biopsychosocial model. **True** False
5. The famous psychologist who authored the preeminent theory of cognitive development was Eric Erickson. True **False**
6. During adolescence physical and psychosocial changes happen at. . . .
   a. **an accelerated rate**
   b. a slower rate
   c. the rate as adults
   d. none of the above
7. Identify a prominent developmental theory of adolescence.
   a. Identity Status
   b. Moral Development Theory

    c. Psychosocial Theory of Human Development

    d. **all of them are prominent developmental theories**

8. Proper nutrition during adolescence . . .

    a. is not as important as it is during other developmental stages

    b. is not able to be tracked because of social factors

    c. **is particularly important to get enough minerals and vitamins**

    d. is not an issue at all for this stage of development

9. The change from prepuberty to full reproductive capacity takes. . . .

    a. **as little as 18 months or as long as 5 years**

    b. up to a year

    c. no time, reproductive capacity begins in a different developmental stage

    d. place when they reach full height

10. The Tanner stages refers to. . . .

    a. skin tone

    b. **sexual maturation**

    c. moral development

    d. none of the above

11. Early-maturing girls have a tendency to have more . . .

    a. emotional problems

    b. a lower self-image

    c. higher rates of depression and anxiety

    d. **all of the above**

12. An important hallmark of changes during adolescence is the maturation of the teen's *abstract thinking capacities*. Abstract thinking is the ability to use . . .

    a. **internal symbols or images to represent reality**

    b. the dictionary

    c. know when to ask for help

    d. peers for guidance

13. Signs of independence can take many forms, such as . . .

    a. choice of music

    b. choice of fashion

c. hobbies and activities

d. **all of the above**

14. A central focus during adolescence is on . . .

a. **identity formation**

b. parents

c. peers

d. values development

15. What psychological term coined by Eric Erickson describes the stage when a teenager is exploring options about self-identity?

a. personhood

b. **identity foreclosure**

c. adolescence

d. psychology

16. Adolescence is a period of cognitive maturity in which the individual demonstrates a higher level the thinking, characterized by the ability of hypothetical and deductive reasoning and to think more deeply about abstract concepts. Piaget (1960) refers to this as . . .

a. **the formal operational stage of cognitive development**

b. the middle stage of cognitive development

c. the end of cognitive development

d. the formal integration stage of cognitive development

17. Urie Bronfenbrenner emphasizes the importance of contextual influences by the environment, such as . . .

a. the family and peers

b. schools and churches

c. the media

d. **all of the above**

18. Experts believe that puberty causes a shift in the timing of one's circadian rhythms. This is important to note for adolescents because. . . .

a. **it impacts sleep by moving the ability to sleep later**

b. it impacts their ability to listen and play music

    c. it is unclear how circadian rhythms impact adolescents

    d. none of the above

CHAPTER 3

1. Brain development between boys and girls is the same. True **False**
2. Sleep has little impact on emotional health. True **False**
3. Adolescent substance use has a significant connection to substance use into adulthood. **True** False
4. Brain plasticity is important for adapting and is a key to learning throughout our lifetime. **True** False
5. A 15-year-old male is more likely to follow a peer's advice than his 8-year-old sister is to listen to her peers for advice. **True** False
6. The neurobiological process of myelination during adolescence....
   a. impedes fast neural connections
   b. **promotes fast neural connections**
   c. has no effect on neural connections
7. How does brain development science provide a reason for why playing soccer as a young person may contribute to greater soccer skill compared to a person who played soccer for the first time as an adult?
   a. The overall mass of the adolescent brain continues to expand in ways not seen during adulthood and this expansion supports all kinds of physical activity.
   b. Pruning during youth brain development will weaken neural connections that interfere with the development of foot and leg coordination.
   c. **Pruning during youth brain development will strengthen neural connections associated with foot and leg coordination.**
8. Which best summarizes the brain maturation process from childhood to late adolescence?
   a. It occurs in a very orderly fashion, from the back of the brain to the front of the brain.

b. **It tends to occur in an uneven fashion, but generally from the back of the brain to the front of the brain.**

c. It occurs in a very orderly fashion, from the front of the brain to the back of the brain.

d. It tends to occur in an uneven fashion, but generally from the front of the brain to the back of the brain.

9. Which below is <u>not</u> a reason discussed in the chapter as a possible source having a deleterious effect on brain maturation?

a. excessive alcohol use

b. excessive exposure to stress

c. excessive marijuana use

d. **excessive video game playing**

10. Which is an accurate statement about brain plasticity?

a. **It describes the ability of the brain's structure and function to adapt in response to the environment.**

b. It's a brain process more relevant to functioning as an adult than during adolescence.

c. It is not affected by hormonal changes during youth.

d. It is most likely a brain maturation process relevant only to youth in Westernized countries.

11. The brake versus accelerator metaphor refers to what?

a. the relative imbalance between the quicker brain maturation process in girls (accelerator) and the slower brain maturation process in boys (brake)

b. the relative imbalance between the quicker brain maturation process in boys (accelerator) and the slower brain maturation process in girls (brake)

c. the relative imbalance between the slower-to-mature limbic brain region (brake) and the earlier developing prefrontal brain region (accelerator)

d. **the relative imbalance between the slower-to-mature prefrontal brain region (brake) and the earlier developing limbic brain region (accelerator)**

12. Which is the following is true about the influence of peers on adolescent risk taking behavior?

  a. **Teenagers are more susceptible to peer influences compared to children and adults.**

  b. Teenagers are less susceptible to peer influences compared to children and adults.

  c. Teenagers are susceptible to peer influences only in school settings.

  d. Teenagers are more susceptible by an older brother or sister than by same-aged peers.

13. The major difference, on average, in brain development between girls and boys is . . .

  a. The influence of improved nutrition has eliminated any gender differences that were once present.

  b. The rate of development by girls is a few months ahead of the rate for boys.

  c. **The rate of development by girls is approximately 2 years ahead of the rate for boys.**

  d. The general principle of brain maturation occurring from back to front of the brain is only characteristic of girls.

14. The authors discuss which two topics regarding brain development and substance use? (mark two)

  a. **Brain development may contribute to risky decisions to use substances.**

  b. Youth with a faster rate of brain development are at higher risk of using substances.

  c. **Substance use during adolescence may impede brain development.**

  d. The brain development differences between boys and girls is a partial explanation for why boys tend to use more substances than girls.

15. In the discussion of data concerning the intersection of brain development and substance use, which two types of study designs were referenced?

    a. cross-lagged and retrospective designs

    b. territorial and longitudinal designs

    c. epidemiological and territorial designs

    d. **cross-sectional and longitudinal designs**

CHAPTER 4

1. The most compelling reason to not use substances during adolescence is that most youth who use any substance during the teenage years will develop a serious substance use disorder. True **False**

2. One major trend of substance use discussed in the chapter is a relatively steady increase in the percent of 12th graders in the U.S. who report no use of any substance lifetime. **True** False

3. The Monitoring Future Survey provides trend data of substance use by high school students in the U.S. **True** False

4. The authors concluded that U.S. adolescents clearly use more substances and at heavier levels than youth in most other Westernized countries. True **False**

5. A type of assisted, clinical interview used to collect detailed alcohol and other drug use information over a specified time period from a client is the Time-Line Follow-Back interview. **True** False

6. Earlier onset of substance use increases the likelihood of . . .

    a. **developing a substance use disorder**

    b. running a marathon

    c. maturing at a faster rate

    d. none of the above

7. The most prevalent non-illicit substance on the list below used by adolescents is . . .

    a. cough medicine

    b. prescription pills

    c. **nicotine**

    d. inhalants

8. A relatively commonly used drug by adolescents is . . .
   a. alcohol
   b. nicotine
   c. marijuana
   d. **all of the above**

9. "Collinearity of drug use" refers to . . .
   a. a teen substance user that is sick often
   b. **a teen substance user that uses all three major drugs of abuse**
   c. nothing to do with teen substance use
   d. teens using substances with the people they are related to

10. Drug use typically occurs in the presence of coexisting problems and disorders. A sizeable proportion of teenagers who use drugs also experience . . .
    a. **one or more co-occurring behavioral or psychological disorders**
    b. being in the top 10% academically
    c. owning their own home at a young age
    d. none of the above

11. Nearly all addictive drugs directly or indirectly target the brain's reward system by flooding this part of the brain with a neurotransmitter, called . . .
    a. estrogen
    b. adrenaline
    c. **dopamine**
    d. a and c

12. Tolerance is . . .
    a. **the need to take larger amounts of the drug to produce the familiar dopamine high**
    b. the ability to work out for long period of time without needing to rest
    c. the brain's response to stopping the use of illicit drugs
    d. the absence of serotonin in the brain when using a substance

13. Signs of caffeine use are . . .
    a. jittery, hyperactive
    b. talkative
    c. anxiety
    d. **all of the above**

14. Long-term effects of cannabis may include . . .
    a. developing a substance use disorder
    b. reduced IQ
    c. heightened immune system
    d. **a and b**

15. Alcohol is a . . .
    a. **depressant**
    b. stimulant
    c. hallucinogen
    d. none of the above

16. Long-term opioid use can result in . . .
    a. **fatal overdose**
    b. infections
    c. breathing problems
    d. all of the above

17. Which is <u>not</u> a sign of using inhalants?
    a. sensitivity to light
    b. have slurred speech
    c. runny nose and/or watery eyes
    d. **hyperactivity**

18. Initiation to substance use peaks at a time when the developing brain may be _____ to the neurotic effect of heavy use, highlighting the importance of efforts to prevent substance use.
    a. combative
    b. reflective
    c. **particularly vulnerable**
    d. resistant

CHAPTER 5

1. It is rare that a youth would come in contact or know someone who experiences a substance use disorder True **False**

2. Alcohol use disorder accounts for the most treatment admissions for adolescents. True **False**

3. Substance use is a moral problem and if teens had a better value system they would not abuse substances. True **False**

4. The authors of the text are very skeptical about prevention programs and think more money should be used for the corrections system to assist with substance use disorders in youth. True **False**

5. Adolescents only reflect what their peers want. It is not that important to include parents in the treatment process. True **False**

6. The DSM-5 is a. . . .
   a. **diagnostic system of mental disorders for all age groups**
   b. diagnostic system pertaining to mental disorders for only adolescents
   c. diagnostic system pertaining to mental disorders for only children and adolescents

7. Which is <u>not</u> a diagnostic criteria for a substance use disorder?
   a. preoccupation
   b. negative consequences
   c. **non-responsive to treatment**
   d. cravings

8. Which is not listed in the chapter as a contributing factor to developing a substance use disorder during adolescence?
   a. peer substance use
   b. family history of a substance use disorder
   c. early onset of use
   d. **residing in a pro-marijuana state**

9. It is estimated that what approximate percent of adolescents with a substance use disorder receives any type of specialty treatment for this disorder?
   a. 33%
   b. 25%

c. <1%

d. **10%**

10. Which below is <u>not</u> one of the four models described to explain the relationship between a co-occurring disorder and a substance use disorder?

    a. **Multi-Path Model**

    b. Self-Medication Model

    c. Disorder Model

    d. Common Factor Model

11. During a comprehensive assessment interview, determining the temporal sequence of multiple disorders requires pinpointing

    a. first the onset and progression of a substance use disorder

    b. first the onset and progression of a behavioral disorder

    c. **the onset and progression of separate disorders**

    d. when first the parents noticed a problem with their teenager

12. Which was <u>not</u> one of several steps that can improve the accuracy of measuring substance use disorder symptoms?

    a. describe the confidentiality guidelines

    b. establish rapport with the adolescent

    c. **use an in-house tool that the clinician is comfortable with**

    d. seek corroboration with several sources

13. Which is true about the differences between a screening and a comprehensive assessment?

    a. Screening is a more valid process than a comprehensive assessment.

    b. Screening is a less valid process than a comprehensive assessment.

    c. Comprehensive assessment determines need for more screening.

    d. **Comprehensive assessment determines need for treatment.**

14. Which statement is accurate about behavioral disorders that coexist with a substance use disorder?

    a. **Several psychiatric or behavioral disorders are relatively frequent.**

    b. No group of psychiatric or behavioral disorders are relatively frequent.

    c. Two disorders account for nearly all mental disorders that coexist with a substance use disorder in boys.

    d. Two disorders account for nearly all mental disorders that coexist with a substance use disorder in girls.

15. Which is true about parents as a source of information in the assessment process?

    a. They are an excellent corroborating source about the teenager's substance use.

    b. **They are not likely to provide detailed reports about the teenager's substance use.**

    c. They rarely can provide useful reports about the teenager's behavioral problems.

    d. Fathers tend be better reporters than mothers.

CHAPTER 6

1. The consequences of emotions can be adaptive because they can serve as an adaptive tool to deal with life's challenges. **True** False

2. A feature common to all anxiety disorder subtypes in the DMS-5 is that the disorder routinely stems from the effects of substance use. True **False**

3. Treating both the co-occurring depression and substance use disorder provides a greater likelihood that both problem areas will improve, although treating only the substance use disorder can be an efficient and effective way to adequately address both. True **False**

4. Agoraphobia is the fear of social situations. **True** False

5. In the case illustration of PTSD, Terry disclosed many symptoms that are characteristic of depression and anxiety disorders. **True** False

6. Emotions during adolescence are . . .

    a. routinely expressed with the same intensities as seen during adulthood

    b. overrated as having a role in an adolescent's mood

    c. a reliable reflection of the adolescent's family situation

    d. **shaped significantly by brain development**

7. The Oregon Adolescent Depression Project found that. . . ..

    a. anxiety and depressive disorders during adolescence were associated with significantly greater odds of abusing opioids during early adulthood

    b. anxiety and depressive disorders during adolescence were associated with a weak odds of abusing cannabis and alcohol during early adulthood

    c. **anxiety and depressive disorders during adolescence were associated with significantly greater odds of abusing cannabis and alcohol during early adulthood**

    d. anxiety and depressive disorders during adolescence were associated with significantly greater odds of abusing cannabis and alcohol during early adulthood for only one gender

8. Which includes a false symptom of a major depressive disorder?

    a. a period of at least 2 weeks of low mood present in most situations; problems with sleep; social withdrawal in many situations

    b. a period of at least 2 weeks of low mood present in limited situations; problems with sleep; social withdrawal in many situations

    c. a period of at least 2 weeks of low mood present in most situations; problems with eating; social withdrawal in limited situations

    d. **b and c**

    e. a and c

9. The value of psychotherapeutic strategies for a major depressive disorder (MDD) is profiled by the authors. What is a point that the authors make about the role of medications?

    a. **Severe cases of MDD may need medication.**

    b. Mild and severe cases of MDD may need medication.

    c. Only atypical cases of MDD may need medication.

    d. A class of medication for MDD is selective serotonin rebalancing initiators (SSRIs).

    e. a and d

10. What is not the case about anxiety disorders?

    a. They are the most common mental disorders across the life span.

    b. Among adolescents with a substance use disorder, they are highly prevalent.

    c. Anxiety disorders are more frequent among female adolescents than in male adolescents.

    d. **Whereas quite common across the life span, anxiety disorders are not all that common among adolescents.**

11. Being phobic about a situation or object means that the person displays ...

    a. unreasonable and excessive fear that leads to immediate anxiety and only occasional avoidance of the object or situation

    b. **unreasonable and excessive fear that leads to immediate anxiety**

    c. unreasonable and excessive fear that leads to delayed anxiety and only occasional avoidance of the object or situation

    d. unreasonable and excessive fear that is the same as regular fear

12. Which below contains a false statement about effective treatments for adolescent anxiety disorders?

    a. **Individual counseling and family modalities are typical; complications are likely if a substance use disorder coexists; CBT and medication approaches have not been shown to be effective.**

    b. Individual counseling and family modalities are typical; complications are likely if a substance use disorder coexists; CBT and medication approaches have been shown to be effective.

    c. Only the individual counseling modality is typical; complications are likely if a substance use disorder coexists; CBT and medication approaches have been shown to be effective.

    d. Only the family counseling modality is typical; complications are likely if a substance use disorder coexists; CBT and medication approaches have been shown to be effective.

13. Which is <u>not</u> the case for bipolar disorder?

    a. defined by periods or episodes of extreme disturbances of a person's mood, thoughts, and behavior

    b. the manic phase often includes the person engaging in risky or reckless behavior

    c. **cannot be reliably diagnosed in adolescents**

    d. behaviors of this disorder can be part of normal adolescence, but do not occur at extreme intensities

14. Which is the case regarding both "acute" trauma and "chronic" trauma?

    a. **Both can lead to PTSD and both are commonly associated with drug abuse.**

    b. Only chronic trauma can lead to PTSD and yet both are commonly associated with drug abuse.

    c. Both can lead to PTSD and yet only chronic PTSD is commonly associated with drug abuse.

    d. Both can lead to PTSD and yet neither is commonly associated with drug abuse among adolescents.

15. Which below contains a false feature of autism?

    a. **It's a spectrum of interrelated disorders that have common symptoms; the symptom of a deficit in social communication is no longer thought to be a core feature; stereotyped or repetitive motor movements are typical.**

    b. It's a spectrum of interrelated disorders that have common symptoms; one core symptom is a deficit in social interaction across numerous and different situations; stereotyped or repetitive motor movements are typical.

c. It's a spectrum of interrelated disorders that have common symptoms; one core symptom is a deficit in social communication; insistence on sameness is a typical feature.

CHAPTER 7

1. ADHD occurs more often in boys than in girls, and behaviors can be different based on gender. **True** False

2. Left untreated, an adolescent with ODD is at risk to develop a CD and additional coexisting disorders. **True** False

3. Schizophrenia occurs at very low rates—approximately 1% of the population. **True** False

4. The risk of developing a substance use disorder among youth with an externalizing disorder is greater than the risk if the youth has an internalizing disorder. **True** False

5. Medication is only one way to treat ADHD. **True** False

6. Regarding the intersection of externalizing disorders and substance use disorders . . .

   a. They are the least common group of co-occurring disorders in adolescents with a substance use disorder.

   b. **They are the most common group of co-occurring disorders in adolescents with a substance use disorder.**

   c. They are an equally common group of co-occurring disorders in adolescents with a substance use disorder.

   d. They are the most common group of co-occurring disorders in female adolescents with a substance use disorder.

7. Which group below contains a disorder <u>not</u> part of the broad domain of externalizing disorders discussed in this chapter?

   a. ADHD, conduct disorder, personality disorders

   b. Oppositional defiant disorder, schizophrenia, ADHD

   c. **Conduct disorder, eating disorders, personality disorders**

8. The authors' view regarding the diagnosis of ADHD is that its. . . .
    a. underdiagnosed
    b. too complex a disorder to be accurately diagnosed
    c. not a valid disorder during adulthood
    d. **overdiagnosed**

9. Psychostimulant medications work for some youth with a diagnosis of ADHD because
    a. they are administered in doses that do not normally pose an addictive threat
    b. they improve brain chemical activity which plays an important role in attention
    c. they are combined with another medication to reduce the likelihood of stimulant addiction
    d. **a and b**
    e. b and c

10. When conduct disorder begins during childhood and includes aggression, the risk
    a. is elevated for persistent delinquent behavior
    b. is not elevated for persistent delinquent behavior but is elevated for severe functioning problems
    c. is elevated for severe functioning problems
    d. **a and c**

11. What did the authors emphasize with respect to treating youth with a diagnosis of oppositional defiant disorder (ODD)?
    a. **Parent counseling is a central focus of treatment.**
    b. Left untreated, an adolescent with ODD is at risk to develop psychosis.
    c. Effective treatment protocols center on group counseling approaches.
    d. Very brief and efficient treatment approaches are equal to long-term approaches.

12. Each personality disorder is characterized by a personality style that
    a. if a late-onset version, it can be just a minor quirk in a person's personality

    b. if an early-onset version, it is much more than a minor quirk in a person's personality

    c. **is so extreme it creates many problems with interpersonal relations**

    d. it creates more internal distress than problems with interpersonal relations

13. Which two forms of treatment are described as possibly useful to address personality disorders?

    a. **cognitive behavior therapy and dialectical behavior therapy**

    b. cognitive behavior therapy and psychiatric medications

    c. dialectical behavior therapy and psychiatric medications

    d. cognitive behavior therapy and family therapy

14. Which symptoms are characteristic of schizophrenia?

    a. delusions, hallucinations, and compulsive behaviors

    b. delusions, hallucinations, and manic episodes

    c. **delusions, hallucinations, and negative symptoms**

    d. hallucinations, compulsive behaviors, and manic episodes

15. Typical treatment for schizophrenia requires . . .

    a. intensive counseling

    b. hospitalization

    c. psychopharmacological medication

    d. **all of the above**

CHAPTER 8

1. Behavioral addictions have many features that are similar to a substance use disorder. **True** False

2. The authors dispute the validity of food addiction and sex addiction because these behaviors represent normal and necessary behaviors. True **False**

3. Whereas many adolescents report to have done some type of gambling, including informal betting with friends, the

prevalence of problem gambling among youth is relatively small.
True False

4. One sign that video gaming addiction is a valid disorder is that the World Health Organization has now identified it as a mental health condition. **True** False

5. Treatment options for adolescents with a behavioral addiction are relatively rare, but there is a growing industry of programs to treat social media indulgence. True **False**

6. Which group of features are true about behavioral addictions?
   a. **They are characterized by compulsive-like behaviors that are similar to a substance use disorder, resulting in negative effects that can impair one's ability to function normally in daily life, and many sufferers need professional treatment.**
   b. They are characterized by compulsive-like behaviors that are not all that similar to a substance use disorder, resulting in negative effects that can impair one's ability to function normally in daily life, and many sufferers need professional treatment.
   c. They are characterized by compulsive-like behaviors that are similar to a substance use disorder, resulting in negative effects that are troublesome but rarely impair one's ability to function normally in daily life, and many sufferers need professional treatment.
   d. They are characterized by compulsive-like behaviors that are not all that similar to a substance use disorder, resulting in negative effects that can impair one's ability to function normally in daily life, but many sufferers do not need professional treatment because self-help groups are sufficient.

7. Why are the behavioral addictions a controversial concept among some researchers?
   a. The DSM does not include any behavioral addictions.
   b. Unless the behavior involves the use of a psychoactive substance, then the behavior cannot be a legitimate addiction.
   c. The underlying behavior represents normal and necessary behaviors.

d. **b and c**

e. a and b

8. Which is <u>not</u> true regarding behavior addictions and the DSM?

a. Sex addiction is not a formal DSM category.

b. Food addiction is not formally featured in DSM-5 but many of its characteristics are part of the definition of a related DSM-5 disorder.

c. Social media addiction is not a formal diagnosis, but many experts are concerned that for youth, this is a problem.

d. **The upcoming edition of the International Classification of Diseases, despite a solid research base, will not include internet gaming disorder as a new disorder.**

9. The research literature on the relationship of adolescence and gambling indicates that . . . . . .

a. **risk factors include being a male and having a history of attention-deficit/hyperactivity disorder**

b. risk factors include being a male and having a history of depression

c. unlike other addictions, family history is not a risk factor

d. early onset of adolescent gambling is not predictive of having an adult gambling problem

10. The authors' main point about the signs and symptoms of substance use disorders and behavioral addictions is. . . .

a. no valid signs and symptoms of behavioral addictions exist, unlike for substance use disorders

b. signs and symptoms of behavioral addictions, except for the "physical-based" features, match many characteristics of substance use disorders

c. **signs and symptoms of behavioral addictions match many features of substance use disorders**

d. only the "physical-based" signs and symptoms of a substance use disorder match the characteristics of behavioral addictions

11. What does <u>not</u> belong as one the authors' points about whether behavioral addictions are valid disorders or not?
    a. The line between what is healthy involvement and unhealthy indulgence is not always clear.
    b. Some overindulgence does not contribute to significant problems in the person's functioning.
    c. Some individuals demonstrate control over the behavior.
    d. **Behavioral addictions are clearly valid for adults but not for adolescents.**

12. What is <u>not</u> among the diagnostic symptoms of a gambling disorder?
    a. **getting in trouble with the law by illegally financing the gambling habit**
    b. placing bets more and more frequently
    c. betting more than originally intended
    d. feeling irritable when unable to gamble or when losing

13. Internet gaming disorder is. . . .
    a. a formal diagnostic category in the WHO's 11th edition of the International Classification of Diseases
    b. a provisional diagnostic category in the DSM-based system
    c. viewed by the DSM authors as a disorder that needs more research
    d. **a, b, and c are true**
    e. a, b, and c are not true

14. Treatment for adolescents with disordered eating is . . . .
    a. in its infancy
    b. **not in its infancy**
    c. only effective for anorexia and not for bulimia
    d. best implemented with adjunct medication

15. Self-help programs for the behavioral addictions are . . .
    a. not growing in popularity
    b. more effective than formal treatment
    c. are just as effective when mixed with AA-based self-help
    d. **rarely specialized for youth**

CHAPTER 9

1. The American Society of Addiction Medicine criteria only prescribes medication and does not have anything to do with identifying services for youth. True **False**
2. The SBIRT approach started in the 1960s and is outdated. True **False**
3. Medically managed hospital-based treatment is the most intensive level of care. **True** False
4. The use of technology in treatment is being phased out. True **False**
5. Exercise may help to strengthen the "naïve" or underdeveloped connections between the brain's brake (frontal/regulatory) and gas pedal (cortical-subcortical) circuitry regions, and thus help shape decision making to be less influenced by the imbalance between these two regions. **True** False
6. Which below includes a factor <u>not noted</u> as reason why there is such a large gap between treatment utilization by youth and those youth with a substance use disorder?
   a. inadequate local treatment options, parents are unsupportive in a treatment option, poor health coverage
   b. inadequate local treatment options, stigma about drug treatment, low motivation by the adolescent to seek help
   c. **inadequate local treatment options, concern by the adolescent of ridicule by peers, low motivation by the adolescent to seek help**
   d. inadequate local treatment options, poor health insurance, low motivation by the adolescent to seek help
7. Which is true regarding research studies that investigated the post-treatment outcomes of youth who received drug abuse treatment?
   a. For some youth, many benefits quickly diminish post-treatment.
   b. Positive treatment benefits exist, including positive changes in substance use and improvement in psychosocial functioning.

    c. Positive treatment benefits exist, but they are limited to positive changes in psychosocial functioning.

    d. **a and b**

    e. b and c

8. Treatment planning and placement should be dictated by the . . .

    a. results of the assessment and health insurance coverage

    b. **results of the assessment and what treatment personalization is needed**

    c. results of the assessment and the parents' recommendation

    d. results of the assessment and the adolescent's recommendation

9. The treatment principles cited by the National Institute on Drug Abuse do <u>not</u> include which one?

    a. developmentally trained staff

    b. **using well-developed, in-house assessment tools and evidence-based treatment strategies**

    c. addressing the disorders that coexist with a substance use disorder

    d. testing for sexually transmitted diseases

10. What are the American Society of Addiction Medicine Criteria?

    a. an emerging system that identifies how to apply evidence-based treatments

    b. an emerging system that identifies a continuum of levels of care

    c. a well-known system that identifies how to apply evidence-based treatments

    d. **a well-known system that identifies a continuum of levels of care**

11. Which below is <u>not</u> one of the basic principles of recovery-oriented services of care?

    a. helps families or support people to understand the challenges faced by the client's treatment program

    b. embraces the possibility of recovery created by the inherent strength and capacity of all clients

    c. **maximizes self-determination and self-management of well-being**

    d. a well-known system that identifies how to apply evidence-based treatments

12. According to the authors, how might physical exercise help adolescents who are seeking to recover from a substance abuse problem?

    a. **It helps to strengthen the brain regions that are involved in decision making.**

    b. It provides a distraction from thinking about using drugs.

    c. It helps to prevent the person from affiliating with drug-using peers.

    d. It fills time that otherwise might be spent using drugs.

13. Brain stimulation (or 'neuromodulation') techniques. . . .

    a. **include various noninvasive ways of stimulating the brain with the aim of treating various neurological and psychiatric disorders**

    b. include various noninvasive ways of stimulating the brain with the aim of preventing various neurological and psychiatric disorders

    c. include various noninvasive ways of stimulating the brain that are not yet viewed as an emerging way to reduce drug craving

14. Which group of behavior change approaches below includes an approach for adolescents <u>not</u> being used by smartphone applications and other digital mental health products (apps)?

    a. cognitive behavioral principles, meditation, mindfulness

    b. social support, mediation, mindfulness

    c. **psychological-based education, mindfulness, psychopharmacology-based education**

    d. psychological-based education, mindfulness, mediation

15. What is the authors' point about the implementation of evidence-based treatment programs?

    a. Delivering treatments with high fidelity is always better than delivering with a tailored approach.

b. Delivering treatments with a tailored approach is always better than delivering with high fidelity.

c. **Delivering treatments with high fidelity may not always be better than delivering with a tailored approach.**

d. Delivering treatments with high fidelity is necessary when treating youth a substance use disorder and a co-occurring disorder.

CHAPTER 10

1. Participatory learning and active cognitive processes are the two core principles of Bandura's social cognitive learning theory. True **False**

2. Modeling when used for adolescent clients could involve teaching the client new coping skills by imitating a healthy peer. **True** False

3. Contingency management involves providing tangible rewards to treatment providers contingent on meeting program standards (e.g., maintaining a high percent of clients that complete treatment). True **False**

4. Dialectical behavior therapy was originally created to treat patients with borderline personality disorder and has since been applied to those with PTSD. **True** False

5. One of the four core skills taught to clients receiving dialectical behavior therapy is mindfulness. **True** False

6. A difference between classical conditioning and operant conditioning is . . .

a. one involves learning and one involves recovery

b. one pairs two stimuli and one pairs behavior and response

c. one always works with involuntary responses and one works with voluntary behaviors

d. one works with involuntary responses in some people and one works with voluntary behaviors in some people

   e. **b and c**

   f. a and d

7. The Cannabis Youth Treatment (CYT) study . . . . . .

   a. highlighted how cognitive behavioral therapy alone is a powerful counseling approach

   b. **showed favorable changes in marijuana use (less use) and some improvement in psychosocial problems**

   c. involved one of the largest stand-alone treatment programs that is now a national model

   d. ironically showed more improvement in alcohol use compared to marijuana use

8. According to Social Cognitive Learning Theory, behavior can be learned from the environment through the process of. . . .

   a. observational learning

   b. active cognitive processes

   c. reactive cognitive processes

   d. **observational learning and active cognitive processes**

   e. observational learning and reactive cognitive processes

9. Cognitive behavioral therapy is organized around which three learning principles that are typically combined into a multicomponent program?

   a. **Classical conditioning, operant conditioning, social learning theory**

   b. Classical conditioning, social learning theory, social behavior theory

   c. Classical operant conditioning, operant conditioning, social learning theory

10. Skinner's point about the weaknesses of the classical conditioning model is that it was . . .

   a. original data based on animals

   b. **too simplistic to explain complex human behavior**

   c. ignored the multidimensionality of involuntary responses

11. Use of cognitive behavioral therapy to address a substance use disorder involves a *functional analysis*, which is. . . .
    a. conducted with the patient after treatment to identify how well the patient is functioning
    b. conducted with both the patient and a parent after treatment to identify how well the patient is functioning
    c. **conducted with the patient at the outset of treatment in order to identify contextual factors linked to the substance use**
    d. conducted with the patient at the outset of treatment in order to identify how the patient functions when intoxicated

12. Dialectical behavior therapy . . .
    a. **is particularly intended for youth with a severe personality disorder**
    b. refers to a therapy that addresses a youth's existential crisis
    c. applies more motivational interviewing techniques than cognitive behavior therapy techniques
    d. is a very effective short-term counseling method

13. Dialectical behavior therapy's emotion regulation component does <u>not</u> involve . . .
    a. **learning about how poor coping skills can lead to dysfunctional emotions**
    b. learning about one's emotions when experiencing extreme emotions
    c. learning about one's vulnerabilities when experiencing extreme emotions
    d. learning about how emotions can make a person feel out of control

14. What is <u>not</u> one of the goals of family therapy that is recommended to be in combination with dialectical behavior therapy?
    a. increase the family's and adolescent's support network
    b. **educate the parents that the cause of the problems are more the adolescent's rather than having roots in the family system**

    c. reduce aggressive interactions

    d. develop parenting skills needed to work with an adolescent with a co-occurring disorder

15. A core similarity of cognitive behavioral therapy and dialectical behavior therapy is that both . . .

    a. are a challenge when applied to adolescents

    b. always involve family counseling as adjunct therapy

    c. require long-term therapy to be successful

    d. **incorporate similar basic theoretical principles**

    e. there are no core similarities

CHAPTER 11

1. There are nine stages of change in Prochaska and Di Clemente's model. True **False**

2. If an adolescent is resistant to treatment services there is nothing to be done, and they should wait for services. True **False**

3. Brief interventions for adolescents are showing promise and are good interventions to consider. **True** False

4. One of the tools in motivational interviewing is OARS. The "A" stands for Acceptance. True **False**

5. Community Reinforcement and Family Training is very confrontational and a strict protocol to follow. True **False**

6. The transtheoretical Stage of Change model posits that the behavioral health change process involves. . . . .

    a. progress through stages both acquiring an addiction and change after the addiction is present

    b. **progress through stages of change after the addiction is present**

    c. progress that differs between adolescents and adults

    d. progress through change while receiving aftercare treatment for addiction

7. What stage is characterized by unawareness that the person's behavior is a problem and an underappreciation of the pros of changing behavior?
   a. **precontemplation**
   b. contemplation
   c. preparation
   d. action
8. What is the main task of the counselor when a client is in the contemplation stage?
   a. increase client's perception of risk
   b. **evoke reasons for change**
   c. help the client prepare for change
   d. help the client take steps toward change
9. William Miller's alternative to the confrontational style often practiced by counselors with alcoholics . . .
   a. addressed resistance and denial in clients via a counselor-centered process
   b. addressed resistance and denial in clients via an evidenced-based process
   c. **combined principles based on Carl Rogers and the Stage of Change model**
   d. combined principles based on Eric Erickson and the Stages of Change model
10. The core MI interviewing skills have been summarized by the acronym OARS. The O stands for . . .
    a. being open to adapting treatment based on the clients preferences
    b. being open-minded with a client
    c. opening lines of communications with the client's family members
    d. **asking open questions rather than closed questions**
11. The use of motivational enhancement treatment in a brief intervention is discussed by the authors as . . .
    a. **teen-friendly with encouraging signs that it's an evidence-based approach**

    b.　teen-friendly but it is way too early to know if it's an evidence-based approach

    c.　because not very teen-friendly, its use needs adjustments by the counselor

    d.　because not very teen-friendly and not evidence-based, other approaches should be used

12.　Based on the operant-based fundamentals of behavioral psychology, the CRAFT model. . . .

    a.　purposely does not pressure reluctant individuals to attend treatment

    b.　involves a trained therapist teaching a concerned significant other (CSO) to be the change agent

    c.　involves giving and withholding rewards, but only after the client is clearly in the action stage

    d.　**a and b**

    e.　b and d

13.　Which of the following is <u>not</u> true about *reflective listening* when applying motivational interviewing?

    a.　**Poor reflective listening is not necessarily bad when used as a reverse psychology technique.**

    b.　This skill is viewed as vital for building trust between you and your client.

    c.　It can acknowledge a client's' point of view without approving it.

    d.　One type is repeating or rephrasing.

14.　Which of the following is <u>not</u> true about *summaries* when applying motivational interviewing?

    a.　It occurs throughout the counseling, with particular application at transition points.

    b.　It can facilitate a new direction in the session.

    c.　It helps to ensure that there is clear communication between the counselor and client.

    d.　**It provides an opportune time for the counselor to assert their directions for behavior change goals.**

15. In the case illustration of Annette, the second session included. . . .
    a. feedback about the importance of the mother seeking treatment
    b. **plans for a follow-up session**
    c. a discussion about the risk of dating an older boyfriend
    d. a psychoeducational component about the impact of using cannabis

CHAPTER 12

1. Family therapy approaches have inconsistently been associated with favorable outcomes. True **False**
2. Despite the changes in divorce rates, the prevalence of the two-parent household has not declined. True **False**
3. Some family therapy models contend that family engagement is the most important component to treatment success. **True** False
4. The functional family therapy approach views adolescent substance abuse as developing in the context of maladaptive peer relationships. True **False**
5. Multisystemic therapy services typically are delivered in the family's home. **True** False
6. What is meant in family therapy by a multisystem approach?
    a. Multiple members of the family are targeted.
    b. **Family factors and multiple non-family factors (e.g., peers and school) are targeted.**
    c. Multiple non-family factors (e.g., peers and school) are targeted.
7. Who below is not one of the pioneers of family therapy to address adolescent substance abuse?
    a. **Marsha Linehan**
    b. Holly Waldron
    c. Howard Liddle
    d. Salvator Minuchin

8. A trend reflecting that nowadays there is no standard family structure is. . . .
   a. nearly 75% of all children in America are being raised together
   b. nearly 10% of all children in America are living in a "nontraditional" family
   c. **higher historical rates of youth in living arrangements of two parents in remarriage**
   d. constantly changing historical rates of youth in living arrangements of two parents in remarriage

9. Ecological family therapy originated from the therapeutic work with substance-abusing adolescents who
   a. **had run away from home**
   b. were chronically truant
   c. had been victims of physical abuse
   d. had failed with individual counseling

10. What is not one of the drug use protective steps noted by the authors that parents can take?
    a. **host a party for teenagers and allow safe levels of drinking under adult supervision**
    b. reduce parental complacency regarding any level of drug use during adolescence
    c. family rules and expectations regarding substance use are clearly defined
    d. monitor affiliation with peers who may be delinquent

11. The authors make a point that the big difference between the various family-based treatment models is . . . . . .
    a. the extent to which they vary on the focus on first and second relatives within the family
    b. **the extent to which they vary on the focus on within the family system or outside of it**
    c. the extent to which they vary on the focus on the parents' drug use
    d. the extent to which they vary on the focus on the adolescents' drug use

12. What is <u>not</u> one of the four core components of family therapy identified by Bobek and colleagues?
    a. family engagement
    b. relational reframing
    c. **rational restructuring**
    d. family restructuring

13. If family treatment were to be administered to an adolescent who is in a juvenile detention center, which approach did the authors recommend?
    a. Brief strategic family therapy
    b. Functional family therapy
    c. Multidimensional family therapy
    d. **none of the above**

14. A unique benefit of family-based treatment is the possibility that . . .
    a. **the siblings of the target adolescent may be positively impacted**
    b. the adolescent's coexisting problems may improve
    c. the parents' marriage may improve
    d. none of the above

15. Family risk factors that are attended to in treatment typically center on. . . .
    a. **weak effective parenting practices**
    b. lack of motivational interviewing skills among parents
    c. lack of family recreational activities
    d. poor parental oversight of the adolescent's schoolwork

CHAPTER 13

1. The overwhelming majority of adolescent treatment programs utilize the basic principles of AA as a component of their treatment approach. **True** False

2. The authors note that a major benefit of mutual-help programs for adolescents is that they provide the opportunity for the

young person to develop new friendships with role-model adults also seeking the same drug-free lifestyle. True **False**

3. Recovery high schools (RHSs), while not yet a routine part of school systems across the U.S., are viewed as so important that some experts call RHS the "13th step." True **False**

4. A major difference between self-help alternatives and 12-step-based self-help is that self-help alternatives are secular and focus on current issues and coping strategies. **True** False

5. The history of the 12-step treatment approach can be traced to the Temperance Movement of the late 1800s and early 1900s. True **False**

6. Which does not belong regarding 12-step programs?
   a. The person works on specific steps toward recovery.
   b. Attendance at self-support groups (e.g., Alcoholic Anonymous and Narcotics Anonymous) is encouraged.
   c. Assistance is provided by a sponsor who is another person in recovery from substance use.
   d. **Assistance can also be provided by a sponsor who is another person that has formal training in addiction counseling.**

7. The language and terminology of the 12-step treatment approach. . . .
   a. were developed with adolescents in mind
   b. have an edge to them that eschews motivational interviewing principles
   c. **have many components that reflect empathy and a nonconfrontational approach**
   d. were originally developed from a science-based framework

8. Which is not true about the history of the 12-step recovery approach?
   a. Its initiator was Bill Wilson ("Bill W").
   b. **Its origins were church-based.**
   c. Its origins were community-based.
   d. Its principles are extended to many other behavioral addictions.

9. The application of the 12-step principles to adolescents. . . ..
   a. is problematic given that it is difficult to adjust the principles to be meaningful for an adolescent
   b. **is not problematic given that it is feasible to adjust the principles to be meaningful for an adolescent**
   c. is problematic because there is no evidence it works for this age group
10. What is the authors' point about a client being religious or not in order to benefit from the 12-step approach?
    a. **Nowadays the term "Higher Power" is used rather than "God."**
    b. A person needs to be religious for the 12-step approach to work.
    c. The term "Higher Power" has always been used rather than "God."
    d. "Higher Power" cannot be interpreted as something of a personal nature.
11. How many of the 12 steps are typically addressed with adolescents during the primary treatment experience?
    a. all of them
    b. just the first two
    c. **five**
    d. there is no typical number; treatment programs vary on this issue
12. Which is not a feature of mutual self-help programs?
    a. Referral to AA/NA groups following adolescent treatment for a substance use disorder is the norm.
    b. AA/NA groups stress that abstinence from drug use is needed.
    c. Participants meet in a group with others in recovery, sharing their experiences.
    d. **Will power as a coping strategy is encouraged.**
13. The responsibility of the sponsor includes. . . ..
    a. making occasional contacts via telephone and e-mail/text
    b. having occasional meetings with the adolescent

    c. **making frequent contacts via telephone and e-mail/text**

    d. having frequent meetings with the adolescent and their parents

14. Experts have identified several factors to consider when referring adolescents to 12-step groups. Which is <u>not</u> one of them?

    a. The referring clinicians should assess the sponsor assigned to their client to evaluate the sponsor's recovery history, stability, and appropriateness to work with adolescents.

    b. **Whereas attending 12-step meetings can be a negative experience, this is not sufficient disincentive to prevent attendance.**

    c. Meetings are led by non-professionals and are open to anyone with a desire to stop using alcohol/drugs, and thus local meetings can vary with respect to their interpersonal climate and cultural orientation.

    d. Adolescents may need to "shop" to find a meeting that is a good fit.

15. Twelve-step facilitation (TSF) is . . . .

    a. **a hybrid of the standard 12-step approach**

    b. only effective when administered in a group setting

    c. clearly more effective than standard 12-step approach

    d. an approach that varies from the core principles of the 12-step model

For the benefit of digital users, indexed terms that span two pages (e.g., 52–53) may, on occasion, appear on only one of those pages.

Tables, figures, and boxes are indicated by *t*, *f*, and *b* following the page number